Clinical Disorders of the Kidney

Editor

JAMES C. CHAN

PEDIATRIC CLINICS
OF NORTH AMERICA

www.pediatric.theclinics.com

Consulting Editor
BONITA F. STANTON

February 2019 • Volume 66 • Number 1

ELSEVIER

1600 John F. Kennedy Boulevard • Suite 1800 • Philadelphia, Pennsylvania, 19103-2899

http://www.theclinics.com

THE PEDIATRIC CLINICS OF NORTH AMERICA Volume 66, Number 1
February 2019 ISSN 0031-3955, ISBN-13: 978-0-323-65509-5

Editor: Kerry Holland
Developmental Editor: Casey Potter

The Pediatric Clinics of North America (ISSN 0031-3955) is published bimonthly by Elsevier Inc., 360 Park Avenue South, New York, NY 10010-1710. Months of issue are February, April, June, August, October, and December. Periodicals postage paid at New York, NY and additional mailing offices. Subscription prices are $229.00 per year (US individuals), $653.00 per year (US institutions), $315.00 per year (Canadian individuals), $868.00 per year (Canadian institutions), $345.00 per year (international individuals), $868.00 per year (international institutions), $100.00 per year (US students and residents), and $165.00 per year (international and Canadian residents and students). To receive students/resident rare, orders must be accompanied by name of affiliated institution, date of term, and the signature of program/residency coordinator on institution letterhead. Orders will be billed at individual rate until proof of status is received. Foreign air speed delivery is included in all Clinics subscription prices. All prices are subject to change without notice. **POSTMASTER:** Send address changes to The Pediatric Clinics of North America, Elsevier Health Sciences Division, Subscription Customer Service, 3251 Riverport Lane, Maryland Heights, MO 63043. **Customer Service: 1-800-654-2452 (US and Canada). From outside of the US and Canada: 1-314-447-8871. Fax: 1-314-447-8029. For print support, E-mail: JournalsCustomerService-usa@elsevier.com. For online support, E-mail: JournalsOnlineSupport-usa@elsevier.com.**

Reprints. For copies of 100 or more, of articles in this publication, please contact the Commercial Reprints Department, Elsevier Inc., 360 Park Avenue South, New York, NY 10010-1710. Tel.: 212-633-3874; Fax: 212-633-3820; E-mail: reprints@elsevier.com.

The Pediatric Clinics of North America is also published in Spanish by McGraw-Hill Inter-americana Editores S.A., Mexico City, Mexico; in Portuguese by Riechmann and Affonso Editores, Rua Comandante Coelho 1085, CEP 21250, Rio de Janeiro, Brazil; and in Greek by Althayia SA, Athens, Greece.

The Pediatric Clinics of North America is covered in MEDLINE/PubMed (Index Medicus), Excerpta Medica, Current Contents, Current Contents/Clinical Medicine, Science Citation Index, ASCA, ISI/BIOMED, and BIOSIS.

PROGRAM OBJECTIVE
The goal of the *Pediatric Clinics of North America* is to keep practicing physicians and residents up to date with current clinical practice in pediatrics by providing timely articles reviewing the state-of-the-art in patient care.

TARGET AUDIENCE
All practicing pediatricians, physicians and healthcare professionals who provide patient care to pediatric patients.

LEARNING OBJECTIVES
Upon completion of this activity, participants will be able to:
1. Review the epidemiology, pathophysiology, clinical features, and treatment options for obesity-related kidney disease in children and adolescents.
2. Discuss recent developments in the field of pediatric chronic kidney disease with a focus on dietary measures to improve outcomes.
3. Recognize the clinical presentation, laboratory evaluation, genetics, pathophysiology, management, and future therapies of Dent disease.

ACCREDITATION
The Elsevier Office of Continuing Medical Education (EOCME) is accredited by the Accreditation Council for Continuing Medical Education (ACCME) to provide continuing medical education for physicians.

The EOCME designates this enduring material for a maximum of 15 *AMA PRA Category 1 Credit*(s)™. Physicians should claim only the credit commensurate with the extent of their participation in the activity.

All other healthcare professionals requesting continuing education credit for this enduring material will be issued a certificate of participation.

DISCLOSURE OF CONFLICTS OF INTEREST
The EOCME assesses conflict of interest with its instructors, faculty, planners, and other individuals who are in a position to control the content of CME activities. All relevant conflicts of interest that are identified are thoroughly vetted by EOCME for fair balance, scientific objectivity, and patient care recommendations. EOCME is committed to providing its learners with CME activities that promote improvements or quality in healthcare and not a specific proprietary business or a commercial interest.

The planning committee, staff, authors and editors listed below have identified no financial relationships or relationships to products or devices they or their spouse/life partner have with commercial interest related to the content of this CME activity:
Oleh M. Akchurin, MD; Robert Todd Alexander, MD, PhD; Brian Becknell, MD, PhD; Martin Bitzan, MD; Denver D. Brown, MD; James C. Chan, MD, DSc; Ellen M. Cody, MD; Lawrence Copelovitch, MD; Bradley P. Dixon, MD; Abdulla M. Ehlayel, MD; Karen W. Eldin, MD; Jeffrey J. Fadrowski, MD, MHS; John W. Foreman, MD; Rosanna Fulchiero, DO; Rouba Garro, MD; Paul R. Goodyer, MD; Monica Guzman-Limon, MD; Kerry Holland; Elizabeth A.K. Hunt, MD; Catherine Kavanagh, MD; Alison Kemp; Rajkumar Mayakrishnan; Rachel Millner, MD; Mark Mitsnefes, MD, MS; Michael L. Moritz, MD, FAAP; Edward Nehus, MD, MS; Oana Nicoara, MD; Rebecca L. Ruebner, MD, MSCE; Joshua Samuels, MD, MPH; Patricia Seo-Mayer, MD; Michael J.G. Somers, MD; Natalie S. Uy, MD; Scott E. Wenderfer, MD, PhD; Pamela D. Winterberg, MD.

The planning committee, staff, authors and editors listed below have identified financial relationships or relationships to products or devices they or their spouse/life partner have with commercial interest related to the content of this CME activity:
Larry A. Greenbaum, MD, PhD: receives research support from Mallinckrodt Pharmaceuticals and is a consultant/advisor for Retrophin, Inc.
Kimberly J. Reidy, MD: receives research support from Complexa.
Katherine Twombley, MD: receives research support from Alexion, Arbor Pharmaceuticals, LLC, Kaneka Pharma America, LLC, Novartis Pharmaceuticals Corporation, and Takeda Pharmaceutical Company Limited.
Chia-shi Wang, MD, MSc: receives research support from Mallinckrodt Pharmaceuticals.

UNAPPROVED/OFF-LABEL USE DISCLOSURE
The EOCME requires CME faculty to disclose to the participants:
1. When products or procedures being discussed are off-label, unlabelled, experimental, and/or investigational (not US Food and Drug Administration [FDA] approved); and

2. Any limitations on the information presented, such as data that are preliminary or that represent ongoing research, interim analyses, and/or unsupported opinions. Faculty may discuss information about pharmaceutical agents that is outside of FDA-approved labelling. This information is intended solely for CME and is not intended to promote off-label use of these medications. If you have any questions, contact the medical affairs department of the manufacturer for the most recent prescribing information.

TO ENROLL

To enroll in the *Pediatric Clinics of North America* Continuing Medical Education program, call customer service at 1-800-654-2452 or sign up online at http://www.theclinics.com/home/cme. The CME program is available to subscribers for an additional annual fee of USD 301.60.

METHOD OF PARTICIPATION

In order to claim credit, participants must complete the following:
1. Complete enrolment as indicated above.
2. Read the activity.
3. Complete the CME Test and Evaluation. Participants must achieve a score of 70% on the test. All CME Tests and Evaluations must be completed online.

CME INQUIRIES/SPECIAL NEEDS

For all CME inquiries or special needs, please contact elsevierCME@elsevier.com

Contributors

CONSULTING EDITOR

BONITA F. STANTON, MD
Founding Dean, Hackensack Meridian School of Medicine at Seton Hall University, President, Academic Enterprise, Hackensack Meridian Health Robert C. and Laura C. Garrett Endowed Chair for the School of Medicine, Dean Professor of Pediatrics, Nutley, New Jersey, USA

EDITOR

JAMES C. CHAN, MD, DSc
Professor of Pediatrics, Tufts University, Director of Research, The Barbara Bush Children's Hospital, Maine Medical Center, Portland, Maine, USA

AUTHORS

OLEH M. AKCHURIN, MD
Assistant Professor of Pediatrics, Pediatric Nephrology, Weill Cornell Medicine, New York, New York, USA

ROBERT TODD ALEXANDER, MD, PhD
Department of Pediatrics and Physiology, Stollery Children's Hospital, Edmonton, Alberta, Canada

BRIAN BECKNELL, MD, PhD
Nephrology Section, Nationwide Children's Hospital, Department of Pediatrics, The Ohio State University College of Medicine, Center for Clinical and Translational Research, The Research Institute at Nationwide Children's Hospital, Columbus, Ohio, USA

MARTIN BITZAN, MD
Associate Professor, Division of Nephrology, Department of Pediatrics, The Montreal Children's Hospital, McGill University Health Centre, Montreal, Quebec, Canada; Kidney Center of Excellence, Al Jalila Children's Hospital, Al Jadaf, Dubai, United Arab Emirates

DENVER D. BROWN, MD
Fellow, Pediatric Nephrology, Children's Hospital at Montefiore, Albert Einstein College of Medicine, Bronx, New York, USA

JAMES C. CHAN, MD, DSc
Professor of Pediatrics, Tufts University, Director of Research, The Barbara Bush Children's Hospital, Maine Medical Center, Portland, Maine, USA

ELLEN M. CODY, MD
Department of Pediatrics, University of Colorado School of Medicine, Aurora, Colorado, USA

LAWRENCE COPELOVITCH, MD
Associate Professor of Pediatrics, Division of Nephrology, The Children's Hospital of Philadelphia, Perelman School of Medicine, University of Pennsylvania, Philadelphia, Pennsylvania, USA

BRADLEY P. DIXON, MD
Associate Professor, Departments of Pediatrics and Medicine, University of Colorado School of Medicine, Aurora, Colorado, USA

ABDULLA M. EHLAYEL, MD
Division of Nephrology, The Children's Hospital of Philadelphia, Philadelphia, Pennsylvania, USA

KAREN W. ELDIN, MD
Department of Pathology and Immunology, Baylor College of Medicine, Texas Children's Hospital, Houston, Texas, USA

JEFFREY J. FADROWSKI, MD, MHS
Associate Professor, Department of Pediatrics, Division of Nephrology, Johns Hopkins School of Medicine, Baltimore, Maryland, USA

JOHN W. FOREMAN, MD
Professor Emeritus, Department of Pediatrics, Duke University School of Medicine, Durham, North Carolina, USA

ROSANNA FULCHIERO, DO
Inova Children's Hospital, Falls Church, Virginia, USA

ROUBA GARRO, MD
Assistant Professor, Division of Pediatric Nephrology, Emory University School of Medicine, Children's Pediatric Institute, Atlanta, Georgia, USA

PAUL R. GOODYER, MD
Professor of Pediatrics and Human Genetics, Departments of Pediatrics, Human Genetics and Experimental Medicine, McGill University, The Montreal Children's Hospital and Research Institute, McGill University Health Centre, Montreal, Quebec, Canada

LARRY A. GREENBAUM, MD, PhD
Marcus Professor of Pediatrics and Division Director of Pediatric Nephrology, Emory University School of Medicine, Children's Healthcare of Atlanta, Atlanta, Georgia, USA

MONICA GUZMAN-LIMON, MD
Division of Pediatric Nephrology and Hypertension, McGovern Medical School, The University of Texas Health Science Center at Houston, Houston, Texas, USA

ELIZABETH A.K. HUNT, MD
Director, Division of Pediatric Nephrology, University of Vermont Children's Hospital, Assistant Professor in Pediatrics, Larner College of Medicine, The University of Vermont Medical Center, Burlington, Vermont, USA

CATHERINE KAVANAGH, MD
Department of Pediatric Nephrology, Columbia University Irving Medical Center, New York, New York, USA

RACHEL MILLNER, MD
University of Arkansas for Medical Sciences Division of Pediatric Nephrology, Arkansas Children's Hospital, Little Rock, Arkansas, USA

MARK MITSNEFES, MD, MS
Professor of Pediatrics, Division of Nephrology and Hypertension, Cincinnati Children's Hospital Medical Center, Cincinnati, Ohio, USA

MICHAEL L. MORITZ, MD, FAAP
Professor of Pediatrics, Clinical Director, Pediatric Nephrology, Medical Director, Pediatric Dialysis, Division of Nephrology, Department of Pediatrics, UPMC Children's Hospital of Pittsburgh, University of Pittsburgh School of Medicine, Pittsburgh, Pennsylvania, USA

EDWARD NEHUS, MD, MS
Assistant Professor of Pediatrics, Division of Nephrology and Hypertension, Cincinnati Children's Hospital Medical Center, Cincinnati, Ohio, USA

OANA NICOARA, MD
Assistant Professor, Department of Pediatrics, Medical University of South Carolina, Charleston, South Carolina, USA

KIMBERLY J. REIDY, MD
Assistant Professor, Pediatric Nephrology, Children's Hospital at Montefiore, Albert Einstein College of Medicine, Bronx, New York, USA

REBECCA L. RUEBNER, MD, MSCE
Assistant Professor, Department of Pediatrics, Division of Nephrology, Johns Hopkins School of Medicine, Baltimore, Maryland, USA

JOSHUA SAMUELS, MD, MPH
Professor, Division of Pediatric Nephrology and Hypertension, McGovern Medical School, The University of Texas Health Science Center at Houston, Houston, Texas, USA

PATRICIA SEO-MAYER, MD
Inova Children's Hospital, Falls Church, Virginia, USA; Division of Nephrology and Hypertension, Pediatric Specialists of Virginia, Fairfax, Virginia, USA; Virginia Commonwealth School of Medicine, Richmond, Virginia, USA

MICHAEL J.G. SOMERS, MD
Associate Chief, Division of Nephrology, Boston Children's Hospital, Associate Professor in Pediatrics, Harvard Medical School, Boston, Massachusetts, USA

KATHERINE TWOMBLEY, MD
Associate Professor, Department of Pediatrics, Medical University of South Carolina, Charleston, South Carolina, USA

NATALIE S. UY, MD
Assistant Professor, Department of Pediatric Nephrology, Columbia University Irving Medical Center, New York, New York, USA

CHIA-SHI WANG, MD, MSc
Assistant Professor of Pediatrics, Emory University School of Medicine, Children's Healthcare of Atlanta, Atlanta, Georgia, USA

SCOTT E. WENDERFER, MD, PhD
Pediatric Nephrology, Department of Pediatrics, Baylor College of Medicine, Texas Children's Hospital, Houston, Texas, USA

PAMELA D. WINTERBERG, MD
Assistant Professor, Division of Pediatric Nephrology, Emory University School of Medicine, Children's Pediatric Institute, Atlanta, Georgia, USA

Contents

> Urinary tract infection (UTI) is the second most common bacterial infection in children and is considered a public health threat given the mounting rates of antibiotic-resistance among uropathogens. This article highlights recent encouraging developments in UTI research. Further work is necessary to translate the discoveries into accessible, cost-effective technologies that will aid clinicians in real-time decision-making.

> The causes of macroscopic and microscopic hematuria overlap; both are often caused by urinary tract infections or urethral/bladder irritation. Coexistent hypertension and proteinuria should prompt investigation for glomerular disease. The most common glomerulonephritis in children is postinfectious glomerulonephritis. In most patients, and especially with isolated microscopic hematuria, the diagnostic workup reveals no clear underlying cause. In those cases whereby a diagnosis is made, the most common causes of persistent microscopic hematuria are thin basement membrane nephropathy, immunoglobulin A nephropathy, or idiopathic hypercalciuria. Treatment and long-term prognosis varies with the underlying disease.

> Obesity is a leading cause of chronic kidney disease. Children with severe obesity have an increased prevalence of early kidney abnormalities and are at high risk to develop kidney failure in adulthood. The pathophysiology of obesity-related kidney disease is incompletely understood, although the postulated mechanisms of kidney injury include hyperfiltration, adipokine dysregulation, and lipotoxic injury. An improved understanding of the long-term effects of obesity on kidney health is essential treat the growing

multisystemic involvement, and a more severe disease course, which includes greater risks for developing nephritis and end-stage kidney disease. Five- and 10-year mortality is lower than in adult-onset SLE. Although patient and renal survival have improved with advances in induction and maintenance immunosuppression, accumulation of irreversible damage is common. Cardiovascular and infectious complications are frequent, as are relapses during adolescence and the transition to adulthood.

with/without syndromic features. Further workup is needed to determine the type of renal tubular acidosis and the presumed etiopathogenesis, which informs treatment choices and prognosis. The risk of nephrolithiasis and calcinosis is linked to the presence (proximal renal tubular acidosis, negligible stone risk) or absence (distal renal tubular acidosis, high stone risk) of urine citrate excretion. New formulations of slow-release alkali and potassium combination supplements are being tested that are expected to simplify treatment and lead to sustained acidosis correction.

Fanconi syndrome, also known as the DeToni, Debré, Fanconi syndrome is a global dysfunction of the proximal tubule characterized by glucosuria, phosphaturia, generalized aminoaciduria, and type II renal tubular acidosis. Often there is hypokalemia, sodium wasting, and dehydration. In children, it typically is caused by inborn errors of metabolism, principally cystinosis. In adults, it is mainly caused by medications, exogenous toxins, and heavy metals. Treatment consists of treating the underlying cause and replacing the lost electrolytes and volume.

Dent disease is an X-linked form of chronic kidney disease characterized by hypercalciuria, low molecular weight proteinuria, nephrocalcinosis, and proximal tubular dysfunction. Clinical presentation is highly variable. Male patients may present with early-onset rickets, recurrent nephrolithiasis, or insidiously with asymptomatic proteinuria or chronic kidney disease. Mutations in both the CLCN5 and OCRL1 genes have been associated with the Dent phenotype and are now classified as Dent-1 and Dent-2, respectively. This article describes the clinical presentation, laboratory evaluation, genetics, pathophysiology, management, and future therapies of Dent disease.

Hypophosphatemic rickets, mostly of the X-linked dominant form caused by pathogenic variants of the PHEX gene, poses therapeutic challenges with consequences for growth and bone development and portends a high risk of fractions and poor bone healing, dental problems and nephrolithiasis/nephrocalcinosis. Conventional treatment consists of PO4 supplements and calcitriol requiring monitoring for treatment-emergent adverse effects. FGF23 measurement, where available, has implications for the differential diagnosis of hypophosphatemia syndromes and, potentially, treatment monitoring. Newer therapeutic modalities include calcium sensing receptor modulation (cinacalcet) and biological molecules targeting FGF23 or its receptors. Their long-term effects must be compared with those of conventional treatments.

The syndrome of inappropriate antidiuresis (SIAD) is a common cause of hyponatremia in hospitalized children. SIAD refers to euvolemic hyponatremia due to nonphysiologic stimuli for arginine vasopressin production in the absence of renal or endocrine dysfunction. SIAD can be broadly classified as a result of tumors, pulmonary or central nervous system disorders, medications, or other causes such as infection, inflammation, and the postoperative state. The presence of hypouricemia with an elevated fractional excretion of urate can aid in the diagnosis. Treatment options include fluid restriction, intravenous saline solutions, oral sodium supplements, loop diuretics, oral urea, and vasopressin receptor antagonists (vaptans).

Nephrogenic diabetes insipidus (NDI) results from the inability of the late distal tubules and collecting ducts to respond to vasopressin. The lack of ability to concentrate urine results in polyuria and polydipsia. Primary and acquired forms of NDI exist in children. Congenital NDI is a result of mutation in AVPR2 or AQP2 genes. Secondary NDI is associated with electrolyte abnormalities, obstructive uropathy, or certain medications. Management of NDI can be difficult with only symptomatic treatment available, using low-solute diet, diuretics, and prostaglandin inhibitors.

Hemolytic uremic syndrome (HUS) is the clinical triad of thrombocytopenia, anemia, and acute kidney injury. Classically associated with enterocolitis from Shiga toxin–producing *Escherichia coli*, HUS is also associated with *Streptococcus pneumoniae* infections; genetic dysregulation of the alternative complement pathway or coagulation cascade; and, rarely, a hereditary disorder of cobalamin C metabolism. These share a common final pathway of a prothrombotic and proinflammatory state on the endothelial cell surface, with fibrin and platelet deposition. Much work has been done to distinguish between the different mechanisms of disease, thereby informing the optimal therapeutic interventions for each entity.

Chronic kidney disease is an ongoing deterioration of renal function that often progresses to end-stage renal disease. Management goals in children include slowing disease progression, prevention and treatment of complications, and optimizing growth, development, and quality of life. Nutritional management is critically important to achieve these goals. Control of blood pressure, proteinuria, and metabolic acidosis with dietary and pharmacologic measures may slow progression of chronic kidney disease. Although significant progress in management has been made, further research is required to resolve many outstanding controversies. We review recent developments in pediatric chronic kidney disease, focusing on dietary measures to improve outcomes.

Pamela D. Winterberg and Rouba Garro

Kidney transplantation is the preferred treatment for end-stage renal disease (ESRD) in children and confers improved survival, skeletal growth, heath-related quality of life, and neuropsychological development compared with dialysis. Kidney transplantation in children with ESRD results in 10-year patient survival exceeding 90%. Therefore, the long-term management of these patients is focused on maintaining quality of life and minimizing long-term side effects of immunosuppression. Optimal management of pediatric kidney transplant recipients includes preventing rejection and infection, identifying and reducing the cardiovascular and metabolic effects of long-term immunosuppressive therapy, supporting normal growth and development, and managing a smooth transition into adulthood.

PEDIATRIC CLINICS OF NORTH AMERICA

SERIES OF RELATED INTEREST

Clinics in Perinatology
https://www.perinatology.theclinics.com/

THE CLINICS ARE AVAILABLE ONLINE!
Access your subscription at:
www.theclinics.com

Foreword

Dealing with the Challenges of the Good Fortune of an Abundance of New Knowledge

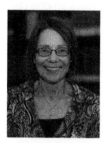

Bonita F. Stanton, MD
Consulting Editor

In this rich update on pediatric kidney disease, James Chan, MD, DSc and his many authors provide a comprehensive update to the vast and growing literature on these disorders. Methods for diagnosis as well as for treatment have changed and expanded rapidly over the last decade. This issue of *Pediatric Clinics of North America* reminds us that renal disorders vary enormously not only in cause and severity but also in their relationship to malfunctioning of other organ systems, as an increasing number of kidney diseases are secondary manifestations of disorders of other organ systems. These articles also underscore that while many of these renal abnormalities occur in both children and adults, their presentations and consequences can be radically different, depending on the age of the host. We learn in this issue about the significant additional considerations to be faced regarding kidney transplants in which the recipients are children compared with those in which they are adults. Finally, the recent changes in our knowledge about these renal disorders described in these articles remind us of the rapid pace at which new knowledge becomes available and the enormous task physicians face to assimilate these changes and advances into their practices. (In 1950, the doubling time of medical knowledge was estimated to be 50 years; by contrast, for 2010, it was estimated to be 3.5 years.[1])

Not only must physicians maintain current knowledge themselves, they must appropriately update their patients and their families. As described so well in this issue of *Pediatric Clinics of North America*, this is the reality that pediatricians face as more children are surviving single-organ and multiorgan disorders longer. Fortunately, modern technology offers some help in this regard. Over that last 10 to 15 years, there has been a proliferation of social media platforms, typically on mobile phones, to provide new knowledge and reaffirm existing knowledge regarding nephrology disorders,

Pediatr Clin N Am 66 (2019) xvii–xviii
https://doi.org/10.1016/j.pcl.2018.10.003
0031-3955/19/© 2018 Published by Elsevier Inc.

both primary and secondary. Physicians have begun to use these platforms to inform their patients. The educational platforms include, but are not limited to, Twitter, videos (especially YouTube), blogs, visual abstracts, online journal clubs, and interactive learning. These platforms appear to vary in popularity depending on the reader (care providers, patients, and families).[2] In short, the information itself about the diseases is new and rapidly expanding and the media hosting this information are new and rapidly expanding. The need for clarity in the presentation of the information, regardless of the audience, appears to be all the more compelling to avoid treatment and diagnostic errors.

In summary, this is a very full and complete issue about renal disorders among children. It is encouraging how much progress has been made in both diagnostics and care and therefore clinical outcomes and survival. But because of longer lifespans, often associated with longer duration of treatment, wider timeframes for the emergence of both short-term and long-term secondary disorders are becoming a reality as well.

Bonita F. Stanton, MD
Hackensack Meridian School of Medicine at Seton Hall University
340 Kingsland Street, Building 123
Nutley, NJ 07110, USA

E-mail address:
bonita.stanton@shu.edu

REFERENCES

1. Densen P. Challenges and opportunities facing medical education. Trans Am Clin Climatol Assoc 2011;122:48–58.
2. Colbert GB, Topf J, Jhaveri KD, et al. The social media revolution in nephrology education. Kidney Int Rep 2018;3(3):519–29.

Preface

Clinical Disorders of the Kidney

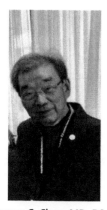

James C. Chan, MD, DSc,
ASPN 50th anniversary,
Toronto. 2018
Editor

It is fulfilling to be a pediatrician because many of our patients will recover fully and have a long and healthful life ahead of them. However, for children with chronic diseases, a healthy future is less certain. Regardless, it is in our nature to strive for the best clinical outcome possible.

One of the perpetual joys and challenges of practice is the pursuit of a better understanding of the underlying disease process with the ultimate aim of improving outcomes. Medical advances in acute and chronic kidney diseases have been remarkable in the past decade. Now we need a reliable update, which this special issue of *Pediatric Clinics of North America* attempts to achieve.

We start with urinary tract infection and other articles to provide a quick reference for the busy pediatrician dealing with these acute illnesses. Then, we move on to perplexing conditions, which a pediatrician may encounter, but often with clinical presentations that are seemingly unconnected to the kidneys. Lastly, we highlight the multisystem impact of acute and chronic kidney disease, with particular emphasis on the challenges of end-stage kidney disease.

Pediatr Clin N Am 66 (2019) xix–xx
https://doi.org/10.1016/j.pcl.2018.10.002
0031-3955/19/© 2018 Published by Elsevier Inc.

pediatric.theclinics.com

Leaders of the American Academy of Pediatrics gave advice on contents, and American Society of Pediatric Nephrology consultants recommended article authors. Finally, all our efforts will be deemed rewarding beyond measure if this issue of *Pediatric Clinics of North America* promotes the joie de vivre of our patients or inspires a medical student, a pediatrician, or another health care professional to choose to go into nephrology.

The following experts gave generously of their time to review the articles. We gratefully acknowledge their contributions: *Carolyn Abitbol, MD, J. Williamson Balfe, MD, FRCP(C), Detlef Bockenhauer, MD, PhD, FRCP, Timothy E. Bunchman, MD, Anna Challa, MMedSc, PhD, Fernando C. Fervenza, DM, PhD, Bethany Joy Foster, MD, Debbie S. Gipson, MD, Jens Goebel, MD, Beatrice Goilav, MD, Gregory H. Gorman, MD, MHS, David Sullivan Hains, MD, Julie R. Ingelfinger, MD, Lada Beara Lasic, MD, MS, Mathieu Lemaire, MD, PhD, FRCP(C), Kevin Lemley, MD, PhD, Deborah P. Jones, MD, Frederick Kaskel, MD, PhD, John D. Mahan, MD, Tej K. Mattoo, MD, DCH, FRCP, Hiren P. Patel, MD, Anthony A. Portale, MD, Fernando Santos, MD, PhD, Steven J. Scheinman, MD, Ekaterini Siomou, MD, PhD, Sangeeta Sule, MD, Alaa Thabet, MB, BS, PhD, Howard M. Trachtman, MD, Rosa Vargas-Poussou, MD, PhD, Steven J. Wassner, MD, and Adam R. Weinstein, MD.*

James C. Chan, MD, DSc
Tufts University
The Barbara Bush Children's Hospital
Maine Medical Center
22 Bramhall Street
Portland, ME 04102-3175, USA

Dedication to Julie Rich Ingelfinger

With this issue, *Pediatric Clinics of North America* honors *Julie R. Ingelfinger, MD*. She is currently a deputy editor at the *New England Journal of Medicine*, professor of pediatrics at Harvard Medical School, and consulting pediatric nephrologist at Massachusetts General Hospital, all in Boston, Massachusetts. To family and colleagues, she is a lot more:

- Her sister, the flutist and author *Eugenia Zukerman*, loves and admires *Julie* for "her brilliance, her kindness, her compassion, and her wicked sense of humor... as well as her ability to take care of patients and family with a devotion seldom seen in others."
- Her fellow nephrology leader *Frederick J. Kaskel, MD, PhD,* Albert Einstein College of Medicine, observes, "*Julie* was able to serve as a mentor for scores of students, residents, fellows, and faculty in all areas of medicine."
- *Joseph T. Flynn, MD*, University of Washington, notes, "Pediatric hypertension research would not be the same without *Julie.*"
- Her many postdoctoral and research associates have benefited from her wisdom in life and work. *Shao-Ling Zhang, PhD,* University of Montreal, cherishes her as "a lifelong friend and idol."

Born in New York City, *Julie Alice Rich* developed her love of nature and poetry as a child, on carefree hikes along the verdant woods and streams of Trout Brook, when the close-knit family moved to West Hartford, Connecticut. Her father, *Stanley Robert Rich*, was an entrepreneur and prolific inventor, famed for developing scanning sonar in submarine detection during World War II. Her mother, *Shirley Cohen Rich*, was the first female student in the Graduate Engineering School of City College of New York and a celebrated performer of modern dance. The parents' diverse achievements must have had an impact on their three daughters' development and accomplishments.

Julie graduated magna cum laude from Radcliffe College/Harvard University, Cambridge, Massachusetts. She earned her MD degree from Albert Einstein College of Medicine, New York City. A student elective in the renal electrolyte laboratory of *Richard M. Hays, MD*, sparked her initial fascination with the working of the kidneys. This interest intensified during her pediatric residency and nephrology fellowship at Washington University, St. Louis Children's Hospital.

Since 1973, *Julie's* academic career has flourished in the environs of the Harvard Medical School, predominantly at the MassGeneral Hospital for Children at Massachusetts General Hospital, where she was Chief of Pediatric

Pediatr Clin N Am 66 (2019) xxi–xxiii
https://doi.org/10.1016/j.pcl.2018.10.004
0031-3955/19/© 2018 Published by Elsevier Inc.

Nephrology (1989-2001). She won the 2009 Barnett Award, the American Academy of Pediatrics' highest honor in nephrology. She served as president of the American Society of Pediatric Nephrology (1993-1994) and received the 2012 Founder's award, in recognition of research achievements in the renal renin-angiotensin system in hypertension, nephrogenesis, and diabetic nephropathy.

Her numerous publications highlight her various scientific contributions. She edited a number of successful textbooks in nephrology and hypertension. She also coauthored a well-received book for the general public: *Coping with Prednisone,* with her sister, Eugenia Zukerman. This came about when Eugenia was found to have a medical condition requiring prednisone and wanted information to avoid side effects. In that book, cowritten from the viewpoint of a patient and a physician, the reader is invited to be part of conversations that too often occur outside of the clinic. Since its first publication in 1998, an update has been published in 2007.

She has been a deputy editor at the *New England Journal of Medicine* since 2001:

- *Jeffrey M. Drazen, MD*, the editor-in-chief, describes her as "a champion for pediatric research in general and pediatric nephology and hypertension in particular. *Julie* brings a passion to everything she does—but most of all she is pediatrician-physician not an editor. She views her work as bringing information to physicians everywhere to help them do a better job of caring for sick kids."
- Her fellow deputy editor, *Caren G. Solomon, MD, MPH*, reflects, "It is remarkable how much Julie manages to do! And no matter how much work she has, she is always the first to volunteer to help her colleagues. It is an honor and a great pleasure to be her colleague and friend."

It is not surprising that *Julie* continues to capture the hearts and minds of people, both at home and around the world.

Not to be overlooked, despite the demands of academic medicine and clinical practice, through all these years, she loved running the Boston Marathon and pursuing her lifelong interests as a classical pianist and published poet. Despite her many accomplishments, *Julie's* greatest joys continue to come from her family, children, and grandchildren:

- Media consultant and author *Laurie Rich* says of her elder sister: "Anyone who knows *Julie*, knows that she keeps an incredibly full schedule ... always making room to see her children and grandchildren play soccer, go skiing, hiking ... She goes to their games, music recitals, and more ... I feel blessed to have *Julie* in my life. We all do." Indeed, *Julie* may say, like her favorite poet, *Emily Dickinson*:

> It's all I have to bring today-
> This, and my heart beside-
> This and my heart, and all the fields-
> And all the meadows wide-
> Be sure you count—should I forget
> Some one the sum could tell-
> This, and my heart, and all the Bees
> Which in the clover dwell.

It is most fitting that we pay tribute to our extraordinary colleague and wonderful friend, *Julie R. Ingelfinger*.

James C. Chan, MD, DSc
Tufts University
The Barbara Bush Children's Hospital
22 Bramhall Street
Portland, ME 04102-3175, USA

Urinary Tract Infections

Rachel Millner, MD[a], Brian Becknell, MD, PhD[b,c,d,*]

KEYWORDS

- Urinary tract infection • Pediatric public health • Prophylactic measures
- Pyelonephritis • Vesicoureteral reflux

KEY POINTS

- UTI should be diagnosed using catheterized specimen for incontinent children, or by clean catch in continent children.
- In children less than 24 months old, renal ultrasound should be performed after first febrile UTI.
- The use of prophylactic antibiotics should be carefully considered in select populations. The benefit in all patients with recurrent UTI is unproven and must be balanced against the increased risk for resistant organisms.
- Additional research is required to identify non-antibiotic treatments of UTI and to identify children at high risk for renal scarring.

BACKGROUND
Epidemiology

Urinary tract infection (UTI) is the second most common bacterial infection in children, affecting 8% of girls and up to 2% of boys within the first 7 years of life.[1,2] The peak incidence of UTI is in infancy, with a second peak in the toddler years and an increased incidence again in adolescence. Of those who develop a UTI in childhood, up to 30% will develop a second UTI.[2] Children with the highest prevalence of UTI include neonates, young infants, toddler girls, and uncircumcised boys less than 1 year of age.[3] Increased risk of UTI is found in special populations, including children with structural and functional urinary tract abnormalities, among others (**Box 1**).

Urinary Tract Infection Classification

Bacteriuria is defined as the presence of bacteria in the urine. This can be associated with infection or urinary tract colonization. Infection is defined by the presence of

[a] UAMS Division of Pediatric Nephrology, Arkansas Children's Hospital, 1 Children's Way, Little Rock, AR 72212, USA; [b] Nephrology Section, Nationwide Children's Hospital, 700 Children's Drive, Columbus, OH 43205, USA; [c] Department of Pediatrics, Ohio State University School of Medicine, 700 Children's Drive, Columbus, OH 43210, USA; [d] Center for Clinical and Translational Research, The Research Institute at Nationwide Children's Hospital, 700 Children's Drive, W308, Columbus, OH 43205, USA
* Corresponding author. Center for Clinical and Translational Research, The Research Institute at Nationwide Children's Hospital, 700 Children's Drive, W308, Columbus, OH 43205.
E-mail address: Brian.becknell2@nationwidechildrens.org

Pediatr Clin N Am 66 (2019) 1–13
https://doi.org/10.1016/j.pcl.2018.08.002
0031-3955/19/© 2018 Elsevier Inc. All rights reserved.

Box 1
Risk factors for urinary tract infections

Bowel and bladder dysfunction

Urinary tract abnormalities
  Structural
  • VUR
  • Posterior urethral valves
  • Prune belly syndrome
  • Ureteropelvic or ureterovesical junction obstruction
  • Megaureter
  • Polycystic kidney disease
  Functional
  • Neurogenic bladder

Indwelling catheter

Immunosuppressed status

Neonates

Uncircumcised boys[3]

---

pathogenic microorganisms in the urinary tract, resulting in a symptomatic inflammatory response, as evidenced by pyuria. Conversely, colonization or asymptomatic bacteriuria (ABU) is the asymptomatic presence of bacteria in the urine without significant pyuria. Cystitis, the most common form of UTI, refers to the presence of inflammation isolated to the bladder. Pyelonephritis occurs when microbes ascend to the upper urinary tract and infect the renal parenchyma. Rarely, pyelonephritis can occur as a consequence of blood-borne infection. UTI can be classified as simple or complicated based on the absence or presence of risk factors, respectively, including structural or functional urinary tract abnormalities, indwelling devices, immunosuppression, or renal transplantation. Additionally, the presence of fever during UTI indicates a higher likelihood of pyelonephritis and increased risk of renal scarring. Defining a UTI as cystitis versus pyelonephritis, or as complicated versus uncomplicated, is helpful in determining prognosis and treatment.

Clinical Impact

UTI is responsible for 500,000 pediatric emergency department visits and more than 1 million clinic visits each year in the United States.[4–6] The overall US health care costs for management and treatment of UTI in 2013 was $630 million.[5,6] UTI carries an acute risk of morbidity and mortality due to urosepsis, renal abscess formation, and acute kidney injury. There is also a chronic risk of morbidity due to acquired renal scars, leading to chronic renal insufficiency, proteinuria, and hypertension. Renal scarring is found on dimercaptosuccinic acid (DMSA) scans on 10% to 40% of children who develop pyelonephritis.[7–9]

Pathogenesis of Urinary Tract Infection

The urinary tract has multiple mechanisms to prevent invasion by uropathogenic bacteria, including unidirectional flow of urine, complete bladder emptying, secretion of antimicrobial proteins and peptides into the urine stream, and urine ionic composition. The urothelium serves as the first line of defense against bacterial infection by preventing bacterial adherence and producing antibacterial peptides and mucous.[10]

Uropathogenic *Escherichia coli* (UPEC) is the most common and best studied pathogen implicated in UTI, accounting for 85% to 90% of episodes.[11,12] Other enteric gram-negative bacteria can cause UTI, including *Klebsiella, Pseudomonas, Proteus, Enterobacter*, and *Citrobacter* spp. Certain gram-positive organisms are also implicated in UTI, such as *Staphylococcus saprophyticus, Enterococcus* sp, and (rarely) *S aureus*. Most uropathogens originate from fecal flora that crosses the perineum to ascend the urethra and infect the bladder. On accessing the urinary tract, UPEC relies on a set of genome-encoded virulence factors to attach to and invade the bladder uroepithelium, as well as to directly interfere with the host immune response. UPEC triggers the host innate immune response, which entails production of inflammatory cytokines, complement activation, antimicrobial peptide secretion, and recruitment of phagocytes.[10,13] Although innate immunity functions effectively to eradicate bacteria, the resulting inflammation also leads to urothelial injury and clinical symptoms of cystitis.

Far less is known regarding the pathogenesis of acute pyelonephritis (APN). In nearly all cases, APN occurs as a consequence of bacterial ascension from the bladder. Thus, the presence of vesicoureteral reflux (VUR) confers increased susceptibility to APN in experimental models. Just as in cystitis, UPEC possesses virulence factors that enhance the likelihood of urinary tract ascent and invasion of the renal parenchyma. UPEC triggers phagocyte recruitment and activation, leading to acute tubulointerstitial nephritis. The collateral damage triggered by the host immune response is self-limited and reversible in most instances but a subset of children experience renal scarring. Emerging studies have identified single nucleotide polymorphisms in genes associated with innate immunity in certain individuals with recurrent APN and/or renal scarring.[7] This represents an area of active research, and the contribution of specific genetic variants to overall APN or renal scarring risk remains unknown.

DIAGNOSIS

The American Academy of Pediatrics (AAP) clinical practice guidelines define UTI based on urine culture and presence of pyuria. Specifically, pyuria is identified by urinalysis (UA): greater than or equal to 10 white blood count (WBC)/mm^3 or greater than or equal to 5 WBC per high-powered field (HPF), or by the presence of leukocyte esterase (LE) on a dipstick. A positive urine culture for UTI is defined by isolation of a single uropathogen at a density of greater than 50,000 colony-forming units (CFUs)/mL for urine specimens collected by catheterization or suprapubic aspiration (SPA), or greater than 100,000 CFU/mL for a midstream, clean-catch urine specimen.[14]

Screening for Urinary Tract Infection in Febrile Infants and Young Children (2–24 Months)

Based on AAP clinical practice guidelines, febrile children 2 to 24 months of age should be screened for UTI based on physician's clinical assessment.[14] The following series of risk factors are used to develop a prediction rule to estimate probability of UTI in infants.[15–17]

Infant girls: presence of more than 2 of the following risk factors increases probability of UTI to greater than 2%
- White race
- Age less than 12 months
- Fever greater than 48 hours
- No other apparent fever source
- Fever greater than or equal to 39°C.

Circumcised infant boys: presence of more than 3 of the following risk factors increases probability of UTI to greater than 2%
- Non-black race
- Fever greater than 24 hours
- No other apparent fever source
- Or fever greater than or equal to 39°C.

In uncircumcised infant boys, the probability of UTI is greater than 2% in the presence of fever greater than 39°C, without additional risk factors.

A probability of greater than or equal to 2% was identified as a screening threshold based on a survey of pediatricians, which showed that most pediatricians considered a probability of 1% to 3% sufficiently high to warrant a urine culture.[14] This screening threshold allows the clinician to place certain febrile infants into a low-likelihood group (probability of <1%–2%) to avoid invasive procedures to collect urine for culture (**Fig. 1**).

Screening for Urinary Tract Infection in Older Children and Specific Populations

Verbal children and adolescents should be screened for UTI if they have symptoms of dysuria, urgency, frequency, cloudy urine, or abdominal or flank pain, with or without fever. In addition, screening should also be done in children of any age with fever without a source if they have known urinary tract abnormalities, such as hydronephrosis, VUR, multicystic dysplastic kidney, neurogenic bladder, and voiding dysfunction, or in nonverbal children with cognitive disabilities.[18–20] In toilet trained children and adolescents, urine should be collected via midstream, clean catch. In children who have not achieved urinary continence, urine should be collected by transurethral catheterization or SPA.

Urine collected via urinary bag placed on the perineum should only be used to rule out a UTI based on UA but should never be used to diagnose a UTI. There is a high likelihood of contamination and false-positive results from bagged urine specimens.[5,14,21] If UTI is suspected based on bag specimen, urine should be recollected via catheterization or SPA. Some studies have suggested that a clean-catch specimen can be obtained from infants and young children using suprapubic and sacral stimulation procedures.[22–24] Although this is an attractive option to avoid invasive procedures and can be done without special equipment in the clinical setting, there is a high risk of culture contamination. A clean-catch urine specimen in infants can be used for screening UA, much like a bag specimen, and may be more reliably obtained (eg, decreased spillage, fecal contamination of bag). However, culture results from this method of collection should be interpreted with caution and, preferably, repeated with a catheterized or SPA urine specimen.

Presence of LE and nitrites on urine dipstick has a combined sensitivity of 93% and specificity 72% for UTI.[14] Urine nitrites are very specific for UTI but are not always present in the setting of UTI.[14] Nitrites are the conversion of dietary nitrates by enteric gram-negative, enteric organisms. It can take up to 4 hours for organisms to reduce nitrates to nitrites, and this can be missed on initial screening UA.[5,25] Furthermore, not all uropathogenic bacteria produce nitrites, giving nitrates a poor sensitivity for ruling out UTI. Alternatively, LE has a high sensitivity for UTI, although a recent study points to a lower incidence of pyuria in children with UTI due to *E* sp, *Klebsiella* sp, and *Pseudomonas aeruginosa* than those with *E coli* UTI.[12] Even so, LE remains a mainstay for UTI diagnosis. Urine microscopy is superior to identify pyuria, bacteriuria, and hematuria but is not always readily available in the clinical setting and is not required for diagnosis of UTI. On urine microscopy, the presence of greater than or equal to 10 WBC/mm^3 or greater than or equal to 5 WBC/HPF is considered significant in raising suspicion for UTI. Of note, the presence of LE is

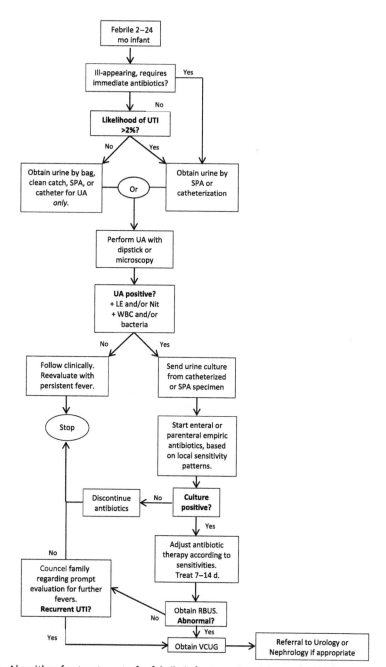

Fig. 1. Algorithm for treatment of a febrile infant age 2 to 24 months. d, day; LE, leukocyte esterase; RBUS, renal bladder ultrasound; SPA, suprapubic aspirate; UA, urinalysis; VCUG, voiding cystourethrogram; WBC, white blood count. (*Data from* Subcommittee on Urinary Tract Infection, Steering Committee on Quality Improvement and Management, Roberts KB. Urinary tract infection: clinical practice guideline for the diagnosis and management of the initial UTI in febrile infants and children 2 to 24 months. Pediatrics 2011;128(3):595–610.)

not specific for UTI because many other conditions can present with sterile pyuria, such as Kawasaki, glomerulonephritis, acute interstitial nephritis, appendicitis, or even intense exercise. In the presence of UTI symptoms, presence of bacteria on a fresh, uncentrifuged specimen in combination with Gram stain is also a reliable test to identify UTI.[12,26] The combined positive predictive value of bacteriuria and pyuria for UTI can be as high as 84%.[27]

As previously noted, urine culture should always be sent from a sample collected by clean catch, catheterization, or SPA, and accompanied by results of UA. Urine culture will show growth within 24 to 48 hours and antimicrobial sensitivities will typically require an additional 24 to 36 hours. Culture may be falsely negative or show a low colony count in children who were treated with antibiotics before urine collection, and this history should be elicited from the parent at the time of urine collection. In this setting, degree of clinical suspicion and findings on UA will likely be most helpful.

In children who perform clean intermittent catheterization, asymptomatic colonization is very common and occurs in almost 50% of children.[28] Cultures can grow up to 10^5 CFU of bacteria and sometimes multiple organisms are isolated. Screening for UTI and defining UTI in these children should follow more stringent criteria to avoid overprescription of antibiotics. Screening UA and urine culture should only be done when suspicion for UTI is high. Madden-Fuentes and colleagues[28] have proposed a stricter definition of UTI in children with spina bifida. This definition requires 2 or more UTI symptoms, greater than 10 WBC/HPF and greater than 100,000 CFU/mL of a single organism before diagnosing and treating a UTI.

Atypical Uropathogens

As noted previously, almost all UTIs are caused by bacteria, chiefly E coli. However, nonbacterial organisms can cause UTI in certain circumstances. Viral cystitis can occur in both immunocompetent and immunocompromised patients. In immunocompetent children, certain adenovirus strains cause a viral cystitis characterized by gross hematuria, dysuria, and abdominal discomfort. In immunocompromised children, polyomaviruses such as BK virus can cause hemorrhagic cystitis. Diagnosis can be made by polymerase chain reaction detection of the viral genome in the urine. Treatment of viral cystitis is often symptomatic. In the setting of severe symptoms or in immunocompromised states, antivirals have been used with variable results and should be considered on a case-by-case basis. Children with urinary schistosomiasis may present with cystitis and terminal hematuria. If such individuals have a history of travel to or immigration from endemic areas, they can be easily screened for urinary schistosomiasis, which is treated with the antiparasitic agent, praziquantel.

Fungal cystitis is rare but can occur in children on chronic antibiotics, with indwelling catheters, or children who are immunocompromised. The most common fungal pathogen is Candida sp.[29] Funguria is identified by presence of fungal elements or budding yeast on microscopy and growth of fungi on culture. Patients with UTI due to Candida sp can rarely develop a kidney fungal ball, usually at the ureteropelvic junction, which is detectable by renal ultrasound.[30]

Asymptomatic Bacteriuria

The clinical significance of ABU in healthy children is controversial. Various studies have shown 0% to 10% of children with ABU will develop a symptomatic UTI.[31–33] One randomized, prospective study of young girls with ABU showed no difference in renal function or renal size between girls treated for ABU and those left untreated.[32,33] ABU is more common in children with urinary tract abnormalities and those who chronically catheterize. ABU is not thought to increase risk of UTI or renal scarring in this population.[31] Screening for ABU is not recommended in any population and bacteriuria should only be treated if there is clinical suspicion for symptomatic infection.

CLINICAL MANAGEMENT
Antimicrobial Treatment

Prompt initiation of empiric antibiotics should occur if clinical suspicion for UTI is high and UA is suggestive of infection (presence of pyuria, with or without nitrites). Empiric antibiotics should be prescribed based on local sensitivity and resistance patterns. Antimicrobial therapy should be tailored to the results of urine culture and sensitivities. Antibiotics should be continued for a total of 7 to 14 days from initiation of appropriate therapy, based on AAP guidelines. Inpatient parenteral therapy should be considered for the first 2 to 4 days in acutely ill children, children who cannot tolerate oral therapy, or when adherence with prescribed regimen is in question. Children with a renal or perinephric abscess should be treated with parenteral therapy and surgical drainage should be considered. Parenteral therapy should also be considered in children who are immunocompromised and those with indwelling devices (eg, catheters, stents).

Commonly used empiric oral antibiotics are detailed in **Table 1**. In 2013, Edlin and colleagues[11] described resistance patterns in pediatric urinary isolates from 192 hospitals throughout the United States and found that up to 24% of E coli cultured were resistant to trimethoprim-sulfamethoxazole (TMP-SMX) and 45% resistant to ampicillin, making these a poor choice for empiric therapy. Furthermore, resistance was found in less than 10% of E coli for cephalosporins, amoxicillin-clavulanate, ciprofloxacin, and nitrofurantoin.[11] Nitrofurantoin is excreted primarily in the urine and can be a good antibiotic choice for isolated, afebrile cystitis. However, it does not achieve adequate concentrations within the blood stream, making it a poor therapy for febrile infants or young children with UTI.[14] In children with recurrent UTI, attention should be paid to culture and susceptibility patterns on previous urine specimens and empiric antibiotics tailored to those results. As soon as culture and sensitivity results are available, antibiotics should be adjusted or narrowed to the specific organism. Empiric antibiotics should be discontinued immediately if the urine culture fails to yield bacterial growth by 48 hours.

The development of infections with multidrug-resistant organisms (MDROs) are more commonly found in hospital-acquired infections, children with urinary tract abnormalities or with indwelling devices, and in children who have received recent antibiotics.[11,34] In the setting of UTI with MDROs, the practitioner should consider consultation with an infectious disease specialist.

Table 1
Common empiric antibiotics and recommended dosing

Antibiotic	Recommended Dosing	Maximum Dose
Amoxicillin-clavulanate	20–40 mg/kg/d divided 3 times daily	500 mg/dose
Trimethoprim (TMP)- sulfamethoxazole	2–24 mo: 6–12 mg TMP/kg/d divided twice daily >24 mo: 8 mg TMP/kg/d divided twice daily	160 mg/dose
Nitrofurantoin	5–7 mg/kg/d divided 4 times daily	100 mg/dose
Cephalexin	50–100 mg/kg/d divided 4 times daily >15 y: 500 mg twice daily	—
Cefpodoxime	10 mg/kg/d divided twice daily	—
Cefixime	8 mg/kg/d once daily	400 mg/d
Cefuroxime	20–30 mg/kg/d divided twice daily	500 mg/dose

Workup After First Febrile Urinary Tract Infection

Renal and bladder ultrasound (RBUS) is recommended after the first febrile UTI in children 2 to 24 months old to evaluate renal parenchyma, renal size, and urinary tract abnormalities that require further evaluation. RBUS can and should be obtained after treatment of UTI because acute infection can alter the size and echogenicity of the renal parenchyma and cause transient hydronephrosis, leading to a falsely abnormal study.[14] However, to rule out abscess or pyonephrosis that would require parenteral antibiotics, RBUS should be considered in the first 48 hours of treatment if illness is more severe than expected or if there is failure to improve with appropriate therapy. Alternatively, guidelines out of the United Kingdom through the National Institutes of Health and Clinical Excellence (NICE) recommend RBUS after first UTI only in children younger than 6 months or in children with atypical UTI (ie, presence of renal injury, atypical organisms, sepsis, or obstructed urine flow). NICE guidelines also recommend DMSA scan in children with atypical or recurrent UTI 4 to 6 months after treatment of acute UTI.

VUR is the most common urinary tract abnormality found after the first febrile UTI in infants and young children. Some degree of VUR is found in up to 40% of children after a first febrile UTI.[1] Based on 2008 data from the North American Pediatric Renal Trials and Collaborative Studies (NAPRTCS), reflux nephropathy is the reported cause of chronic kidney disease in up to 8.4% of children.[35] Current guidelines recommend obtaining voiding cystourethrogram (VCUG) only if RBUS is abnormal or after a second febrile UTI. RBUS abnormalities include hydronephrosis, scarring, or other findings suggestive of high grade VUR or obstructive uropathy (ie, abnormal bladder thickening, uroepithelial thickening in the renal pelvis, or hydroureter).[14] Notably, RBUS has poor sensitivity and specificity for clinically significant VUR. One study showed 40% sensitivity and 76% specificity for VUR on a positive RBUS.[36] Lack of hydronephrosis on RBUS does not rule out VUR. Therefore, if clinical suspicion is high or if the patient develops a second febrile UTI in the absence of RBUS abnormalities, VCUG should be strongly considered. Patients with VUR and febrile UTI should be evaluated and followed by a pediatric nephrologist or urologist.

In some cases, a VCUG should be considered after a first febrile UTI. The likelihood of an underlying urinary tract abnormality is higher in infants younger than 2 months of age with a first febrile UTI, and VCUG should be performed without waiting for a second febrile UTI. The practitioner may also consider a VCUG after a first febrile UTI in a circumcised boy, due to concerns for underlying obstructive uropathy not identified on ultrasonography.

A DMSA scan is a nuclear imaging study used to identify alterations in radiotracer uptake within the renal parenchyma. In the early phase of an acute UTI, DMSA is highly sensitive for identifying APN. Up to 57% of children with a febrile UTI have findings of APN on DMSA.[37,38] According to the Randomized Intervention for Children with Vesicoureteral Reflux (RIVUR) study data, DMSA done 4 to 6 months following treatment of a UTI revealed renal scarring in up to 15% of children who had radiologic evidence of pyelonephritis.[1,37] Different studies show widely varying results on renal scarring following UTI, ranging from 10% to 40%.[7–9] DMSA is more sensitive than RBUS in identifying renal scarring. If DMSA is unavailable, emerging studies suggest that magnetic resonance urography is a suitable alternative modality for detection of renal scars.[39,40] Some nephrology societies recommend obtaining nuclear renal scanning with technetium-labelled DMSA following the first febrile UTI in the setting of an atypical UTI or abnormal RBUS or VCUG.[5,41,42] However, AAP guidelines do not recommend DMSA scan as part of the initial workup of first febrile UTI. This is based on a lack of evidence that these findings will alter acute management of UTI.

All children should have a thorough physical examination to look for findings that would suggest a complicated UTI. Physical examination should focus on the abdomen and pelvis, assessing for abdominal masses, palpable stool, or bladder. A careful genitourinary examination should be performed assessing for abnormalities of the urethral opening, genital adhesions, or vulvovaginitis. An examination of the spine is important to rule out sacral dimples or hair tufts indicate occult spinal lesions.

Recurrent Urinary Tract Infection

Recurrent UTI (rUTI) is defined as 2 discrete UTI episodes, using the previously mentioned UTI definition criteria. One observational study identified risk factors for rUTI as age (3–5 years, typical toilet training age), white race, and higher grade VUR.[2] A prospective study identified grade III to IV VUR associated with female gender to be a risk factor for UTI recurrence.[43] Bowel and bladder dysfunction (BBD) is also a risk factor for the development of rUTI. BBD can be diagnosed formally through the use of a validated questionnaire.[38] Data collected from the RIVUR and CUTIE (Careful Urinary Tract Infection Evaluation) studies showed that there was an increased risk of development of rUTI in children with both BBD and VUR.[1,18,44] In adolescents, a sexual history should be obtained to identify postcoital UTIs or to differentiate from sexually transmitted infections.

A careful history and physical examination are integral to the workup of rUTI. Past medical history should be carefully reviewed to identify possibly underdiagnosed or falsely diagnosed UTIs. The clinician should elucidate whether previous UTIs have been febrile. Additional history should focus on evaluation of baseline voiding and stooling behaviors. The practitioner should ask parents and children about use of over-the-counter laxatives, stool softeners, and enemas. The child or parent should be questioned about stooling habits to assess for constipation or stool withholding and history of urinary accidents during the day or night. If available, past abdominal imaging can be reviewed to assess stool burden. Patients and families should be asked about gait disturbances and alterations in lower extremity sensation or movement to assess for underlying spinal cord abnormalities. Thorough examination for neurologic deficits, sacral dimples, tufts of hair, or genitourinary abnormalities is required.

Imaging should start with an RBUS to assess for hydronephrosis, hydroureter, or bladder abnormalities. VCUG should be obtained in children with recurrent febrile UTIs to assess for VUR and other bladder defects. When reviewing these studies, special attention should be paid to bladder capacity, postvoid residual, and bladder wall thickening that may suggest bladder dysfunction. Referral to urology for assessment of bladder dynamics may be beneficial in these patients. Children and adolescents with BBD benefit from aggressive bowel management with laxatives and stool softeners, timed voiding, and biofeedback exercises to improve bladder emptying. Sometimes, urology referral is required to assist with treatment of BBD, particularly when workup is negative and patient is refractory to treatment.

Prophylactic Antibiotics

The role of continuous antibiotic prophylaxis (CAP) in pediatric UTI prevention has been hotly debated over the past several decades. Most of the evidence regarding the use of CAP stems from studies in subjects with VUR and rUTI. Craig and colleagues[45] identified a moderate reduction in rUTI among subjects ages 0 to 18 years on CAP with TMP-SMX. Although VUR status was unknown in 17% of subjects, Garin and colleagues[46] concluded that neither CAP nor grade I to III VUR significantly influenced rUTI in children 3 months to 18 years. The Swedish Reflux Trial concluded that girls with high-grade VUR experienced reduced rates of rUTI and renal scarring compared with placebo controls over a 2-year period.[47,48] In the United States, the

RIVUR trial demonstrated a 50% reduction in rUTI among patients on CAP between the ages of 2 to 71 months with grade I to IV VUR.[49] The benefit of CAP was particularly evident in girls, patients with febrile index UTI, and those with BBD.[18] However, CAP was associated with a 3-fold increase in antibiotic resistance among stool *E coli* isolates. There was no significant impact of CAP on new renal scarring in the RIVUR study, which was relatively infrequent (8.3%) over the 24-month study period.[49] The apparent benefit of CAP in selected patient populations has led some investigators to advocate a selective prophylaxis approach in children with VUR.[50]

Other Prophylactic Measures

Therapies such as methenamine, cranberry juice, and probiotics have been studied as prophylactic agents in patients with rUTI. Recent, comprehensive reviews of these therapies have concluded that there is insufficient evidence to assign significant benefit to these agents.[51–53] Cranberry juice and supplements may provide benefit as prophylactic agents by acidifying the urine due to increased excretion of hippuric acid and/or by preventing adhesion of UPEC to urothelial cells. Studies using cranberry products in children have led to conflicting results, and they differ widely in cranberry dosing and frequency.[54] Larger, carefully-designed trials are required before recommendations for cranberry dosing can be confidently made in the pediatric population.

Perspectives for the Future Management of Pediatric Urinary Tract Infection

Given the enormity of UTI as a public health threat in children and the mounting rates of antibiotic-resistance among uropathogens, this article concludes by highlighting several recent, encouraging developments in UTI research. Emerging technologies point to the role of mass spectrometry and nucleic acid testing in improving the speed and accuracy of UTI diagnosis.[55] Implementing platforms based on these technologies in clinical laboratories will help limit antibiotic overuse. From a therapeutic viewpoint, recent studies point to the validity of disrupting host-pathogen interactions as a novel approach to UTI prevention and treatment. In this regard, the development of mannosides is highlighted. This is a novel class of antibiotics that disrupts high-affinity binding interactions between type I piliated *E coli* and mannosylated receptors on the bladder mucosal surface.[56] A recent study found that mannosides can abrogate experimental UTI and eradicate intestinal reservoirs of UPEC, offering a promising approach to long-term UTI prevention.[57] Finally, the potential value of leveraging rapidly evolving genomics approaches is emphasized, including analysis of gene copy number variation and whole genome sequencing as prognostic tools to identify patients at risk for UTI recurrence. Specifically, a recent landmark paper demonstrated the role of low *DEFA1A3* gene copy number in identifying patients at risk for breakthrough UTI while on antibiotic prophylaxis in the RIVUR study.[58] In summary, the fields of basic and applied UTI research are rapidly evolving. Further work is required to translate these discoveries into accessible, cost-effective technologies that aid clinicians in real-time decision-making at the bedside.

REFERENCES

1. Chesney RW, Carpenter MA, Moxey-Mims M, et al. Randomized intervention for children with vesicoureteral reflux (RIVUR): background commentary of RIVUR investigators. Pediatrics 2008;122(Suppl 5):S233–9.
2. Keren R, Shaikh N, Pohl H, et al. Risk factors for recurrent urinary tract infection and renal scarring. Pediatrics 2015;136(1):e13–21.

3. Schoen EJ, Colby CJ, Ray GT. Newborn circumcision decreases incidence and costs of urinary tract infections during the first year of life. Pediatrics 2000; 105(4 Pt 1):789–93.
4. Spencer JD, Schwaderer A, McHugh K, et al. Pediatric urinary tract infections: an analysis of hospitalizations, charges, and costs in the USA. Pediatr Nephrol 2010; 25(12):2469–75.
5. Korbel L, Howell M, Spencer JD. The clinical diagnosis and management of urinary tract infections in children and adolescents. Paediatr Int Child Health 2017; 37(4):273–9.
6. Freedman AL, Urologic Diseases in America Project. Urologic diseases in North America Project: trends in resource utilization for urinary tract infections in children. J Urol 2005;173(3):949–54.
7. Montini G, Tullus K, Hewitt I. Febrile urinary tract infections in children. N Engl J Med 2011;365(3):239–50.
8. Montini G, Zucchetta P, Tomasi L, et al. Value of imaging studies after a first febrile urinary tract infection in young children: data from Italian renal infection study 1. Pediatrics 2009;123(2):e239–46.
9. Shaikh N, Craig JC, Rovers MM, et al. Identification of children and adolescents at risk for renal scarring after a first urinary tract infection: a meta-analysis with individual patient data. JAMA Pediatr 2014;168(10):893–900.
10. Spencer JD, Schwaderer AL, Becknell B, et al. The innate immune response during urinary tract infection and pyelonephritis. Pediatr Nephrol 2014;29(7): 1139–49.
11. Edlin RS, Shapiro DJ, Hersh AL, et al. Antibiotic resistance patterns of outpatient pediatric urinary tract infections. J Urol 2013;190(1):222–7.
12. Shaikh N, Shope TR, Hoberman A, et al. Association Between Uropathogen and Pyuria. Pediatrics 2016;138(1). https://doi.org/10.1542/peds.2016-0087.
13. Becknell B, Schwaderer A, Hains DS, et al. Amplifying renal immunity: the role of antimicrobial peptides in pyelonephritis. Nat Rev Nephrol 2015;11(11):642–55.
14. Subcommittee on Urinary Tract Infection, Steering Committee on Quality Improvement and Management, Roberts KB. Urinary tract infection: clinical practice guideline for the diagnosis and management of the initial UTI in febrile infants and children 2 to 24 months. Pediatrics 2011;128(3):595–610.
15. Downs SM. Technical report: urinary tract infections in febrile infants and young children. The urinary tract subcommittee of the American Academy of Pediatrics committee on quality improvement. Pediatrics 1999;103(4):e54.
16. Gorelick MH, Hoberman A, Kearney D, et al. Validation of a decision rule identifying febrile young girls at high risk for urinary tract infection. Pediatr Emerg Care 2003;19(3):162–4.
17. Shaw KN, Gorelick M, McGowan KL, et al. Prevalence of urinary tract infection in febrile young children in the emergency department. Pediatrics 1998;102(2):e16.
18. Shaikh N, Hoberman A, Keren R, et al. Recurrent urinary tract infections in children with bladder and bowel dysfunction. Pediatrics 2016;137(1). https://doi.org/10.1542/peds.2015-2982.
19. Atiyeh B, Husmann D, Baum M. Contralateral renal abnormalities in patients with renal agenesis and noncystic renal dysplasia. Pediatrics 1993;91(4):812–5.
20. Atiyeh B, Husmann D, Baum M. Contralateral renal abnormalities in multicystic-dysplastic kidney disease. J Pediatr 1992;121(1):65–7.
21. Becknell B, Schober M, Korbel L, et al. The diagnosis, evaluation and treatment of acute and recurrent pediatric urinary tract infections. Expert Rev Anti Infect Ther 2015;13(1):81–90.

22. Altuntas N, Tayfur AC, Kocak M, et al. Midstream clean-catch urine collection in newborns: a randomized controlled study. Eur J Pediatr 2015;174(5):577–82.

23. Kaufman J, Fitzpatrick P, Tosif S, et al. Faster clean catch urine collection (Quick-Wee method) from infants: randomised controlled trial. BMJ 2017;357:j1341.

24. Ramage IJ, Chapman JP, Hollman AS, et al. Accuracy of clean-catch urine collection in infancy. J Pediatr 1999;135(6):765–7.

25. Powell HR, McCredie DA, Ritchie MA. Urinary nitrite in symptomatic and asymptomatic urinary infection. Arch Dis Child 1987;62(2):138–40.

26. Whiting P, Westwood M, Watt I, et al. Rapid tests and urine sampling techniques for the diagnosis of urinary tract infection (UTI) in children under five years: a systematic review. BMC Pediatr 2005;5(1):4.

27. Hoberman A, Wald ER. Urinary tract infections in young febrile children. Pediatr Infect Dis J 1997;16(1):11–7.

28. Madden-Fuentes RJ, McNamara ER, Lloyd JC, et al. Variation in definitions of urinary tract infections in spina bifida patients: a systematic review. Pediatrics 2013; 132(1):132–9.

29. Fisher JF, Sobel JD, Kauffman CA, et al. Candida urinary tract infections–treatment. Clin Infect Dis 2011;52(Suppl 6):S457–66.

30. Karlowicz MG. Candidal renal and urinary tract infection in neonates. Semin Perinatol 2003;27(5):393–400.

31. Ottolini MC, Shaer CM, Rushton HG, et al. Relationship of asymptomatic bacteriuria and renal scarring in children with neuropathic bladders who are practicing clean intermittent catheterization. J Pediatr 1995;127(3):368–72.

32. Lindberg U, Claesson I, Hanson LA, et al. Asymptomatic bacteriuria in schoolgirls. VIII. Clinical course during a 3-year follow-up. J Pediatr 1978;92(2):194–9.

33. Kemper KJ, Avner ED. The case against screening urinalyses for asymptomatic bacteriuria in children. Am J Dis Child 1992;146(3):343–6.

34. Uzodi AS, Lohse CM, Banerjee R. Risk factors for and outcomes of multidrug-resistant Escherichia coli infections in children. Infect Dis Ther 2017;6(2):245–57.

35. Smith JM, Stablein DM, Munoz R, et al. Contributions of the Transplant Registry: the 2006 Annual Report of the North American Pediatric Renal Trials and Collaborative Studies (NAPRTCS). Pediatr Transplant 2007;11(4):366–73.

36. Mahant S, Friedman J, MacArthur C. Renal ultrasound findings and vesicoureteral reflux in children hospitalised with urinary tract infection. Arch Dis Child 2002;86(6):419–20.

37. Mattoo TK, Chesney RW, Greenfield SP, et al. Renal Scarring in the Randomized Intervention for Children with Vesicoureteral Reflux (RIVUR) trial. Clin J Am Soc Nephrol 2016;11(1):54–61.

38. Farhat W, Bagli DJ, Capolicchio G, et al. The dysfunctional voiding scoring system: quantitative standardization of dysfunctional voiding symptoms in children. J Urol 2000;164(3 Pt 2):1011–5.

39. Freeman CW, Altes TA, Rehm PK, et al. Unenhanced MRI as an alternative to (99m)Tc-labeled dimercaptosuccinic acid scintigraphy in the detection of pediatric renal scarring. AJR Am J Roentgenol 2018;210(4):869–75.

40. Kocyigit A, Yuksel S, Bayram R, et al. Efficacy of magnetic resonance urography in detecting renal scars in children with vesicoureteral reflux. Pediatr Nephrol 2014;29(7):1215–20.

41. Baumer JH, Jones RW. Urinary tract infection in children, National Institute for Health and Clinical Excellence. Arch Dis Child Educ Pract Ed 2007;92(6):189–92.

42. Ammenti A, Cataldi L, Chimenz R, et al. Febrile urinary tract infections in young children: recommendations for the diagnosis, treatment and follow-up. Acta Paediatr 2012;101(5):451–7.
43. Olbing H, Smellie JM, Jodal U, et al. New renal scars in children with severe VUR: a 10-year study of randomized treatment. Pediatr Nephrol 2003;18(11):1128–31.
44. Cara-Fuentes G, Gupta N, Garin EH. The RIVUR study: a review of its findings. Pediatr Nephrol 2015;30(5):703–6.
45. Craig JC, Simpson JM, Williams GJ, et al. Antibiotic prophylaxis and recurrent urinary tract infection in children. N Engl J Med 2009;361(18):1748–59.
46. Garin EH, Olavarria F, Garcia Nieto V, et al. Clinical significance of primary vesicoureteral reflux and urinary antibiotic prophylaxis after acute pyelonephritis: a multicenter, randomized, controlled study. Pediatrics 2006;117(3):626–32.
47. Brandstrom P, Esbjorner E, Herthelius M, et al. The Swedish reflux trial in children: III. Urinary tract infection pattern. J Urol 2010;184(1):286–91.
48. Brandstrom P, Neveus T, Sixt R, et al. The Swedish reflux trial in children: IV. Renal damage. J Urol 2010;184(1):292–7.
49. Investigators RT, Hoberman A, Greenfield SP, et al. Antimicrobial prophylaxis for children with vesicoureteral reflux. N Engl J Med 2014;370(25):2367–76.
50. Mattoo TK, Carpenter MA, Moxey-Mims M, et al. The RIVUR trial: a factual interpretation of our data. Pediatr Nephrol 2015;30(5):707–12.
51. Schwenger EM, Tejani AM, Loewen PS. Probiotics for preventing urinary tract infections in adults and children. Cochrane Database Syst Rev 2015;(12):CD008772.
52. Lee BS, Bhuta T, Simpson JM, et al. Methenamine hippurate for preventing urinary tract infections. Cochrane Database Syst Rev 2012;(10):CD003265.
53. Jepson RG, Williams G, Craig JC. Cranberries for preventing urinary tract infections. Cochrane Database Syst Rev 2012;(10):CD001321.
54. Durham SH, Stamm PL, Eiland LS. Cranberry products for the prophylaxis of urinary tract infections in pediatric patients. Ann Pharmacother 2015;49(12):1349–56.
55. Davenport M, Mach KE, Shortliffe LMD, et al. New and developing diagnostic technologies for urinary tract infections. Nat Rev Urol 2017;14(5):296–310.
56. Cusumano CK, Pinkner JS, Han Z, et al. Treatment and prevention of urinary tract infection with orally active FimH inhibitors. Sci Transl Med 2011;3(109):109ra15.
57. Spaulding CN, Klein RD, Ruer S, et al. Selective depletion of uropathogenic E. coli from the gut by a FimH antagonist. Nature 2017;546(7659):528–32.
58. Schwaderer AL, Wang H, Kim S, et al. Polymorphisms in alpha-defensin-encoding DEFA1A3 associate with urinary tract infection risk in children with vesicoureteral reflux. J Am Soc Nephrol 2016;27(10):3175–86.

Approach to the Child with Hematuria

Denver D. Brown, MD, Kimberly J. Reidy, MD*

KEYWORDS

- Hematuria • Red blood cells • Macroscopic • Gross hematuria
- Microscopic hematuria • Glomerulonephritis • Hypercalciuria
- Thin basement membrane nephropathy

KEY POINTS

- Infection is a frequent cause of both gross and microscopic hematuria.
- Coexistent Hypertension and proteinuria should prompt investigation for glomerular disease.
- Microscopic hematuria is often transient and work-up will not identify the cause.
- The most common causes of persistent microscopic hematuria are thin basement membrane nephropathy, immunoglobulin A nephropathy, or idiopathic hypercalciuria.

OVERVIEW

Red blood cells (RBCs) in the urine are required for a diagnosis of hematuria. Hematuria can be either macroscopic or microscopic. Macroscopic hematuria (**Fig. 1**A) is visible as red or brown discoloration of the urine. Changing the color of urine from yellow to pink or red requires only a small amount of blood, as little as 1 mL of blood per 1000 mL of urine.[1] Besides hematuria, urinary color change can be caused by the presence of other substances: (1) medications (eg, rifampin, nitrofurantoin, metronidazole, triamterene, propofol, senna), (2) foods (eg, food dyes, beets/beetroot, blackberries, rhubarb, fava beans), or (3) presence of heme (eg, hemoglobin/myoglobinuria). Thus, for a diagnosis of hematuria, the presence of RBCs should always be confirmed by urine microscopy examination of freshly voided urine; more than 3 to 5 RBC/high-power field is considered abnormal. A freshly voided urine limits RBC lysis, and, therefore, false negative results. Urine microscopy may also reveal urinary sediment with RBC casts (**Fig. 1**B, C) or dysmorphic RBCs, suggesting glomerulonephritis. Exogenous blood, as with Munchhausen syndrome or contamination with menstruation, needs to be excluded.

Pediatric Nephrology, Children's Hospital at Montefiore, Albert Einstein College of Medicine, 3415 Bainbridge Avenue, Bronx, NY 10467, USA
* Corresponding author.
E-mail address: kreidy@montefiore.org

Pediatr Clin N Am 66 (2019) 15–30
https://doi.org/10.1016/j.pcl.2018.08.003
0031-3955/19/© 2018 Elsevier Inc. All rights reserved.

pediatric.theclinics.com

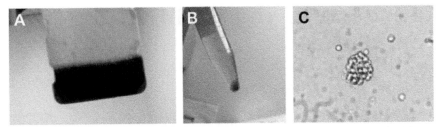

Fig. 1. Macroscopic hematuria: (*A*) gross hematuria, (*B*) urine sediment, (*C*) RBC cast.

MACROSCOPIC HEMATURIA
Epidemiology and Cause

In children, gross hematuria occurs relatively rarely with an incidence in the United States estimated at 1.3 of 1000 outpatient visits.[2] Blood in the urine can originate from either the upper urinary tract (kidneys and ureters) or the lower urinary tract (bladder and urethra). Typically, features of hematuria due to upper urinary tract pathologic condition include painless brown/cola-colored urine. Conversely, signs of hematuria originating from the lower urinary tract include dysuria, bright red blood, and the appearance of clots. Although macroscopic hematuria itself presents in both male and female children equally, some causes of gross hematuria (see **Box 1**) have a sex predilection; for example, urinary tract infections (UTI) are more common in girls.[2–4] The most common causes of gross hematuria in children include UTI, trauma, and perineal irritation. Less common causes include sickle cell disease/trait, nephrolithiasis, glomerulonephritides, malignancy, urologic abnormalities (including ureteral pelvic junction obstruction), coagulopathies, and drug-induced cystitis.

WorkUp

Determination of the source of hematuria and underlying cause requires a thorough history and physical examination. The source of hematuria may be suggested by timing during micturition: hematuria at voiding onset indicates urethral bleeding; hematuria present throughout the urinary stream indicates bleeding anywhere

---

Box 1
Differential diagnosis

Agents that can change urine color (foods, dyes, medications)

Red diaper syndrome (gastroenteritis due to *Serratia marcescens*)

Hemoglobinuria

Myoglobinuria

Upper urinary tract
  Glomerular
  Vascular
  Interstitial

Lower urinary tract
  Cyst
  Stone
  Obstruction
  Infection (viral, bacterial, parasite)
  Trauma
  Malignancy

along the urinary tract, whereas terminal hematuria indicates a bladder or urethral origin. Dysuria, urgency, frequency, and enuresis are suggestive of UTI. Abdominal and flank pain are suggestive of nephrolithiasis; however, flank pain may be present with other causes of hematuria as well. History should include assessment for recent infections (eg, throat or skin infections that may precede postinfectious glomerulonephritis), personal or family history of hemoglobinopathies/coagulopathies, drug exposures, and trauma. Systemic illnesses associated with gross hematuria (such as vasculidities) may present with extrarenal symptoms; these include rashes, joint pain, hair loss, mouth ulcers, weight loss, and fever. Family history of hematuria, renal disease, and deafness suggests hereditary nephropathies. On physical examination, hypertension and edema are suggestive of glomerulonephritis.

The most likely differential diagnosis (**Fig. 2**) should guide laboratory and radiologic testing. The workup of gross hematuria should include a renal bladder ultrasound with Doppler. Rare but important causes of gross hematuria are renal tumors. Renal neoplasms include Wilm tumor, renal cell carcinoma (RCC), and medullary RCC. Of these, Wilm tumor occurs most commonly in children less than 15 years of age; in up to 20%, gross hematuria may be the presenting symptom.[5] Although medullary RCC is rare, children with sickle cell trait have higher tumor risk. Renal ultrasound with Doppler also identifies renal arterial or venous thrombosis. Thrombosis should be high on the differential diagnosis for gross hematuria presenting in either a nephrotic child or a newborn infant.

Common and/or important causes of gross hematuria in children
Upper urinary tract

Postinfectious glomerulonephritis As suggested by its name, postinfectious glomerulonephritis (PIGN) classically presents with red-brown or cola-colored urine, edema, proteinuria, and hypertension, nephritic syndrome. In the developing world, PIGN accounts for one-fifth of acute renal failure hospitalizations[6,7] with poststreptococcal GN (PSGN) being the most common. PSGN is preceded by beta-hemolytic streptococcal infection of the throat, upper respiratory tract, or skin. The onset of PSGN varies by infection site: symptoms begin 1 to 2 weeks following throat infection versus 3 to 5 weeks following skin infections.[8,9]

In addition to streptococcus, numerous other infectious agents (including staphylococcal, gram-negative bacteria, viral, fungal, and parasitic agents) cause PIGN.[9–12] The pathogenesis of PIGN is thought to result from molecular mimicry: the infection triggers production of antibodies capable of cross-reacting with host antigens. In support of this concept, sera from patients with PSGN contained circulating antibodies to both collagen and laminin components of the glomerular basement membrane.[6] Certain strains of streptococcus are more likely to cause PSGN, likely due to the presence of nephritogenic antigens. In PSGN, 2 primary nephritogenic antigens are nephritis-associated plasmin receptor and streptococcal pyrogenic exotoxin B.[7] In addition to these antigens, streptococcal neuraminidases enzymatically alter host immunoglobulins. This enzymatic modification may induce autoimmune reactivity leading to formation of immunoglobulin antibodies.[6] Antigen-antibody complexes then form either in the circulation or in situ by binding antigen already in the glomerulus. Antigen-antibody immune complex deposition on the glomerular capillary wall activates both the complement cascade and the coagulation pathways.[6,13]

The age of onset for PSGN is approximately 4–14 years, and it preferentially affects boys.[9] At the time of infection, children may experience low-grade fever, malaise, and poor appetite. Following a latent period, up to 70% present with gross hematuria,

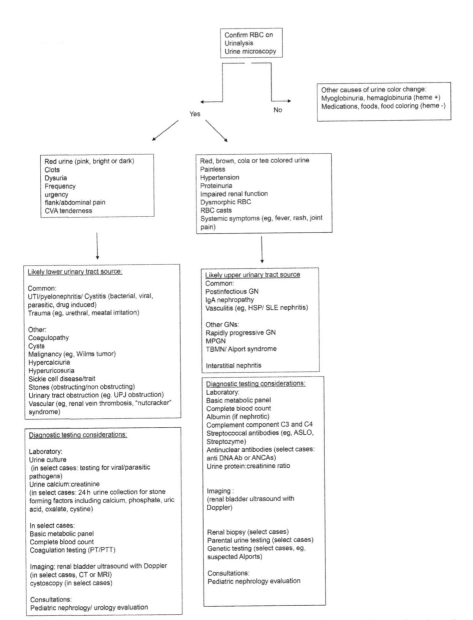

Fig. 2. Gross hematuria workup. Abs, antibodies; ANCAs, antineutrophil cytoplasmic antibodies; CT, computed tomography; CVA, cerebrovascular accident; HSP/SLE, Henoch-Schönlein purpura/systemic lupus erythematosus; MPGN, membranoproliferative glomerulonephritis; PT/PTT, prothrombin time/partial thromboplastin time; UPJ, ureteropelvic junction.

whereas microscopic hematuria is present in all patients.[8] The urine is often dark, typically described as "rusty," "tea," or "cola" colored.[14] Patients may also present with either localized edema or anasarca as a result of salt and water retention.[15] This sodium and water retention may also manifest as hypertension, which can escalate into hypertensive crisis.[14,16] In some cases of PSGN, patients are asymptomatic.[15]

Classic laboratory findings of PSGN include (1) decreased renal function (elevated serum creatinine); (2) RBC casts on urine microscopy; (3) subnephrotic proteinuria; (4) decreased complement component C3; and (5) positive streptococcal (antistreptolysin and Anti-DNase B) antibodies. A minority will present with overt renal failure and/or nephrotic range proteinuria.[17–19]

These clinical features typically establish a PSGN diagnosis. However, renal biopsy should be considered in cases of atypical presentation with significant renal impairment and/or persistent hypocomplementemia.[20,21] In classic PSGN, light microscopy reveals widespread proliferation of endothelial cells and mesangial cells and neutrophilic infiltration of the glomerulus, a diffuse exudative proliferative glomerulonephritis. Although rare, a crescentic PSGN will often result in severe renal dysfunction.[21,22] In electron microscopy of classic PSGN, subepithelial deposits (or "humps") are visualized. Less frequently, subendothelial and intramembranous deposits may be present.[23] These subepithelial deposits consist predominantly of immunoglobulin G (IgG) and C3 and, on immunofluorescence, these deposits produce a granular "starry-sky" pattern.[24]

PSGN treatment is supportive; the disease course is most often self-limited with symptoms beginning to resolve within 1 week. Hypocomplementemia may take up to 8 to 12 weeks to resolve.[25] Edema and hypertension are treated initially by sodium restriction and diuretic therapy. In some cases, persistent hypertension may be treated with calcium channel blockers. Antiproteinuric agents may be helpful but used with caution when there is evidence of renal insufficiency or in cases of hyperkalemia. In rare cases of severe renal impairment, refractory fluid overload or electrolyte derangement, renal replacement therapy may be needed. Although randomized controlled trials are lacking, severe crescentic PSGN is often treated with immunosuppression.[21,26]

Immunoglobulin A nephropathy Immunoglobulin A nephropathy (IgAN) is the most common primary glomerulonephritis worldwide.[27–29] Although prevalence varies, it is highest in East Asian and Caucasian populations. In China, it accounts for up to 45% of primary glomerulonephritis. Susceptibility to IgAN is likely affected by genetic factors.[30] IgAN is rare among black populations.[31] It preferentially affects men and boys.[29,32] It can affect patients of various ages but often presents in the second to third decades of life.[33] There is a subset of people, estimated to be 3% to 16%, who have IgAN histologically but lack any clinical symptoms of nephritis.[34,35]

The pathophysiology of IgAN is complex. Abnormal IgA1 subclass glycosylation is an important predisposing factor. Normally, galactose is attached to the hinge region of the IgA1 heavy chain; patients with IgAN have higher quantities of galactose-deficient IgA1. IgA1 antibodies contribute to normal immune response to mucosal antigens; in IgAN, this mucosal response leads to galactose-deficient IgA1 antibody production.[36] Circulating galactose-deficient IgA1 forms immune complexes with IgG and IgM, which then deposit in the renal mesangium.[37,38] In addition to forming circulating immune complexes, deposition of galactose-deficient IgA1 in glomeruli may lead to in situ mesangial complex formation.[39] In response to mesangial complex deposition, mesangial cells proliferate, secrete increased matrix, and release proinflammatory factors.[40,41] These proinflammatory factors may contribute to tubular damage.[40,42] IgA1 deposition may also activate the alternative complement pathway leading to further renal damage.[43,44]

The most common clinical presenting symptom of IgAN is recurrent gross hematuria, which is present in 40% to 55% of patients.[29] Gross hematuria is commonly triggered by an upper respiratory or gastrointestinal (mucosal) infection. Unlike PSGN, hematuria is usually evident within days of the infection, making it a "synpharyngitic hematuria." Rather than gross hematuria, 30% to 40% of patients present with microscopic hematuria with nonnephrotic range proteinuria.[45,46] A small percentage of patients develop nephrotic syndrome or rapidly progressive glomerulonephritis (RPGN).

IgAN diagnosis is confirmed by renal biopsy, by mesangial IgA immunofluorescence deposits. Less commonly, IgA deposits can also be found in the subendothelial capillary wall.[47] Deposits of IgG and/or IgM may also be present, but IgA must be dominant for the diagnosis.[28,29,48] Codeposition with IgG and subendothelial capillary wall infiltration are both associated with poor prognoses.[47,48] C3 is present in more than 90% of biopsy specimens.[49] In IgAN, the most common light microscopy finding is mesangial hypercellularity and matrix expansion.[49] Other potential patterns include segmental glomerulosclerosis, glomerular crescents, and tubulointerstitial atrophy/fibrosis.[49]

The prognosis for patients with IgAN varies. As many as 40% of patients progress to end-stage renal disease (ESRD) in 10 to 20 years.[50] Clinical predictors of progression include proteinuria exceeding 1 g/d, hypertension, severe histologic pathologic condition, and elevated serum creatinine at the time of diagnosis.[45,51,52]

There are no specific treatments for IgAN. Treatment of hypertension and proteinuria with angiotensin-converting enzyme inhibitors (ACEIs)/angiotensin II receptor blockers (ARBs) can be beneficial in slowing progression. Although clinical trials have not been conclusive, fish oil/omega-3 fatty acids have been used for their anti-inflammatory properties.[53,54] Glucocorticoid therapy use is controversial but may be beneficial in the case of persistent heavy proteinuria, despite antiproteinurics, RPGN, or histologically active disease.[55,56] There are a paucity of studies evaluating the role of other immunosuppressive agents, as monotherapy or in combination with glucocorticoids. For crescentic IgAN, cyclophosphamide in combination with glucocorticoids has been used.[57,58] In cases of ESRD, renal transplantation is the treatment of choice. However, IgA deposition may recur in the graft, with or without clinically significant disease. Recurrence has been reported to be as high as 58% of cases.[59,60] Currently no intervention exists for preventing disease recurrence in the transplanted allograft.

Vasculitides Vasculitides are rare in the pediatric population: the estimated incidence of primary vasculitis in children less than 17 years old is approximately 23 per 100,000.[61] However, the most common pediatric vasculitides overall are Kawasaki disease and immunoglobulin A vasculitis (IgAV), which is also known as Henoch-Schönlein purpura. Although the most common renal manifestation of Kawasaki disease is sterile pyuria, it occasionally results in gross hematuria with a hypocomplementemic glomerulonephritis.[62]

IgAV is a small-vessel vasculitis.[63] It is more common in men and boys and Caucasians. IgAV often presents in the winter and spring months. The classic triad of symptoms is abdominal pain, arthritis/arthralgias, and nonthrombocytopenic palpable purpura of the buttocks and lower extremities.[64] A variable percentage, 20% to 54%, also has renal involvement; this is more frequent among older-aged children.[65–67] Renal manifestations can present concurrently with systemic symptoms or may develop months later. Renal manifestations may include hematuria (microscopic more often than macroscopic) and subnephrotic range proteinuria. Less commonly, patients may also have nephrotic syndrome, hypertension, and renal insufficiency.[68,69]

The pathogenesis of IgAV is not fully understood and may overlap with IgAN with elevations in circulating abnormally glycosylated IgA1, IgA1-circulating immune complexes, and IgA-rheumatoid factors.[70] In those who develop nephritis, large-molecular-mass (vs small) IgA1-IgG circulating immune complexes appear to play a pivotal role.[71] On skin or renal biopsy, IgA, complement (C3 in particular), and fibrin deposits on capillary walls are seen. Renal biopsy findings are indistinguishable from IgAN. Diagnosis of IgAV is often made by clinical presentation but can be confirmed by biopsy. Kidney biopsy is typically reserved for cases of clinical uncertainty or patients with significant renal involvement.

IgAV often resolves spontaneously and requires only supportive care consisting of rest, hydration, and oral analgesics. Hospitalization may be required for severe symptoms, especially in cases of renal impairment. Although evidence suggests glucocorticoids may not significantly alter the disease course, they may decrease the duration of abdominal pain.[72–75] Currently, there is a lack of consensus on the best management of IgAV nephritis. The 2012 Kidney Disease: Improving Global Outcomes guidelines recommended a 3- to 6-month course of ACEIs/ARBs therapy for patients with proteinuria greater than 0.5 g/d before a trial of glucocorticoids.[76] However, others argue for earlier use of glucocorticoids in pediatric patients with more severe renal compromise. It has been suggested that patients with proteinuria >1 g/d, nephrotic syndrome, or crescentic GN receive intravenous pulse and then oral steroids.[77]

Although IgAV may recur, an overwhelming majority of pediatric patients undergo complete recovery. Subsequent relapses tend to be milder. For those children with renal involvement, female patients are 2.5 times more likely to have long-term renal impairment.[68] Presentation with nephrotic-range proteinuria, elevated serum creatinine, and/or hypertension portends a poorer prognosis. In one study, 20% developed long-term renal impairment.[68] IgAV with crescentic GN has an even worse prognosis. In one study, 37% progressed to ESRD, and an additional 18% developed chronic kidney disease.[78]

Lower urinary tract hematuria

Nephrolithiasis Although not as common as in adults, the incidence of pediatric nephrolithiasis is increasing. A recent retrospective study found that it accounted for as many as 1 in 685 US hospital admissions.[79] In general, stones are slightly more common in boys than girls. However, this varies with age and other stone-forming risk factors. Young boys have more congenital abnormalities, whereas older-aged girls have higher rates of UTI.[80–82] Stones are more common in Caucasian children than other racial groups. Nephrolithiasis is rare in children of African descent.[79,81] Recently, antibiotic (including sulfa, cephalosporin, fluoroquinolone, nitrofurantoin/methenamine, and broad-spectrum penicillin) exposure was identified as a risk factor for pediatric stone.[83,84] Antibiotic-induced intestinal microbiome (eg, *Oxalobacter formigene*) alterations are a plausible biologic mechanism for this increased risk. Indeed, rising stone disease rates may be due in part to increased antibiotic exposure.

Stone formation is affected by multiple factors, including the urinary ion distribution, solute supersaturation, urinary volume, and pH. As many as 86% of children have an underlying risk factor.[85] These risk factors include (1) lithogenic urine (hypercalciuria; hypocitraturia; or increased supersaturation of calcium phosphates or oxalates); (2) drug exposure (eg, furosemide or antibiotic exposure); (3) UTI; and (4) genitourinary malformations leading to stasis.[80,85] Genetic causes of stone formation include hereditary forms of renal tubular acidosis, primary hyperoxaluria, and cystinuria. Stones can develop anywhere along the genitourinary tract, but renal stones are more common in younger patients.[86]

Macroscopic hematuria and abdominal/flank pain are the most common presenting symptoms for children with renal stones. Up to 55% of children may present with gross hematuria.[87] Other common symptoms include dysuria and urgency.

Concomitant UTI may also occur with obstructing, bladder, or urethral stones. It is not uncommon for nephrolithiasis to be asymptomatic and diagnosed incidentally during a workup for an unrelated complaint.

Workup of nephrolithiasis should include urinalysis and urine culture to rule out infection. In addition, crystals may be visualized on microscopic examination. A 24-hour urine collection for "stone-risk profile" can be used to assess urinary volume, to assess pH, and to quantify urine ions and solutes along with a saturation index to determine the potential for stone formation. Ultrasonography is effective in visualizing radiolucent stones and can demonstrate the presence of urinary obstruction. Because of its low radiation exposure, it is recommended as the first-line imaging technique.[88] Computed tomography without contrast is a more sensitive modality for detecting small renal and ureteral stones but should be used judiciously given high radiation exposure.[88,89]

Most often, treatment is supportive. Hydration and pain control can allow for spontaneous stone passage. Alpha blockade agents may improve stone passage.[90,91] Extracorporeal shock wave lithotripsy or surgical stone removal may be needed for large stones, uncontrollable pain, urinary obstruction, or renal compromise. Long-term medical management for stone prevention includes maintaining oral hydration, a low salt and moderate protein diet as well as the use of medications, including potassium citrate and/or thiazide diuretics when indicated by the stone risk profile.

Renal cysts Renal cysts may be (1) congenital (eg, multicystic dysplastic kidneys); (2) monogenic renal cystic disease (eg, autosomal recessive polycystic kidney disease or autosomal dominant polycystic kidney disease [ADPKD]); (3) associated with genetic syndromes (eg, tuberous sclerosis); (4) acquired (eg, in chronic dialysis); or (5) isolated.[92,93] Isolated cysts can be simple and benign or complex; complex cysts require monitoring given their malignant potential.[94] Clinically, cystic disease of any kind may present with abdominal pain, especially in cases of renomegaly. Macroscopic hematuria may occur from cyst rupture. Although all cysts have the potential to bleed, gross hematuria is a common complication of ADPKD and tuberous sclerosis. Renal cysts may also lead to UTI/pyelonephritis from urinary stasis and infection. In some cases, cystic disease results in hypertension. Diagnosis of the underlying cystic disease may include genetic studies to evaluate for mutations.

ADPKD, also known as adult polycystic kidney disease, is of autosomal dominant inheritance and is the most common inherited renal disease. An estimated 4 to 7 million people worldwide suffer from ADPKD.[95] ADPKD results from mutations in either (1) *PKD1*, located on chromosome 16 encoding for polycystin 1, or (2) *PKD2* gene on chromosome 4, which encodes polycystin 2. Polycystins localize to renal tubular epithelia primary cilia and regulate cell signaling. ADPKD results in macrocysts and enlarged kidneys. The number and size of cysts increase with age. Thus, during childhood, ADPKD may have mild manifestations.

ADPKD management and outcome depends on disease severity. Antihypertensive treatment targeting the renin-angiotensin system is used for blood pressure control. Recently, tolvaptan (a vasopressin V2 receptor inhibitor) was approved for treatment of adults with ADPKD to delay GFR decline. Fifty percent of patients with ADPKD progress to ESRD, and ADPKD accounts for up to 15% of the US adult dialysis population.[96]

Renal venous thrombosis Renal venous thrombosis (RVT) is a rare thromboembolic condition that is associated with significant morbidity.[97] RVT results from a reduction in blood flow and an increase in blood viscosity, promoting a coagulopathic state. Associated risk factors in the newborn period include prematurity, maternal diabetes, dehydration, polycythemia, sepsis, birth asphyxia, umbilical catheters, and congenital renal vein defects.[98,99] In older children, prothrombotic conditions such as nephrotic syndrome as well as renal transplantation are risk factors.[100,101] In infants, it appears to affect more male infants than female infants and is often unilateral, occurring more often on the left side.[98] Genetic mutations that result in hypercoagulable states, such as Factor V Leiden mutation, are risk factors for RVT. The classic triad of RVT symptoms is gross hematuria, thrombocytopenia, and a palpable abdominal mass.[98] Renal ultrasound with Doppler is the preferred modality for diagnosis. Most commonly, it will demonstrate decreased renal blood flow and an enlarged kidney with loss of corticomedullary differentiation, rather than an overt thrombus. Gross hematuria can also result from renal arterial thrombosis. Umbilical artery catheters increase this risk; in these cases, the thrombus is more often visualized by ultrasound.

Anticoagulation or fibrinolytic therapy may be needed with renal arterial or venous thrombosis, especially with bilateral disease. Long-term follow-up is indicated, because there is high risk for long-term renal impairment.[102]

MICROSCOPIC HEMATURIA
Epidemiology and Cause

In contrast to gross hematuria, microscopic hematuria is common: microscopic hematuria is present in 3% to 5% of healthy children on screening urinalysis. This microscopic hematuria is most often transient and resolves spontaneously. On repeat testing, only 1% to 2% of children will have persistent microscopic hematuria. Although there is much overlap between the causes of macroscopic and microscopic hematuria, the most common causes differ. The top 3 causes are thin basement membrane nephropathy (TBMN), IgAN, and hypercalciuria.[103]

Workup
The workup for microscopic hematuria starts with a thorough history and physical examination. A key element is to determine if there are associated signs or symptoms. Symptomatic microscopic hematuria (with complaints of dysuria, urgency, or frequency) suggests underlying infection or urethral/bladder irritation. As with macroscopic hematuria, other signs or symptoms associated with microscopic hematuria will guide the initial workup (see **Fig. 2**).

Less commonly (an estimated 0.7% of school-aged children) is the finding of microscopic hematuria in association with proteinuria. The presence of both microscopic hematuria and proteinuria portends higher risk for renal disease. A repeat urinalysis should be sent with a simultaneous urine protein:creatinine ratio. Persistent hematuria with a urine protein:creatinine ratio greater than 0.2 mg/mg (or >0.5 mg/mg in an infant) should prompt an immediate pediatric nephrology referral.

Screening of asymptomatic children is not currently recommended by the American Academy of Pediatrics. If a urinalysis in an asymptomatic patient results in isolated microscopic hematuria, the initial step is to repeat urinalyses (every 1–2 weeks). Repeat urinalysis from patients with positive screening urinalyses is most often normal by the third repeat test.[104] If the urinalysis does not normalize, further workup (**Fig. 3**) may be initiated. Workup in most children with isolated asymptomatic proteinuria will not lead to a diagnosis. However, continued long-term follow-up with monitoring for proteinuria or hypertension may be warranted. In an Israeli study, persistent isolated microscopy hematuria was associated with an increased risk of ESRD.[105]

Common causes of microscopic hematuria in children
Thin basement membrane nephropathy and Alport syndrome Genetic alterations in type IV collagen chains result in TBMN. TBMN typically presents with isolated persistent

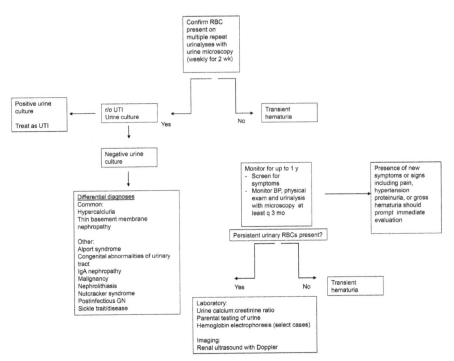

Fig. 3. Isolated asymptomatic microscopic hematuria workup. BP, blood pressure; q, every; r/o, rule out.

microscopic hematuria. Often, there is a family history of microscopic hematuria. In some patients, TBMN can result in episodes of gross hematuria. Definitive diagnosis of TBMN requires a renal biopsy in which electron microcopy reveals diffuse thinning of the glomerular basement membrane. However, a renal biopsy is rarely performed in the absence of significant proteinuria or recurrent gross hematuria.

Although often a benign disease, a subset of patients with TBMN develops progressive proteinuria and renal failure. This variability in disease severity has led to the concept of a spectrum of hereditary nephropathy linked to type IV collagen genetic variants. The most severe loss of function mutations in collagen type IV result in Alport syndrome. X-linked Alport syndrome results from collagen IV alpha 5 mutations. The autosomal recessive form of Alport syndrome results from mutations in either collagen IV alpha 3 or alpha 4 chains. The rarer form, autosomal dominant, similarly results from aberrant alpha 3 or alpha 4 chains. Like TBMN, Alport syndrome may present with microscopic or gross hematuria. Hearing loss or otic defects are additional associated findings. Long-term prognosis is poor, with ESRD likely.

Hypercalciuria Although prevalence depends on the population studied, 7% of childhood onset persistent isolated microscopic hematuria can be attributed to idiopathic hypercalciuria (IH).[103] In addition to microscopic hematuria, IH increases the risk of both nephrolithiasis and osteoporosis. Children with IH frequently have a family history of IH or nephrolithiasis. Nevertheless, IH has neither an identified monogenic cause nor a single pathogenic factor. Increased urinary calcium excretion occurs secondary to both increased intestinal calcium absorption and impaired renal urinary absorption. IH and nephrolithiasis require treatment, which should include high water intake, low sodium diet, as well as potassium citrate- if there is associated hypocitra-turia- and/or thiazide diuretics. Because of an increased risk of osteoporosis, dietary restriction of calcium is NOT recommended.

SUMMARY

The causes of macroscopic and microscopic hematuria overlap (**Box 1**); both are often caused by UTIs or urethral/bladder irritation. Coexistent hypertension and/or proteinuria should prompt investigation for glomerular disease. The most common glomerulonephritis in children is PIGN. In most patients, and especially with isolated microscopic hematuria, the diagnostic workup reveals no clear underlying cause. In those cases whereby a diagnosis is made, the most common causes of persistent microscopic hematuria are TBMN, IgAN, or IH. Treatment and long-term prognosis vary with the underlying disease.

ACKNOWLEDGMENTS

DB is supported by NIH NIDDK T32 DK007110. KR is supported by NIH R03 DK105242.

REFERENCES

1. Phadke KD, Vijayakumar M, Sharma J, et al. Consensus statement on evaluation of hematuria. Indian Pediatr 2006;43(11):965–73.
2. Ingelfinger JR, Davis AE, Grupe WE. Frequency and etiology of gross hematuria in a general pediatric setting. Pediatrics 1977;59(4):557–61.
3. Youn T, Trachtman H, Gauthier B. Clinical spectrum of gross hematuria in pediatric patients. Clin Pediatr 2006;45(2):135–41.
4. Greenfield SP, Williot P, Kaplan D. Gross hematuria in children: a ten-year review. Urology 2007;69(1):166–9.
5. Irtan S, Ehrlich PF, Pritchard-Jones K. Wilms tumor: "state-of-the-art" update, 2016. Semin Pediatr Surg 2016;25(5):250–6.
6. Rodriguez-Iturbe B, Batsford S. Pathogenesis of poststreptococcal glomerulonephritis a century after Clemens von Pirquet. Kidney Int 2007;71(11): 1094–104.
7. Rodriguez-Iturbe B, Musser JM. The current state of poststreptococcal glomerulonephritis. J Am Soc Nephrol 2008;19(10):1855–64.
8. Tasic V. Postinfectious glomerulonephritis. In: Schaefer F, Geary DF, editors. Comprehensive pediatric nephrology. The Netherlands: Elsevier; 2008. p. 309–17.
9. Balasubramanian R, Marks SD. Post-infectious glomerulonephritis. Paediatr Int Child Health 2017;37(4):240–7.
10. Nasr SH, Markowitz GS, Stokes MB, et al. Acute postinfectious glomerulonephritis in the modern era: experience with 86 adults and review of the literature. Medicine 2008;87(1):21–32.
11. Nasr SH, D'Agati VD. IgA-dominant postinfectious glomerulonephritis: a new twist on an old disease. Nephron Clin Pract 2011;119(1):c18–25 [discussion: c26].
12. Stratta P, Musetti C, Barreca A, et al. New trends of an old disease: the acute post infectious glomerulonephritis at the beginning of the new millenium. J Nephrol 2014;27(3):229–39.
13. Kambham N. Postinfectious glomerulonephritis. Adv Anat Pathol 2012;19(5): 338–47.

14. Sanjad S, Tolaymat A, Whitworth J, et al. Acute glomerulonephritis in children: a review of 153 cases. South Med J 1977;70(10):1202–6.
15. Sagel I, Treser G, Ty A, et al. Occurrence and nature of glomerular lesions after group A streptococci infections in children. Ann Intern Med 1973;79(4):492–9.
16. Fux CA, Bianchetti MG, Jakob SM, et al. Reversible encephalopathy complicating post-streptococcal glomerulonephritis. Pediatr Infect Dis J 2006;25(1):85–7.
17. Baldwin DS, Gluck MC, Schacht RG, et al. The long-term course of poststreptococcal glomerulonephritis. Ann Intern Med 1974;80(3):342–58.
18. Cameron JS, Vick RM, Ogg CS, et al. Plasma C3 and C4 concentrations in management of glomerulonephritis. Br Med J 1973;3(5882):668–72.
19. Eison TM, Ault BH, Jones DP, et al. Post-streptococcal acute glomerulonephritis in children: clinical features and pathogenesis. Pediatr Nephrol 2011;26(2): 165–80.
20. Dedeoglu IO, Springate JE, Waz WR, et al. Prolonged hypocomplementemia in poststreptococcal acute glomerulonephritis. Clin Nephrol 1996;46(5):302–5.
21. Roy S 3rd, Murphy WM, Arant BS Jr. Poststreptococcal crescenteric glomerulonephritis in children: comparison of quintuple therapy versus supportive care. J Pediatr 1981;98(3):403–10.
22. Lewy JE, Salinas-Madrigal L, Herdson PB, et al. Clinico-pathologic correlations in acute poststreptococcal glomerulonephritis. A correlation between renal functions, morphologic damage and clinical course of 46 children with acute poststreptococcal glomerulonephritis. Medicine 1971;50(6):453–501.
23. Tejani A, Ingulli E. Poststreptococcal glomerulonephritis. Current clinical and pathologic concepts. Nephron 1990;55(1):1–5.
24. Sorger K, Gessler M, Hubner FK, et al. Follow-up studies of three subtypes of acute postinfectious glomerulonephritis ascertained by renal biopsy. Clin Nephrol 1987;27(3):111–24.
25. Ahn SY, Ingulli E. Acute poststreptococcal glomerulonephritis: an update. Curr Opin Pediatr 2008;20(2):157–62.
26. Wong W, Morris MC, Zwi J. Outcome of severe acute post-streptococcal glomerulonephritis in New Zealand children. Pediatr Nephrol 2009;24(5):1021–6.
27. Berger J. IgA glomerular deposits in renal disease. Transplant Proc 1969;1(4): 939–44.
28. Wyatt RJ, Julian BA. IgA nephropathy. N Engl J Med 2013;368(25):2402–14.
29. Galla JH. IgA nephropathy. Kidney Int 1995;47(2):377–87.
30. Kiryluk K, Julian BA, Wyatt RJ, et al. Genetic studies of IgA nephropathy: past, present, and future. Pediatr Nephrol 2010;25(11):2257–68.
31. Jennette JC, Wall SD, Wilkman AS. Low incidence of IgA nephropathy in blacks. Kidney Int 1985;28(6):944–50.
32. Li LS, Liu ZH. Epidemiologic data of renal diseases from a single unit in China: analysis based on 13,519 renal biopsies. Kidney Int 2004;66(3):920–3.
33. D'Amico G, Colasanti G, Barbiano di Belgioioso G, et al. Long-term follow-up of IgA mesangial nephropathy: clinico-histological study in 374 patients. Semin Nephrol 1987;7(4):355–8.
34. Waldherr R, Rambausek M, Duncker WD, et al. Frequency of mesangial IgA deposits in a non-selected autopsy series. Nephrol Dial Transplant 1989;4(11):943–6.
35. Suzuki K, Honda K, Tanabe K, et al. Incidence of latent mesangial IgA deposition in renal allograft donors in Japan. Kidney Int 2003;63(6):2286–94.
36. Smith AC, Molyneux K, Feehally J, et al. O-glycosylation of serum IgA1 antibodies against mucosal and systemic antigens in IgA nephropathy. J Am Soc Nephrol 2006;17(12):3520–8.

37. Tomana M, Novak J, Julian BA, et al. Circulating immune complexes in IgA nephropathy consist of IgA1 with galactose-deficient hinge region and antiglycan antibodies. J Clin Invest 1999;104(1):73–81.
38. Suzuki H, Fan R, Zhang Z, et al. Aberrantly glycosylated IgA1 in IgA nephropathy patients is recognized by IgG antibodies with restricted heterogeneity. J Clin Invest 2009;119(6):1668–77.
39. Glassock RJ. Analyzing antibody activity in IgA nephropathy. J Clin Invest 2009; 119(6):1450–2.
40. Lai KN, Leung JC, Chan LY, et al. Podocyte injury induced by mesangial-derived cytokines in IgA nephropathy. Nephrol Dial Transplant 2009;24(1):62–72.
41. Barratt J, Feehally J, Smith AC. Pathogenesis of IgA nephropathy. Semin Nephrol 2004;24(3):197–217.
42. Lai KN, Leung JC, Chan LY, et al. Activation of podocytes by mesangial-derived TNF-alpha: glomerulo-podocytic communication in IgA nephropathy. Am J Physiol Renal Physiol 2008;294(4):F945–55.
43. McCoy RC, Abramowsky CR, Tisher CC. IgA nephropathy. Am J Pathol 1974; 76(1):123–44.
44. Maillard N, Wyatt RJ, Julian BA, et al. Current understanding of the role of complement in IgA nephropathy. J Am Soc Nephrol 2015;26(7):1503–12.
45. Hall CL, Bradley R, Kerr A, et al. Clinical value of renal biopsy in patients with asymptomatic microscopic hematuria with and without low-grade proteinuria. Clin Nephrol 2004;62(4):267–72.
46. Topham PS, Harper SJ, Furness PN, et al. Glomerular disease as a cause of isolated microscopic haematuria. Q J Med 1994;87(6):329–35.
47. Bellur SS, Troyanov S, Cook HT, et al. Immunostaining findings in IgA nephropathy: correlation with histology and clinical outcome in the Oxford classification patient cohort. Nephrol Dial Transplant 2011;26(8):2533–6.
48. Shin DH, Lim BJ, Han IM, et al. Glomerular IgG deposition predicts renal outcome in patients with IgA nephropathy. Mod Pathol 2016;29(7):743–52.
49. Roberts IS. Pathology of IgA nephropathy. Nat Rev Nephrol 2014;10(8):445–54.
50. D'Amico G. Natural history of idiopathic IgA nephropathy: role of clinical and histological prognostic factors. Am J Kidney Dis 2000;36(2):227–37.
51. Berthoux F, Mohey H, Laurent B, et al. Predicting the risk for dialysis or death in IgA nephropathy. J Am Soc Nephrol 2011;22(4):752–61.
52. Wakai K, Kawamura T, Endoh M, et al. A scoring system to predict renal outcome in IgA nephropathy: from a nationwide prospective study. Nephrol Dial Transplant 2006;21(10):2800–8.
53. Donadio JV, Grande JP. The role of fish oil/omega-3 fatty acids in the treatment of IgA nephropathy. Semin Nephrol 2004;24(3):225–43.
54. Reid S, Cawthon PM, Craig JC, et al. Non-immunosuppressive treatment for IgA nephropathy. Cochrane Database Syst Rev 2011;(3):CD003962.
55. Kobayashi Y, Hiki Y, Kokubo T, et al. Steroid therapy during the early stage of progressive IgA nephropathy. A 10-year follow-up study. Nephron 1996;72(2): 237–42.
56. Lv J, Xu D, Perkovic V, et al. Corticosteroid therapy in IgA nephropathy. J Am Soc Nephrol 2012;23(6):1108–16.
57. McIntyre CW, Fluck RJ, Lambie SH. Steroid and cyclophosphamide therapy for IgA nephropathy associated with crescenteric change: an effective treatment. Clin Nephrol 2001;56(3):193–8.

58. Tumlin JA, Lohavichan V, Hennigar R. Crescentic, proliferative IgA nephropathy: clinical and histological response to methylprednisolone and intravenous cyclophosphamide. Nephrol Dial Transplant 2003;18(7):1321–9.
59. Moroni G, Longhi S, Quaglini S, et al. The long-term outcome of renal transplantation of IgA nephropathy and the impact of recurrence on graft survival. Nephrol Dial Transplant 2013;28(5):1305–14.
60. Odum J, Peh CA, Clarkson AR, et al. Recurrent mesangial IgA nephritis following renal transplantation. Nephrol Dial Transplant 1994;9(3):309–12.
61. Gardner-Medwin JM, Dolezalova P, Cummins C, et al. Incidence of Henoch-Schonlein purpura, Kawasaki disease, and rare vasculitides in children of different ethnic origins. Lancet 2002;360(9341):1197–202.
62. Watanabe T. Kidney and urinary tract involvement in kawasaki disease. Int J Pediatr 2013;2013:831834.
63. Piram M, Mahr A. Epidemiology of immunoglobulin A vasculitis (Henoch-Schonlein): current state of knowledge. Curr Opin Rheumatol 2013;25(2):171–8.
64. Weiss PF. Pediatric vasculitis. Pediatr Clin North Am 2012;59(2):407–23.
65. Stewart M, Savage JM, Bell B, et al. Long term renal prognosis of Henoch-Schonlein purpura in an unselected childhood population. Eur J Pediatr 1988;147(2):113–5.
66. Trapani S, Micheli A, Grisolia F, et al. Henoch Schonlein purpura in childhood: epidemiological and clinical analysis of 150 cases over a 5-year period and review of literature. Semin Arthritis Rheum 2005;35(3):143–53.
67. Jauhola O, Ronkainen J, Koskimies O, et al. Renal manifestations of Henoch-Schonlein purpura in a 6-month prospective study of 223 children. Arch Dis Child 2010;95(11):877–82.
68. Narchi H. Risk of long term renal impairment and duration of follow up recommended for Henoch-Schonlein purpura with normal or minimal urinary findings: a systematic review. Arch Dis Child 2005;90(9):916–20.
69. Chang WL, Yang YH, Wang LC, et al. Renal manifestations in Henoch-Schonlein purpura: a 10-year clinical study. Pediatr Nephrol 2005;20(9):1269–72.
70. Lau KK, Suzuki H, Novak J, et al. Pathogenesis of Henoch-Schonlein purpura nephritis. Pediatr Nephrol 2010;25(1):19–26.
71. Levinsky RJ, Barratt TM. IgA immune complexes in Henoch-Schonlein purpura. Lancet 1979;2(8152):1100–3.
72. Dudley J, Smith G, Llewelyn-Edwards A, et al. Randomised, double-blind, placebo-controlled trial to determine whether steroids reduce the incidence and severity of nephropathy in Henoch-Schonlein Purpura (HSP). Arch Dis Child 2013;98(10):756–63.
73. Weiss PF, Feinstein JA, Luan X, et al. Effects of corticosteroid on Henoch-Schonlein purpura: a systematic review. Pediatrics 2007;120(5):1079–87.
74. Rosenblum ND, Winter HS. Steroid effects on the course of abdominal pain in children with Henoch-Schonlein purpura. Pediatrics 1987;79(6):1018–21.
75. Hahn D, Hodson EM, Willis NS, et al. Interventions for preventing and treating kidney disease in Henoch-Schonlein Purpura (HSP). Cochrane Database Syst Rev 2015;(8):CD005128.
76. Kidney Disease: Improving Global Outcomes (KDIGO) Chapter 11: Henoch-Schonlein purpura nephritis. Kidney Int Suppl 2012;2:218–20.
77. Niaudet P, Habib R. Methylprednisolone pulse therapy in the treatment of severe forms of Schonlein-Henoch purpura nephritis. Pediatr Nephrol 1998;12(3):238–43.

78. Habib RNP, Levy M. Schönlein-Henoch purpura nephritis and IgA nephropathy. In: Tisher CCBB, editor. Renal pathology with clinical and functional correlations. Philadelphia: Lippincott; 1993. p. 472.
79. Bush NC, Xu L, Brown BJ, et al. Hospitalizations for pediatric stone disease in United States, 2002-2007. J Urol 2010;183(3):1151–6.
80. Diamond DA. Clinical patterns of paediatric urolithiasis. Br J Urol 1991;68(2): 195–8.
81. Stapleton FB, McKay CP, Noe HN. Urolithiasis in children: the role of hypercalciuria. Pediatr Ann 1987;16(12):980–1, 984-992.
82. Novak TE, Lakshmanan Y, Trock BJ, et al. Sex prevalence of pediatric kidney stone disease in the United States: an epidemiologic investigation. Urology 2009;74(1):104–7.
83. Tasian GE, Jemielita T, Goldfarb DS, et al. Oral antibiotic exposure and kidney stone disease. J Am Soc Nephrol 2018;29(6):1731–40.
84. Nazzal L, Blaser MJ. Does the receipt of antibiotics for common infectious diseases predispose to kidney stones? a cautionary note for all health care practitioners. J Am Soc Nephrol 2018;29(6):1590–2.
85. Gearhart JP, Herzberg GZ, Jeffs RD. Childhood urolithiasis: experiences and advances. Pediatrics 1991;87(4):445–50.
86. Kalorin CM, Zabinski A, Okpareke I, et al. Pediatric urinary stone disease–does age matter? J Urol 2009;181(5):2267–71 [discussion: 2271].
87. Coward RJ, Peters CJ, Duffy PG, et al. Epidemiology of paediatric renal stone disease in the UK. Arch Dis Child 2003;88(11):962–5.
88. Colleran GC, Callahan MJ, Paltiel HJ, et al. Imaging in the diagnosis of pediatric urolithiasis. Pediatr Radiol 2017;47(1):5–16.
89. Passerotti C, Chow JS, Silva A, et al. Ultrasound versus computerized tomography for evaluating urolithiasis. J Urol 2009;182(4 Suppl):1829–34.
90. Mokhless I, Zahran AR, Youssif M, et al. Tamsulosin for the management of distal ureteral stones in children: a prospective randomized study. J Pediatr Urol 2012; 8(5):544–8.
91. Tasian GE, Cost NG, Granberg CF, et al. Tamsulosin and spontaneous passage of ureteral stones in children: a multi-institutional cohort study. J Urol 2014; 192(2):506–11.
92. Acquired cystic kidney disease in children undergoing continuous ambulatory peritoneal dialysis. Kyushu Pediatric Nephrology Study Group. Am J Kidney Dis 1999;34(2):242–6.
93. Franchi-Abella S, Mourier O, Pariente D, et al. Acquired renal cystic disease after liver transplantation in children. Transplant Proc 2007;39(8):2601–2.
94. Wallis MC, Lorenzo AJ, Farhat WA, et al. Risk assessment of incidentally detected complex renal cysts in children: potential role for a modification of the Bosniak classification. J Urol 2008;180(1):317–21.
95. Akoh JA. Current management of autosomal dominant polycystic kidney disease. World J Nephrol 2015;4(4):468–79.
96. Badani KK, Hemal AK, Menon M. Autosomal dominant polycystic kidney disease and pain - a review of the disease from aetiology, evaluation, past surgical treatment options to current practice. J Postgrad Med 2004;50(3):222–6.
97. Schmidt B, Andrew M. Neonatal thrombosis: report of a prospective Canadian and international registry. Pediatrics 1995;96(5 Pt 1):939–43.
98. Kosch A, Kuwertz-Broking E, Heller C, et al. Renal venous thrombosis in neonates: prothrombotic risk factors and long-term follow-up. Blood 2004;104(5): 1356–60.

99. Kuhle S, Massicotte P, Chan A, et al. A case series of 72 neonates with renal vein thrombosis. Data from the 1-800-NO-CLOTS registry. Thromb Haemost 2004; 92(4):729–33.

100. Tinaztepe K, Buyan N, Tinaztepe B, et al. The association of nephrotic syndrome and renal vein thrombosis: a clinicopathological analysis of eight pediatric patients. Turk J Pediatr 1989;31(1):1–18.

101. Harmon WE, Stablein D, Alexander SR, et al. Graft thrombosis in pediatric renal transplant recipients. A report of the North American Pediatric Renal Transplant Cooperative Study. Transplantation 1991;51(2):406–12.

102. Moudgil A. Renal venous thrombosis in neonates. Curr Pediatr Rev 2014;10(2): 101–6.

103. Clark M, Aronoff S, Del Vecchio M. Etiologies of asymptomatic microscopic hematuria in children - systematic review of 1092 subjects. Diagnosis (Berl) 2015; 2(4):211–6.

104. Iitaka K, Igarashi S, Sakai T. Hypocomplementaemia and membranoproliferative glomerulonephritis in school urinary screening in Japan. Pediatr Nephrol 1994; 8(4):420–2.

105. Vivante A, Afek A, Frenkel-Nir Y, et al. Persistent asymptomatic isolated microscopic hematuria in Israeli adolescents and young adults and risk for end-stage renal disease. JAMA 2011;306(7):729–36.

Childhood Obesity and the Metabolic Syndrome

Edward Nehus, MD, MS*, Mark Mitsnefes, MD, MS

KEYWORDS

- Obesity-related kidney disease • Obesity-related glomerulopathy
- Metabolic syndrome • Bariatric surgery

KEY POINTS

- Obesity and the metabolic syndrome are significant risk factors for the development of chronic kidney disease.
- The pathophysiology of obesity-related kidney disease is multifactorial and includes hemodynamic factors (hypertension and hyperfiltration), inflammation, and renal lipotoxicity.
- Children with severe obesity have an increased prevalence of early kidney abnormalities, although the natural history and clinical spectrum of obesity-related kidney disease in children are not known.
- Treatment options for obesity-related kidney disease include conservative weight loss strategies, angiotensin-converting enzyme inhibitors, and bariatric surgery.
- Strategies to promote the early identification and prompt management of obesity-related kidney disease are needed to improve outcomes in children with this condition.

INTRODUCTION

Childhood obesity has become a worldwide epidemic.[1] The prevalence of obesity in US school age children and adolescents tripled from 1980 to 2000 and remains high at 17%.[2] Childhood obesity is frequently associated with the metabolic syndrome, which now affects approximately 10% of US adolescents.[3] Obesity and the obesity-related metabolic syndrome are recognized as significant risk factors for chronic kidney disease (CKD) and end-stage renal disease (ESRD), with recent estimates indicating that 24% to 33% of all kidney disease in the United States is related to obesity.[4] Children with obesity are likely to remain obese in adulthood[5] and experience an increased risk of adverse clinical outcomes, including kidney disease.[6,7] Therefore, it is fundamental that pediatricians are informed of the effects of childhood

Financial Disclosure: There are no conflicts of interest to disclose.
Division of Nephrology and Hypertension, Cincinnati Children's Hospital Medical Center, 3333 Burnet Avenue, MLC 7022, Cincinnati, OH 45229, USA
* Corresponding author.
E-mail address: edward.nehus@cchmc.org

Pediatr Clin N Am 66 (2019) 31–43
https://doi.org/10.1016/j.pcl.2018.08.004
0031-3955/19/© 2018 Elsevier Inc. All rights reserved.

pediatric.theclinics.com

obesity on long-term kidney outcomes. This article reviews the epidemiology, pathophysiology, clinical features, and management of obesity-related kidney disease in children and adolescents.

DEFINITIONS OF OBESITY AND THE METABOLIC SYNDROME IN CHILDREN
Childhood Obesity

Childhood adiposity is commonly measured using body mass index (BMI), defined as the weight in kilograms divided by the square of the height in meters. Because the distribution of BMI changes with age, BMI levels must be interpreted relative to age- and gender-specific normative distributions. Therefore, expert recommendations to identify elevated BMI in children are based on percentile cutoffs rather than absolute values. In 2005, a committee composed of representatives from the American Medical Association, the Health Resources and Service Administration, and the Centers for Disease Control and Prevention provided consensus guidelines for practitioners to identify childhood obesity. According to these recommendations, "overweight" is defined when BMI is greater than or equal to the 85th percentile and less than 95th percentile, and "obesity" is defined by a BMI of greater than or equal to the 95th percentile.[8] These cutoffs accurately identify children with increased risk to remain overweight and obese as adults[9] and develop cardiovascular risk factors (high blood pressure, dyslipidemia, and insulin resistance).[10,11] More recently, children and adolescents with severe obesity have been identified as a subgroup with a much more adverse cardiometabolic risk profile.[12,13] Severe obesity now represents the fastest growing subcategory of pediatric obesity and affects between 4% and 6% of children in the United States. Although the definition of severe obesity does not have universal agreement, the American Heart Association recently issued a consensus statement providing guidelines for the identification and management of this condition. They recommend severe obesity be defined as a BMI of 120% or greater of the 95th percentile or an absolute BMI of greater than or equal to 35 kg/m^2, whichever is lower based on age and sex.[14]

The Metabolic Syndrome in Children

The term the metabolic syndrome has generally referred to a clustering of risk factors for cardiovascular disease, including abdominal obesity, dyslipidemia, glucose intolerance, and hypertension. The presence of these risk factors in childhood increases the likelihood of developing the metabolic syndrome, type 2 diabetes, and cardiovascular disease in adulthood.[15,16] However, a consensus definition of the metabolic syndrome in children has not been universally accepted. Prevalence rates of the metabolic syndrome in a representative sample of US adolescents varied from 2.0% to 9.8% in all teens and 12.4% to 44.2% in obese teens, depending on the definition used.[3,17] In response to this, the International Diabetes Federation suggested a definition of childhood and adolescent metabolic syndrome that incorporated age-related developmental differences unique to the pediatric population (**Table 1**).[18] According to these guidelines, children less than 10 years of age cannot be diagnosed with the metabolic syndrome owing to insufficient data in this age group. As with adults, waist circumference remains the main component owing to its strong association with insulin resistance, hyperlipidemia, and blood pressure. Waist circumference percentiles, rather than absolute values, are used in children 10 to less than 16 years of age to compensate for developmental variation. For children 10 years and older, the metabolic syndrome is defined by abdominal obesity and the presence of 2 or more other risk factors.

Table 1
The International Diabetes Federation consensus definition of the metabolic syndrome in children and adolescents

Age Group (y)	Waist Circumference	Triglycerides	HDL-C	Blood Pressure	Glucose
6–<10	≥90th percentile	Metabolic syndrome cannot be diagnosed			
10–<16	≥90th percentile	≥150 mg/dL	<40 mg/dL	SBP ≥130 or DBP ≥85 mm Hg	≥100 mg/dL or known T2DM
≥16	≥94 cm for Europoid men[a] ≥80 cm for Europoid women	≥150 mg/dL[b]	<40 mg/dL in males[b] <50 mg/dL in females	SBP ≥130[b] or DBP ≥85 mm Hg	≥100 mg/dL or known T2DM

Abbreviations: DBP, diastolic blood pressure; HDL-C, high-density lipoprotein cholesterol; SBP, systolic blood pressure; T2DM, type 2 diabetes mellitus.

[a] Specific values exist for other ethnicities; in the United States, the Third Adult Treatment Panel (ATP III) values of 102 cm for males and 88 cm for females are likely to continue to be used for clinical purposes.

[b] Includes these who are receiving treatment for these conditions (ie, dyslipidemia or hypertension).

THE EPIDEMIC OF OBESITY, THE METABOLIC SYNDROME, AND CHRONIC KIDNEY DISEASE

There has been increasing interest in the association of obesity with CKD, in part generated by a parallel increase in obesity and kidney disease over recent decades. Concurrent with the increase in obesity from 1980 to 2000, the incidence of ESRD nearly quadrupled.[19] Epidemiologic studies have confirmed obesity is a strong, independent risk factor for developing CKD and ESRD.[20–22] Vivante and colleagues[7] investigated the incidence of ESRD in 1.2 million adolescents followed for a mean of 25 years. They reported that being obese at age 17 was associated with a 6-fold increased risk of developing ESRD and a 19-fold increased risk of developing diabetic ESRD, confirming that childhood obesity is a significant risk factor for the future development of kidney disease.

Clinical studies have also linked kidney injury to obesity. Since the first report of obesity-related kidney disease in 1974,[23] the disease now termed obesity-related glomerulopathy (ORG) has reached epidemic proportions. From 1986 to 2000, the incidence of proteinuria and renal dysfunction attributable to obesity increased 10-fold.[24] ORG is characterized histologically by increased glomerular size and glomerular sclerosis.[24,25] The prognosis of ORG is poor, with up to 50% of patients progressing to ESRD within 10 years of diagnosis.[25] This condition, however, likely only represents those with the most advanced clinical disease. The full spectrum of obesity-related kidney disease, including those with less severe forms of kidney injury, is yet to be determined.

Comorbid conditions related to obesity have been implicated in the development of kidney disease, including diabetes and hypertension. However, evidence suggests that obesity and the obesity-related metabolic syndrome are primarily responsible for the epidemic of kidney disease previously attributed to these comorbid conditions.[26] Obesity and the metabolic syndrome are independently associated with the development of CKD, including among those without diabetes and hypertension.[27–30] Compared with those who are lean and metabolically healthy, both metabolically healthy obese patients and those who are nonobese but metabolically unhealthy have an increased risk of CKD. Not surprisingly, metabolically unhealthy obese individuals have the highest risk of developing CKD.[31] Histologic findings in patients with the metabolic syndrome and severe obesity corroborate the epidemiologic studies linking these conditions with CKD. Pathologic changes, including thickening of the glomerular basement membrane, glomerular sclerosis, and interstitial fibrosis are present in patients with severe obesity and the metabolic syndrome before the onset of proteinuria and decreased kidney funciton.[32–35] Taken together, these findings indicate that obesity and the metabolic syndrome per se are direct causes of kidney injury, and their combined presence poses the highest risk for developing CKD.

MECHANISMS OF KIDNEY DISEASE IN OBESITY AND THE METABOLIC SYNDROME

Despite the burgeoning evidence linking obesity with CKD, the mechanism of obesity-related kidney disease has remained largely elusive. Proposed pathways of kidney injury in obesity and the metabolic syndrome include hemodynamic factors, inflammatory/metabolic effects, and lipotoxicity (**Fig. 1**).

Hemodynamic Factors

An increased glomerular filtration rate (GFR), or hyperfiltration, is an early manifestation of kidney disease in obesity and the metabolic syndrome. Clinical studies have confirmed that hyperfiltration is strongly associated with BMI, insulin resistance, hypertension, and dyslipidemia.[36,37] Although a universal definition of hyperfiltration does not exist, the most commonly used threshold is a GFR value of greater than 135 mL/min/1.73 m^2.[38] This increase in GRF is thought to be caused by a maladaptive hemodynamic response at the single nephron level that results in glomerular hypertension and increased capillary hydraulic pressure.[39] The exact mechanisms by which obesity and the metabolic syndrome cause altered renal hemodynamics remain unknown, although several factors are likely involved. Obese subjects demonstrate increased sodium retention by the proximal tubule, which may cause decreased sodium delivery to the macula densa, afferent arteriolar vasodilation, and hyperfiltration. Increased sympathetic activation and upregulation of the renin-angiotensin-aldosterone system may also contribute to hyperfiltration by inducing sodium retention and hypertension.[40] Histologically, hyperfiltration is evident by increased glomerular size, which may be accompanied by glomerular sclerosis, particularly in the perihilar region. These hemodynamic changes cause progressive kidney damage, manifested by an increase in proteinuria and subsequent decrease in kidney function. Several studies have demonstrated that obesity-associated hyperfiltration improves after marked weight loss, indicating that hyperfiltration represents a reversible physiologic adaptation.[41]

Inflammatory and Metabolic Effects

Obesity and the metabolic syndrome are now recognized as conditions of chronic inflammation, which may mediate insulin resistance and contribute to kidney injury.[42] Although the mechanistic links between obesity, inflammation, and kidney injury are not fully elucidated, adipose tissue itself likely plays a central role. Adipocytes function as an endocrine organ by secreting bioactive substances, called adipokines, that may mediate obesity-related metabolic effects and kidney disease.[43] The adipokines that have been most extensively studied include adiponectin and leptin.

Adiponectin is an antiinflammatory adipokine that protects against obesity-related metabolic dysfunction, insulin resistance, and free fatty acid accumulation.[44]

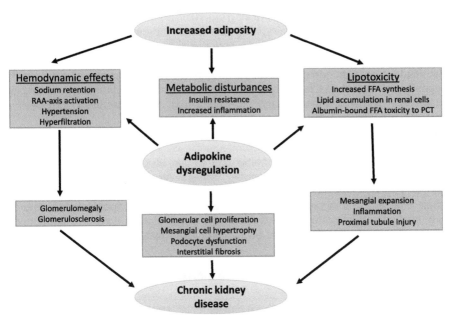

Fig. 1. Potential mechanisms of kidney injury in obesity. FFA, free fatty acids; PCT, proximal convoluted tubule; RAA, renin-angiotensin-aldosterone.

Adiponectin levels are decreased in obesity,[45] and recent evidence suggests that this is a direct cause of obesity-related kidney disease. Low plasma adiponectin levels correlate with increased proteinuria in obese subjects[46,47] and predict progression of kidney disease in patients with type 2 diabetes.[48,49] Animal studies have implicated that adiponectin has a protective role in preventing glomerular and interstitial kidney disease. Adiponectin-deficient mice exhibit increased proteinuria, podocyte dysfunction, and interstitial fibrosis, all of which improve with administration of adiponectin.[46,50]

Leptin is a proinflammatory adipokine that is increased in obesity.[44,51] The primary role of leptin is to signal satiety, increase energy expenditure, and improve lipid metabolism; therefore, obesity has been interpreted as a state of leptin resistance. Leptin is strongly correlated with insulin resistance and inflammation,[52,53] both of which increase the risk of developing CKD.[27,54] Leptin directly affects kidney function by stimulating glomerular cell proliferation[55] and mesangial cell hypertrophy.[56] Leptin also mediates obesity-related hypertension, presumably through activation of the sympathetic nervous system.[57]

Obesity is, therefore, characterized as a state of adipokine dysregulation that is likely a central mediator of kidney disease in obesity. Emerging evidence indicates this process occurs by directly promoting glomerular and interstitial injury, and indirectly through metabolic and hemodynamic pathways.

Lipotoxicity

Obesity is a state of dysregulated lipid metabolism, wherein increased free fatty acid synthesis and decreased free fatty acid oxidation lead to the intracellular accumulation of lipids and lipoproteins. This process can cause cellular dysfunction in a variety of tissues, including cardiac myocytes, hepatocytes, and pancreatic beta cells. Renal lipotoxicity occurs when this abnormal lipid metabolism results in the accumulation of triglycerides and cholesterol in renal glomerular and tubulointerstitial cells. Free fatty acids, cholesterol, and their metabolites cause increased expression of proinflammatory cytokines including vascular endothelial growth factor, interleukin-6, and transforming growth factor-β.[58,59] Recent evidence suggests that lipid accumulation also leads to mitochondrial damage, which contributes to ongoing cellular injury.[60] Together, these intracellular metabolic and inflammatory effects lead to mesangial expansion, glomerulosclerosis, and proteinuria that are characteristic of obesity-related kidney disease.[58,61]

Renal lipotoxicity may also occur indirectly by exposure of proximal tubule cells to albumin-bound free fatty acids in the glomerular filtrate. This toxicity occurs as a result of increased glomerular filtration of albumin that can accompany hyperfiltration and glomerular injury in obesity-related kidney disease. Albumin-bound free fatty acids are then endocytosed into the proximal tubule, where they can exert a variety of pathologic effects, including promoting inflammation and cellular apoptosis.[62,63] Therefore, lipotoxic effects of free fatty acids in the glomerular filtrate may contribute to ongoing tubulointerstitial injury that occurs in obesity-related kidney disease.[64]

CLINICAL PRESENTATION, EVALUATION, AND MANAGEMENT
Presentation and Disease Course

Obesity-related kidney disease often presents as isolated proteinuria with or without renal insufficiency. Proteinuria may be discovered incidentally or as part of an evaluation for other obesity-related comorbidities. Because kidney disease is often asymptomatic and may be present for years before detection, targeted screening for microalbuminuria in obese children at higher risk for kidney disease is a reasonable approach. This screening should include those with insulin resistance, diabetes, or hypertension and children with severe obesity, especially those for whom surgical intervention is being considered. However, owing to the relatively low prevalence of microalbuminuria in the general population of obese children (0.3%),[65] universal screening is not indicated at this time.

The clinical presentation of obesity-related kidney disease can be quite variable, ranging from mild proteinuria (urinary protein-to-creatinine [UPC] ratio of >0.2 but <2 mg/g) to nephrotic range proteinuria (UPC of >2 mg/g) with functional renal impairment (increased serum creatinine). Nephrotic range proteinuria with or without increased creatinine generally indicates the presence of significant glomerular injury on renal biopsy (segmental or globally sclerotic lesions). However, even children with advanced disease rarely present with the typical findings of nephrotic syndrome, such as hypoalbuminemia and edema. The reasons for this finding are not completely clear, but may be related to the different etiologies between obesity-related kidney injury and primary nephrotic syndrome. The putative cause of obesity-related kidney disease is secondary to the systemic effects of obesity, rather than owing to direct immunologic injury to the kidney, as is thought to occur in primary glomerular kidney disease.

The clinical course of obesity-related kidney disease is not known with certainty. The most severe form of this condition (ORG with significant glomerulosclerosis) is associated with a poor prognosis. In 1 study of 15 adult patients with obesity and biopsy-proven glomerulosclerosis, 5 patients progressed to ESRD over a mean follow-up of 6.8 years.[25] In another series of 71 patients with ORG, 14% had a progression of kidney disease over a mean follow-up of 27 months.[24] Risk factors for disease progression included severity of proteinuria and increased serum creatinine at presentation. However, these studies included patients who had clinically indicated biopsies and therefore are not representative of patients with less severe disease, who may have a more indolent course.

To evaluate the prevalence of early kidney abnormalities in adolescents with severe obesity, we recently performed a cross-sectional analysis of the Teen-Longitudinal Assessment of Bariatric Surgery (Teen-LABS) cohort. This study was a prospective observational study of 242 adolescents, ages 13 to 19, who underwent bariatric surgery. Before surgery, 17% had proteinuria (defined as an albumin-to-creatinine ratio of >30 mg/g), and 3% had an estimated GFR of less than 60 mL/min/1.73 m^2. These numbers were significantly elevated compared with healthy cohorts, indicating that a concerning amount of severely obese adolescents have evidence of early kidney disease.[66] Considering adolescent obesity is associated with a 13-fold risk of developing ESRD,[7] progression of kidney disease in these adolescents is a concern. However, long-term kidney outcomes in this population are not known.

Clinical Evaluation

Children with obesity and evidence of kidney disease require a comprehensive evaluation to determine the etiology of kidney disease. Clinical evaluation should begin with a careful history, specifically eliciting any history of gross hematuria, edema, or change in urinary habits or color. These symptoms are typically absent in obesity-related kidney disease, and their presence suggests an alternative diagnosis (eg, glomerulonephritis or urinary tract infection). A complete medical history should be obtained with a particular emphasis on obesity-related comorbidities, including diabetes, nonalcoholic fatty liver disease, kidney stones, sleep apnea, and inappropriate dietary practices. Inquiry should be made into the family history, specifically asking about kidney disease and other related comorbidities, including diabetes and hypertension. Physical examination should begin with calculation of BMI, measurement of the waist circumference, and assessing growth percentile. Blood pressure should be taken twice in the right arm with an appropriately sized cuff. Other physical examination findings that should be assessed include the presence of edema and acanthosis nigricans. Any dysmorphic features should be noted, because these factors may indicate an underlying genetic cause for obesity, particularly in those with short stature.

Laboratory analysis begins with a urinalysis with microscopy. The presence of red blood cell casts on microscopy suggests a primary glomerulonephritis rather than obesity-related kidney disease. Glucosuria may indicate the presence of diabetes mellitus or severe tubular damage and CKD. A UPC ratio or 24-hour urine collection should be obtained to quantify the severity of proteinuria. Further laboratory testing should include a renal profile, serum albumin level, complete blood count, C3/C4 levels, thyroid-stimulating hormone, lipid profile, insulin level, and hemoglobin A1c. In obesity-related kidney disease, complement levels are normal and a low C3 is consistent with primary glomerulonephritis. Serum albumin levels are typically normal or only mildly decreased. An albumin of less than 2.5 mg/dL should raise suspicion for nephrotic syndrome secondary to primary glomerular disease (eg, minimal change disease or focal segmental glomerulosclerosis). If the serum creatinine is elevated, a serum cystatin C level may also be obtained as another measurement of kidney function. Additional diagnostic evaluation includes a renal ultrasound evaluation to determine the presence of any anatomic abnormalities or findings suggestive of chronic kidney injury, such as increased renal echogenicity. If hypertension is present, an echocardiogram should be performed to assess cardiac structure and function.

The diagnosis of ORG is confirmed with a kidney biopsy. Indications for biopsy include elevated serum creatinine and/or persistent significant proteinuria (a UPC ratio of >1 or >1 g of protein in a 24-hour collection). Globally enlarged glomeruli with segmental sclerotic lesions, in particular occurring in the perihilar region, confirms the diagnosis. In severe forms, significant interstitial fibrosis is present and portends a poor prognosis.

Treatment

The treatment of obesity-related kidney disease requires prompt recognition and a multidisciplinary approach to prevent disease progression. Weight loss remains the cornerstone of therapy, which begins with conservative measures including dietary management and exercise. Caloric restriction, with or without exercise programs, has resulted in a modest decrease in proteinuria ranging from 30% to 50%, and some patients may even achieve complete remission.[67,68] However, poor adherence to dietary restrictions is commonly encountered and is a limiting factor to the therapeutic effectiveness.[68] Treatment with angiotensin-converting enzyme inhibitors is also indicated, which has been shown to improve proteinuria and prevent the progression of kidney disease.[69]

Particular attention is needed to identify and treat obesity-related comorbidities, including hypertension and dyslipidemia. Patients with hypertension should be counseled to adhere to a salt-restricted diet, most commonly the Dietary Approaches to Stop Hypertension (DASH) diet. This diet limits sodium intake through a diet that emphasizes fruits, vegetables, and low-fat milk products. If blood pressure remains uncontrolled, angiotensin-converting enzyme inhibitors are generally used as a first-line pharmacologic treatment. The treatment of dyslipidemia in children with CKD begins with dietary management to reduce total saturated fat and cholesterol intake. Additional treatment with lipid-lowering medications, most notably statins, is controversial. The 2013 Kidney Disease Improving Global Outcomes (KDIGO) guidelines recommend that statins should not be initiated in children with CKD, owing to a lack of evidence in clinically meaning outcomes.[70] However, the 2011 Expert Panel on Integrated Guidelines for Cardiovascular Health and Risk Reduction in Children and Adolescents recommend the initiation of statins in children 10 to 21 years of age with persistently elevated low-density lipoprotein cholesterol levels despite a 6-month trial of dietary management. This recommendation is based on the association of childhood dyslipidemia with progression of atherosclerotic lesions in pathology and imaging studies.[71] Considering that obesity and the metabolic syndrome are presumed mediators of kidney injury in obesity-related kidney disease, it is reasonable to initiate statin therapy in this population for dyslipidemia that is not controlled with conservative measures.

Considering the limited efficacy of lifestyle and pharmacologic interventions to treat severe obesity, bariatric surgery has become an accepted treatment option for this population. Bariatric surgical procedures include Roux-en-Y gastric bypass, adjustable gastric banding, and vertical sleeve gastrectomy. All 3 procedures have proven efficacy and are becoming increasingly used for severely obese adolescents with significant obesity-related comorbidities.[14] Short-term outcomes are excellent, including a 25% to 35% weight loss after surgery and improvement in obesity-related comorbidities, including dyslipidemia, hypertension, and type 2 diabetes mellitus.[72–78] Accordingly, evidence-based best practice guidelines recommend that severely obese adolescents with comorbid conditions be strongly considered for weight loss surgery.[79]

Bariatric surgery also has beneficial effects on kidney outcomes. Improvements in albuminuria and kidney function after bariatric surgery have been consistently reported in adult literature.[41,80,81] To investigate kidney outcomes in adolescents after bariatric surgery, we recently performed a 3-year longitudinal study of the Teen-LABS cohort.[82] In participants with decreased kidney function preoperatively, estimated GFR improved from 76 mL/min/1.73 m^2 to 102 mL/min/1.73 m^2 at 3 years. Similarly, in those with increased albuminuria at baseline (albumin/creatinine ratio of $\geq$30 mg/ g), the albumin/creatinine ratio improved from 74 mg/g to 17 mg/g. In participants without any evidence of preoperative kidney disease, kidney function and albuminuria remained stable during the 3-year follow-up period. This study indicated that early kidney injury associated with severe obesity is reversible after bariatric surgery, which should therefore be considered as a treatment option in children who fail conventional management.

SUMMARY

Obesity and the obesity-related metabolic syndrome are now recognized as significant causes of CKD. The injurious renal effects of severe obesity are present in childhood, although the natural history and clinical spectrum of obesity-related kidney disease in children are not known. Treatment options include weight loss and angiotensin-converting enzyme inhibitors, although kidney disease may progress despite these measures. Future research efforts aimed at early identification and novel preventive strategies are essential to improving clinical outcomes in obese children with kidney disease.

REFERENCES

1. Wang Y, Lobstein T. Worldwide trends in childhood overweight and obesity. Int J Pediatr Obes 2006;1(1):11–25.
2. Ogden CL, Carroll MD, Kit BK, et al. Prevalence of childhood and adult obesity in the United States, 2011-2012. JAMA 2014;311(8):806–14.
3. Lee AM, Gurka MJ, DeBoer MD. Trends in metabolic syndrome severity and lifestyle factors among adolescents. Pediatrics 2016;137(3):e20153177.
4. Wang Y, Chen X, Song Y, et al. Association between obesity and kidney disease: a systematic review and meta-analysis. Kidney Int 2008;73(1):19–33.
5. Singh AS, Mulder C, Twisk JW, et al. Tracking of childhood overweight into adulthood: a systematic review of the literature. Obes Rev 2008;9(5):474–88.
6. Juonala M, Magnussen CG, Berenson GS, et al. Childhood adiposity, adult adiposity, and cardiovascular risk factors. N Engl J Med 2011;365(20):1876–85.
7. Vivante A, Golan E, Tzur D, et al. Body mass index in 1.2 million adolescents and risk for end-stage renal disease. Arch Intern Med 2012;172(21):1644–50.
8. Barlow SE, Expert C. Expert committee recommendations regarding the prevention, assessment, and treatment of child and adolescent overweight and obesity: summary report. Pediatrics 2007;120(Suppl 4):S164–92.
9. Whitaker RC, Wright JA, Pepe MS, et al. Predicting obesity in young adulthood from childhood and parental obesity. N Engl J Med 1997;337(13):869–73.
10. Freedman DS, Dietz WH, Srinivasan SR, et al. The relation of overweight to cardiovascular risk factors among children and adolescents: the Bogalusa Heart Study. Pediatrics 1999;103(6 Pt 1):1175–82.
11. Freedman DS, Khan LK, Dietz WH, et al. Relationship of childhood obesity to coronary heart disease risk factors in adulthood: the Bogalusa Heart Study. Pediatrics 2001;108(3):712–8.
12. Calcaterra V, Klersy C, Muratori T, et al. Prevalence of metabolic syndrome (MS) in children and adolescents with varying degrees of obesity. Clin Endocrinol 2008;68(6):868–72.

13. Freedman DS, Mei Z, Srinivasan SR, et al. Cardiovascular risk factors and excess adiposity among overweight children and adolescents: the Bogalusa Heart Study. J Pediatr 2007;150(1):12–7.e12.

14. Kelly AS, Barlow SE, Rao G, et al. Severe obesity in children and adolescents: identification, associated health risks, and treatment approaches: a scientific statement from the American Heart Association. Circulation 2013;128(15): 1689–712.

15. Morrison JA, Friedman LA, Gray-McGuire C. Metabolic syndrome in childhood predicts adult cardiovascular disease 25 years later: the Princeton Lipid Research Clinics Follow-up Study. Pediatrics 2007;120(2):340–5.

16. Morrison JA, Friedman LA, Wang P, et al. Metabolic syndrome in childhood predicts adult metabolic syndrome and type 2 diabetes mellitus 25 to 30 years later. J Pediatr 2008;152(2):201–6.

17. Cook S, Auinger P, Li C, et al. Metabolic syndrome rates in United States adolescents, from the national health and nutrition examination survey, 1999-2002. J Pediatr 2008;152(2):165–70.

18. Zimmet P, Alberti G, Kaufman F, et al. The metabolic syndrome in children and adolescents. Lancet 2007;369(9579):2059–61.

19. Collins AJ, Foley RN, Chavers B, et al. US renal data system 2013 annual data report. Am J Kidney Dis 2014;63(1 Suppl):A7.

20. Fox CS, Larson MG, Leip EP, et al. Predictors of new-onset kidney disease in a community-based population. JAMA 2004;291(7):844–50.

21. Hsu CY, McCulloch CE, Iribarren C, et al. Body mass index and risk for end-stage renal disease. Ann Intern Med 2006;144(1):21–8.

22. Kramer H, Luke A, Bidani A, et al. Obesity and prevalent and incident CKD: the hypertension detection and follow-up program. Am J Kidney Dis 2005;46(4): 587–94.

23. Weisinger JR, Kempson RL, Eldridge FL, et al. The nephrotic syndrome: a complication of massive obesity. Ann Intern Med 1974;81(4):440–7.

24. Kambham N, Markowitz GS, Valeri AM, et al. Obesity-related glomerulopathy: an emerging epidemic. Kidney Int 2001;59(4):1498–509.

25. Praga M, Hernandez E, Morales E, et al. Clinical features and long-term outcome of obesity-associated focal segmental glomerulosclerosis. Nephrol Dial Transplant 2001;16(9):1790–8.

26. Bakker SJ, Gansevoort RT, de Zeeuw D. Metabolic syndrome: a fata morgana? Nephrol Dial Transplant 2007;22(1):15–20.

27. Chen J, Muntner P, Hamm LL, et al. Insulin resistance and risk of chronic kidney disease in nondiabetic US adults. J Am Soc Nephrol 2003;14(2):469–77.

28. Kurella M, Lo JC, Chertow GM. Metabolic syndrome and the risk for chronic kidney disease among nondiabetic adults. J Am Soc Nephrol 2005;16(7):2134–40.

29. Chen J, Muntner P, Hamm LL, et al. The metabolic syndrome and chronic kidney disease in U.S. adults. Ann Intern Med 2004;140(3):167–74.

30. Chang Y, Ryu S, Cho J, et al. Metabolically healthy obesity and development of chronic kidney disease. Ann Intern Med 2016;165(10):744–5.

31. Jung CH, Lee MJ, Kang YM, et al. The risk of chronic kidney disease in a metabolically healthy obese population. Kidney Int 2015;88(4):843–50.

32. Alexander MP, Patel TV, Farag YM, et al. Kidney pathological changes in metabolic syndrome: a cross-sectional study. Am J Kidney Dis 2009;53(5):751–9.

33. Serra A, Romero R, Lopez D, et al. Renal injury in the extremely obese patients with normal renal function. Kidney Int 2008;73(8):947–55.

34. Goumenos DS, Kawar B, El Nahas M, et al. Early histological changes in the kidney of people with morbid obesity. Nephrol Dial Transplant 2009;24(12):3732–8.
35. Ohashi Y, Thomas G, Nurko S, et al. Association of metabolic syndrome with kidney function and histology in living kidney donors. Am J Transplant 2013;13(9): 2342–51.
36. Palatini P. Glomerular hyperfiltration: a marker of early renal damage in pre-diabetes and pre-hypertension. Nephrol Dial Transplant 2012;27(5):1708–14.
37. Tomaszewski M, Charchar FJ, Maric C, et al. Glomerular hyperfiltration: a new marker of metabolic risk. Kidney Int 2007;71(8):816–21.
38. Cachat F, Combescure C, Cauderay M, et al. A systematic review of glomerular hyperfiltration assessment and definition in the medical literature. Clin J Am Soc Nephrol 2015;10(3):382–9.
39. Brenner BM, Lawler EV, Mackenzie HS. The hyperfiltration theory: a paradigm shift in nephrology. Kidney Int 1996;49(6):1774–7.
40. D'Agati VD, Chagnac A, de Vries AP, et al. Obesity-related glomerulopathy: clinical and pathologic characteristics and pathogenesis. Nat Rev Nephrol 2016; 12(8):453–71.
41. Bolignano D, Zoccali C. Effects of weight loss on renal function in obese CKD patients: a systematic review. Nephrol Dial Transplant 2013;28(Suppl 4):iv82–98.
42. Navarro-Diaz M, Serra A, Lopez D, et al. Obesity, inflammation, and kidney disease. Kidney Int Suppl 2008;(111):S15–8.
43. Briffa JF, McAinch AJ, Poronnik P, et al. Adipokines as a link between obesity and chronic kidney disease. Am J Physiol Renal Physiol 2013;305(12):F1629–36.
44. Ouchi N, Parker JL, Lugus JJ, et al. Adipokines in inflammation and metabolic disease. Nat Rev Immunol 2011;11(2):85–97.
45. Ryo M, Nakamura T, Kihara S, et al. Adiponectin as a biomarker of the metabolic syndrome. Circ J 2004;68(11):975–81.
46. Sharma K, Ramachandrarao S, Qiu G, et al. Adiponectin regulates albuminuria and podocyte function in mice. J Clin Invest 2008;118(5):1645–56.
47. Yano Y, Hoshide S, Ishikawa J, et al. Differential impacts of adiponectin on low-grade albuminuria between obese and nonobese persons without diabetes. J Clin Hypertens 2007;9(10):775–82.
48. Kacso I, Lenghel A, Bondor CI, et al. Low plasma adiponectin levels predict increased urinary albumin/creatinine ratio in type 2 diabetes patients. Int Urol Nephrol 2012;44(4):1151–7.
49. Kacso IM, Bondor CI, Kacso G. Plasma adiponectin is related to the progression of kidney disease in type 2 diabetes patients. Scand J Clin Lab Invest 2012;72(4): 333–9.
50. Ohashi K, Iwatani H, Kihara S, et al. Exacerbation of albuminuria and renal fibrosis in subtotal renal ablation model of adiponectin-knockout mice. Arterioscler Thromb Vasc Biol 2007;27(9):1910–7.
51. Considine RV, Sinha MK, Heiman ML, et al. Serum immunoreactive-leptin concentrations in normal-weight and obese humans. N Engl J Med 1996;334(5):292–5.
52. Ruige JB, Dekker JM, Blum WF, et al. Leptin and variables of body adiposity, energy balance, and insulin resistance in a population-based study. The Hoorn Study. Diabetes Care 1999;22(7):1097–104.
53. Shamsuzzaman AS, Winnicki M, Wolk R, et al. Independent association between plasma leptin and C-reactive protein in healthy humans. Circulation 2004; 109(18):2181–5.

54. Shankar A, Sun L, Klein BE, et al. Markers of inflammation predict the long-term risk of developing chronic kidney disease: a population-based cohort study. Kidney Int 2011;80(11):1231–8.

55. Wolf G, Hamann A, Han DC, et al. Leptin stimulates proliferation and TGF-beta expression in renal glomerular endothelial cells: potential role in glomerulosclerosis [see comments]. Kidney Int 1999;56(3):860–72.

56. Lee MP, Orlov D, Sweeney G. Leptin induces rat glomerular mesangial cell hypertrophy, but does not regulate hyperplasia or apoptosis. Int J Obes 2005;29(12):1395–401.

57. Simonds SE, Pryor JT, Ravussin E, et al. Leptin mediates the increase in blood pressure associated with obesity. Cell 2014;159(6):1404–16.

58. Jiang T, Wang Z, Proctor G, et al. Diet-induced obesity in C57BL/6J mice causes increased renal lipid accumulation and glomerulosclerosis via a sterol regulatory element-binding protein-1c-dependent pathway. J Biol Chem 2005;280(37):32317–25.

59. Nishida Y, Yorioka N, Oda H, et al. Effect of lipoproteins on cultured human mesangial cells. Am J Kidney Dis 1997;29(6):919–30.

60. Szeto HH, Liu S, Soong Y, et al. Protection of mitochondria prevents high-fat diet-induced glomerulopathy and proximal tubular injury. Kidney Int 2016;90(5):997–1011.

61. Sun L, Halaihel N, Zhang W, et al. Role of sterol regulatory element-binding protein 1 in regulation of renal lipid metabolism and glomerulosclerosis in diabetes mellitus. J Biol Chem 2002;277(21):18919–27.

62. Arici M, Chana R, Lewington A, et al. Stimulation of proximal tubular cell apoptosis by albumin-bound fatty acids mediated by peroxisome proliferator activated receptor-gamma. J Am Soc Nephrol 2003;14(1):17–27.

63. Weinberg JM. Lipotoxicity. Kidney Int 2006;70(9):1560–6.

64. Kamijo A, Kimura K, Sugaya T, et al. Urinary free fatty acids bound to albumin aggravate tubulointerstitial damage. Kidney Int 2002;62(5):1628–37.

65. Nguyen S, McCulloch C, Brakeman P, et al. Being overweight modifies the association between cardiovascular risk factors and microalbuminuria in adolescents. Pediatrics 2008;121(1):37–45.

66. Xiao N, Jenkins TM, Nehus E, et al. Kidney function in severely obese adolescents undergoing bariatric surgery. Obesity (Silver Spring) 2014;22(11):2319–25.

67. Morales E, Valero MA, Leon M, et al. Beneficial effects of weight loss in overweight patients with chronic proteinuric nephropathies. Am J Kidney Dis 2003;41(2):319–27.

68. Shen WW, Chen HM, Chen H, et al. Obesity-related glomerulopathy: body mass index and proteinuria. Clin J Am Soc Nephrol 2010;5(8):1401–9.

69. Mallamaci F, Ruggenenti P, Perna A, et al. ACE inhibition is renoprotective among obese patients with proteinuria. J Am Soc Nephrol 2011;22(6):1122–8.

70. Wanner C, Tonelli M, Kidney Disease: Improving Global Outcomes Lipid Guideline Development Work Group Members. KDIGO Clinical Practice Guideline for Lipid Management in CKD: summary of recommendation statements and clinical approach to the patient. Kidney Int 2014;85(6):1303–9.

71. Expert Panel on Integrated Guidelines for Cardiovascular Health and Risk Reduction in Children and Adolescents, National Heart, Lung, and Blood Institute. Expert panel on integrated guidelines for cardiovascular health and risk reduction in children and adolescents: summary report. Pediatrics 2011;128(Suppl 5):S213–56.

72. Alqahtani AR, Antonisamy B, Alamri H, et al. Laparoscopic sleeve gastrectomy in 108 obese children and adolescents aged 5 to 21 years. Ann Surg 2012;256(2): 266–73.
73. Boza C, Viscido G, Salinas J, et al. Laparoscopic sleeve gastrectomy in obese adolescents: results in 51 patients. Surg Obes Relat Dis 2012;8(2):133–7 [discussion: 137–9].
74. Inge TH, Courcoulas AP, Jenkins TM, et al. Weight loss and health status 3 years after bariatric surgery in adolescents. N Engl J Med 2016;374(2):113–23.
75. Nadler EP, Reddy S, Isenalumhe A, et al. Laparoscopic adjustable gastric banding for morbidly obese adolescents affects android fat loss, resolution of comorbidities, and improved metabolic status. J Am Coll Surg 2009;209(5):638–44.
76. O'Brien PE, Sawyer SM, Laurie C, et al. Laparoscopic adjustable gastric banding in severely obese adolescents: a randomized trial. JAMA 2010;303(6):519–26.
77. Olbers T, Gronowitz E, Werling M, et al. Two-year outcome of laparoscopic Roux-en-Y gastric bypass in adolescents with severe obesity: results from a Swedish Nationwide Study (AMOS). Int J Obes 2012;36(11):1388–95.
78. Schauer PR, Bhatt DL, Kirwan JP, et al. Bariatric surgery versus intensive medical therapy for diabetes–3-year outcomes. N Engl J Med 2014;370(21):2002–13.
79. Pratt JS, Lenders CM, Dionne EA, et al. Best practice updates for pediatric/adolescent weight loss surgery. Obesity (Silver Spring) 2009;17(5):901–10.
80. Chang AR, Chen Y, Still C, et al. Bariatric surgery is associated with improvement in kidney outcomes. Kidney Int 2016;90(1):164–71.
81. Imam TH, Fischer H, Jing B, et al. Estimated GFR before and after bariatric surgery in CKD. Am J Kidney Dis 2017;69(3):380–8.
82. Nehus EJ, Khoury JC, Inge TH, et al. Kidney outcomes three years after bariatric surgery in severely obese adolescents. Kidney Int 2017;91(2):451–8.

Pediatric Hypertension
Diagnosis, Evaluation, and Treatment

Monica Guzman-Limon, MD, Joshua Samuels, MD, MPH*

KEYWORDS

- Blood pressure • Hypertension • Pediatrics • Guidelines

KEY POINTS

- Early identification and appropriate management of hypertension in children and adolescents is important to prevent the development of hypertensive end organ disease.
- The etiology of hypertension in children and adolescents is varied; however, the prevalence of pediatric primary hypertension is increasing.
- The 2017 American Academy of Pediatrics Clinical Practice Guidelines for the Screening and Management of High Blood Pressure in Children and Adolescents provide a comprehensive reference for evaluation and management of hypertension in this age group and should be used when assessing patients with elevated blood pressure and hypertension.

PHYSIOLOGY OF NORMAL BLOOD PRESSURE

New guidelines for the detection, evaluation, and management of hypertension in children and adolescents have recently been published by the American Academy of Pediatrics.[1] Consequently, a review of normal blood pressure (BP) and hypertension and its management is warranted. BP is the pressure exerted by circulating blood on arterial blood vessel walls during both cardiac contraction and relaxation, which is represented as the systolic and diastolic BP, respectively. The BP level at any given moment is determined by a complex interaction of various physiologic mechanisms that regulate cardiac output, vascular tone, and the quantity and distribution of blood volume. Abnormalities in BP can be idiopathic or not yet understood, or can be attributed to a disturbance of one of these regulating factors of BP. An understanding of normal physiology can aid the clinician in the evaluation of hypertensive patients.

The following well-recognized formula is derived from the basic concept that flow equals pressure times resistance: BP = cardiac output × total peripheral resistance. Numerous circulating and vasoactive factors contribute to total peripheral resistance, or vasoconstriction, such as activation of sympathetic nervous system, releasing catecholamines, as well as increased levels of angiotensin II, which is influenced by renin

Division of Pediatric Nephrology and Hypertension, McGovern Medical School at the University of Texas Health Science Center, 6431 Fannin Street, MSB 3-121, Houston, TX 77030, USA
* Corresponding author.
E-mail address: Joshua.A.Samuels@uth.tmc.edu

Pediatr Clin N Am 66 (2019) 45–57
https://doi.org/10.1016/j.pcl.2018.09.001
0031-3955/19/© 2018 Elsevier Inc. All rights reserved.

release. Changes in total blood volume are mediated by factors such as renal sodium handling through the actions of aldosterone, natriuretic hormone, and other vasoactive substances; the glomerular filtration rate; and intrarenal blood flow and tubular functional integrity.[2,3] Changes in cardiac output also occur through changes in sympathetic and parasympathetic tone and consequent changes heart rate and stroke volume. The circulating renin–angiotensin–aldosterone system is an important mediator of both vascular tone and regulation of total body volume, and thus is key in the development and maintenance of hypertension.[3,4] Renin is a proteolytic enzyme synthesized in juxtaglomerular cells of the renal afferent arterioles and is released in response to decreased renal blood flow, which may occur either owing to obstruction of renal arterial flow or from decreased effective arterial blood volume. Renin cleaves angiotensinogen (from the liver) to form angiotensin I, which is then converted to angiotensin II by the angiotensin-converting enzyme (ACE). Angiotensin II stimulates adrenal aldosterone secretion, which increases sodium reabsorption in the distal convoluted tubule, thereby increasing total body blood volume. Additionally, angiotensin II is a potent vasoconstrictor that increases total peripheral resistance.[4]

DEFINITION AND DIAGNOSIS OF HYPERTENSION IN CHILDREN AND ADOLESCENTS

The long-term consequences of undetected hypertension in children remains unclear,[5] but adults with unrecognized hypertension are at increased risk of cardiovascular and cerebrovascular disease.[6,7] Because the vascular biology of hypertension is likely similar in youth, sustained hypertension in the young may represent an early phenotype of vasculopathy; thus, the diagnosis of hypertension in children is important and must be accurate.[7] The definitions and techniques for the diagnosis of hypertension are discussed herein.

Casual Blood Pressure: Methods and Norms

Casual BP describes measurement of BP in a noncontinuous fashion, as in an outpatient clinic settings. Devices used for office BP measurement include auscultatory BP measurement with mercury and aneroid sphygmomanometers and automatic oscillometric devices.[8] Mercury manometers, once the gold standard for BP measurement, do not require calibration but require routine maintenance including cleaning of the bulb, tubing, and release valve. However, the use of mercury manometers has decreased owing to concern over mercury exposure; in many settings, the use of mercury manometers is not permissible. Aneroid sphygmomanometers rely on bellows, springs, and gauges to measure BP. Aneroid manometers can provide very accurate BPs, but need to be calibrated regularly. Oscillometric sphygmomanometers are increasing in use primarily owing to ease of use and may be appropriate for screening purposes.[9] Aside from patient positioning and incorrect application of the cuff, operator-dependent error is minimized by oscillometric devices. Unlike auscultatory devices, which measure systolic and diastolic BP by Korotkoff sounds, oscillometric devices measure mean arterial BP and use proprietary algorithms to calculate a systolic and diastolic BP.[10] Further, all pediatric norms are derived from auscultatory measurements; thus, oscillometric measurements are not validated.

Factors that can affect BP in children include activity level, intake of substances such as caffeine, certain medications, and substances, or anxiety with measurement.[11] Three measures of BP should be obtained both within each visit and repeated over multiple visits because BP often can vary both within visits and across visits.[12,13] Although sometimes difficult to achieve in younger children, it is important to adhere as closely as possible to good BP measurement techniques as outlined in **Table 1**.[1,14]

Table 1 Technique for blood pressure measurement	
Ideal conditions	1. No stimulant medications or foods before measurement. 2. Blood pressure should be measured in a relaxed environment. 3. Allow a 5-minute rest period before measurement.
Positioning	1. Patient should be seated with back supported. 2. Feet on the floor. 3. Right arm supported. 4. Antecubital fossa at the level of the heart.
Method	1. Perform measurement by auscultatory method. 2. Stethoscope should be placed over the brachial artery pulse, proximal and medial to the cubital fossa, below the bottom edge of the cuff.
Cuff	1. Cuff should be applied to bare skin. 2. Bladder width should be ≥40% of arm circumference. 3. Bladder length should cover 80%–100% of the arm circumference.
Confirm	1. Take blood pressure in all 4 limbs. 2. Recheck blood pressure on repeated visits. 3. Consider ambulatory blood pressure monitoring.

The definition of hypertension in younger children is statistical, in which the patient's BP is compared with a compilation of approximately 50,000 BPs of normal weight children from ages 1 through 17, categorized by age, sex and height. For children under the age of 13, a normal BP is defined as a measurement that falls below the 90th percentile (matched for age, sex and height); elevated BP is defined as 90th or greater percentile but less than the 95th percentile; stage I hypertension is defined as s BP that is greater than or equal to the 95th percentile; and stage II hypertension is defined as BP that is greater than or equal to the 95th percentile plus 12 mm Hg.[1] Reference tables for BP are used to find the 50th, 90th, 95th, and 95th + 12 cutoffs specific to the sex, age and height of the child. Additional normative tables with the 95th and 99th percentiles are available for patients 26 to 44 weeks postmenstrual age and for infants up to 1 year of age.[15,16]

In teens[1] and adults,[17] the newer thresholds used to define hypertension are static, with a normal BP defined as less than 120/80 mm Hg, an elevated BP as greater than or equal to 120/less than 80 mm Hg, and hypertension as greater than or equal to 130/greater than 80 mm Hg. Stage II hypertension is defined as a BP of greater than or equal to 140/greater than or equal to 90 (**Table 2**).

Ambulatory Blood Pressure: Methods and Norms

Ambulatory BP monitoring (ABPM) devices measure BP outside the office setting over an entire circadian day. The technique can be useful in assessing the degree of hypertension throughout the day, as well as in identifying patients with white coat hypertension and those with masked hypertension. ABPM devices consist of a BP cuff and tubing that connects the cuff to a monitor that is approximately the size of a deck of cards. The device measures BP throughout both day and night and can be programmed to intervals, generally between 20 and 60 minutes. The patient is instructed to record wake and sleep time as well as the timing of medications or any unusual occurrences or symptoms. A minimum of 1 recording per hour over a 24-hour period is considered adequate for interpretation of the study.[18]

Analysis of ABPM data in children should be done according to the American Heart Association guidelines as published in the 2014 update on ABPM in children and

Table 2
New blood pressure classifications

BP Classification	Children Aged 1–12 y (Percentile)	Everyone ≥13 y Old (mm Hg)
Normotensive	<90th and <120/80	<120/<80
Elevated blood pressure	≥90th or ≥120/80 mm Hg (lower) to <95th	120–129/<80
Stage 1 hypertension	≥95th to <95th + 12 mm Hg or 130/80–139/89 (lower)	130–139/80–89
Stage 2 hypertension	≥95th + 12 mm Hg or ≥140/90 (lower)	≥140/90

Data from Flynn JT, Kaelber DC, Baker-Smith CM, et al. Clinical practice guideline for screening and management of high blood pressure in children and adolescents. Pediatrics 2017;140(3). [pii:e20171904]; and Whelton PK, Carey RM, Aronow WS, et al. 2017 ACC/AHA/AAPA/ABC/ACPM/AGS/APhA/ASH/ASPC/NMA/PCNA guideline for the prevention, detection, evaluation, and management of high blood pressure in adults: executive summary: a report of the American College of Cardiology/American Heart Association Task Force on Clinical Practice Guidelines. Hypertension 2018;71(6):1269–324.

adolescents.[18] Reference standards most commonly used are from data collected in Germany from 1141 Caucasian children.[19,20] Those data are stratified by sex and height to a minimum height of 120 cm. The lack of ethnic diversity and data on children less than 120 cm in height renders use of these data as normative data for all children problematic.[19,20] Interpretation of ABPM begins with classification of BP based on casual auscultatory BP. Identification of elevated mean BP or what is termed elevated BP load from ABPM data allows the patients' BP pattern to be categorized as normal, white coat hypertension, masked hypertension, prehypertension, ambulatory hypertension, or severe ambulatory hypertension.[18,21]

The following is the suggested classification of ABPM in children:

- Normal blood pressure is <90th percentile in office BP with <95th percentile mean ABPM and < 25 percent ambulatory blood pressure (ABP) load.
- White coat hypertension is ≥ 95th percentile in office BP, <95th percentile mean ABPM and < 25 percent ABP load.
- Prehypertension is ≥ 90th percentile in office BP with <95th percentile mean ABPM and ≥ 25 percent ABP load.
- Masked hypertension is <95th percentile in office BP with ≥ 95th percentile mean ABPM and ≥ 25 percent ABP load.
- Ambulatory hypertension is ≥ 95th percentile in office BP, with ≥ 95th percentile mean ABPM and 25–50 percent ABP load.
- Severe ambulatory hypertension is ≥ 95th percentile in office BP, with ≥ 95th percentile mean ABPM and ≥ 50 percent ABP load.

EPIDEMIOLOGY, RISK FACTORS, AND ETIOLOGY OF HYPERTENSION IN CHILDREN AND ADOLESCENTS
Epidemiology

The prevalence of hypertension in children and adolescents (as reported in studies that used the 2004 4th Working Group definitions) in the United States has been estimated to be approximately 3% in numerous studies.[22–24] Although the worldwide prevalence of pediatric hypertension is not known, international studies from Iceland and China have demonstrated similar prevalence figures.[25,26] Prevalence using the 2017 guidelines, once available, are likely to be higher than the previously estimated 3%. Normative data from the 2017 guidelines are derived from normal weight children with cutoffs for the diagnosis of hypertension lower than previous cutoffs[1,27]; however, currently there are no studies that provides such statistics.

Tracking

Numerous studies suggest that BP in childhood predicts BP level in adulthood. A systematic review and metaregression analysis that included 50 cohort studies showed a strong association of high BP in childhood to high BP in adulthood.[28] In The Childhood Determinants of Adult Health Study, children with elevated BP were 35% more likely to have elevated BP as adults compared with those who had had normal BP as children.[29] Additionally, the group identified modifiable risk factors contributing to resolution of elevated BP, for example, increased vegetable intake and decreased alcohol consumption.[29]

Risk Factors

Risk factors for hypertension can be divided into those that are nonmodifiable such as family history and genetic predisposition, and those that are modifiable, which are numerous.

The heritability of BP has been extensively studied in monozygotic and dizygotic twin studies including both pediatric and adult patients. The heritability in many such studies was between 50% and 60% both in twin pairs within a shared environment as well as in adult pairs who no longer shared the same environment.[30-32] Studies in non-white persons and studies that differentiated between male and female persons found heritability to be similar, suggesting neither ethnicity nor gender significantly affects heritability.[30-36] Newer North American studies suggest there is variability with the prevalence of obesity among different ethnicities, with higher rates of hypertension in Hispanic and African American adolescents.[24]

Obesity is a well-known modifiable risk factor that has been associated with a higher prevalence of hypertension in children and adolescents. UTHealth Houston Pediatric and Adolescent Hypertension Program school screening data from Houston, Texas, reported that the prevalence of overweight and obesity was nearly 30% for both boys and girls. Cheung and colleagues[24] found that hypertension was more common in obese teens of all ethnicities; among white adolescents, those who were obese had a 3-fold increase in the prevalence of hypertension.[23] BP in Hispanic students was even more affected by excess weight. Obese adolescent girls have been found to have a 6-fold increase in the prevalence of hypertension when compared with their nonobese counterparts.[37]

Other modifiable risk factors associated with hypertension include high salt intake and low intake of potassium. Numerous observational and interventional studies, although varied in methodology, suggest that higher sodium intake is associated with higher BP in children and adolescents.[38] Additionally, a metaanalysis of 10 controlled trials in children with a minimum of a 2-week intervention supports the notion that a modest decrease in salt intake (42%–54%) is associated with a decrease in systolic BP.[39] There are fewer studies examining the relation between potassium intake and BP levels, but some observational studies in children using casual BP measurements suggest that high potassium intake is beneficial.[38,40]

Etiology of Hypertension in Children

Primary hypertension

Primary hypertension in children was previously thought to be a diagnosis of exclusion. More recent studies[41,42] note increasing rates of primary hypertension that parallel the obesity epidemic. As many as 91% of hypertensive patients seen at tertiary referral centers are found to have primary hypertension; 89% of such patients were overweight or obese (body mass index of >85%).[42] Characteristics of pediatric patients with primary hypertension include not only obesity, but also older children and family history of hypertension.[41] In 1 cohort, stage of hypertension did not predict hypertension etiology.[42] Given the changing epidemiology of hypertension in youth, the 2017 Clinical Practice Guidelines for the Screening and Management of High Blood Pressure in Children and Adolescents states that extensive workup for secondary cause of hypertension is not required for children greater than 6 years of age who are obese, have a family history of hypertension, and lack physical examination findings suggestive of secondary hypertension and have no evidence of end-organ damage.[1]

Secondary hypertension
Secondary hypertension, of which there are many potential causes, is more common in children with hypertension as compared with adults. Some forms of secondary hypertension are obvious by history or clinical examination, whereas others are obscure. The important causes of secondary hypertension are discussed herein.

Secondary hypertension: renal disease
Renal parenchymal disease and renovascular hypertension are a common cause of secondary hypertension in children, accounting for more than one-half of all cases of secondary hypertension in 1 study.[43] An abnormal plasma creatinine level or abnormal renal ultrasound examination was found to be predictive of secondary hypertension in another single-center study.[44] Forms of renal parenchymal disease leading to hypertension include glomerulonephritis, polycystic kidney disease, congenital abnormalities of the kidneys and urinary tract and chronic kidney disease. Renovascular disease refers to obstruction of the renal arteries and veins and is a major cause of secondary hypertension. Some etiologies include atherosclerosis, fibromuscular dysplasia, vasculitis, and extrinsic compression of the renal vasculature.

Secondary hypertension: coarctation of the aorta
Coarctation of the aorta is a narrowing of the aorta that is classically associated with an upper to lower extremity BP difference of 20 mm Hg or more, a systolic murmur with radiation to the back, and other congenital cardiac malformations. Both congenital and arteriosclerotic changes in patients with coarctation predispose such patients to the development of hypertension, even after successful surgical correction.[45] Additionally, nearly one-half of patients who have previously undergone successful repair of their coarctation have been found to have masked hypertension.[46]

Endocrine forms of secondary hypertension
Endocrinopathies are a rare but important cause of secondary hypertension.[44] Making an accurate diagnosis has the potential to provide curative treatment such as surgery or directed medical treatment of the underlying condition. Most forms of endocrine hypertension involve the adrenal gland, because adrenal hormones are key to the maintenance of BP.

The adrenal medulla produces dopamine, norepinephrine and epinephrine in chromaffin cells, also called pheochromocytes. In addition to the adrenal medulla, chromaffin cells migrate to form paraganglionic collections on both sides of the aorta.[47] Tumors arising from these cells, such as pheochromocytomas and paragangliomas, generally produce excess amounts of catecholamines leading to severe, episodic, or sustained secondary hypertension with associated symptoms of diaphoresis, headaches, palpitations, and tremors.[47] Details on the workup for chromaffin cell tumors are beyond the scope of this article; however, clinical practice guidelines are available through the Endocrine Society.[48]

The adrenal cortex produces mineralocorticoids (aldosterone, deoxycorticosterone), glucocorticoids (cortisol and corticosterone), and sex steroids (androgens). The dysregulation of hormone synthesis from the adrenal cortex can lead to hypertension from excess mineralocorticoids or excess glucocorticoids.[49] Low renin activity level, high aldosterone levels, and hypertension characterize the syndrome of primary aldosteronism.[47] Rare forms of monogenic hypertension most commonly involve genes that impact mineralocorticoid production. Patients with familial hyperaldosteronism typically have abnormal serum potassium levels and early-onset hypertension. In hypertensive patients with low renin and low aldosterone levels, other mineralocorticoids such as deoxycorticosterone can be high from deoxycorticosterone-producing tumors or congenital adrenal hyperplasia. These mineralocorticoids activate the aldosterone receptor to retain sodium and water and excrete potassium.[47] Impaired activity of the microsomal enzyme responsible for inactivating cortisol, HSD11B2, can also lead to hypertension from excess cortisol, which acts as a potent mineralocorticoid.[47]

Iatrogenic Cushing syndrome results from exogenous glucocorticoid use and is common, whereas Cushing disease is caused by endogenous cortisol production and is rare. Hypertension related to excess glucocorticoids in Cushing syndrome or disease is mediated by excess deoxycorticosterone, cortisol action on the mineralocorticoid receptor, and enhanced pressor activity to endogenous vasoconstrictors.[50]

Secondary hypertension: medications

Over-the-counter drugs such as pseudoephedrine, phenylpropanolamine, caffeine, and nonsteroidal antiinflammatory drugs can cause or exacerbate hypertension in some patients.[1] Prescribed drugs such as central nervous system stimulants used for attention deficit hyperactivity disorder have also been shown to have negative cardiovascular effects, often increasing diastolic BP and heart rate.[51]

Although beyond the scope of this article, there are many other secondary causes of hypertension in children that can be reviewed elsewhere.[52]

EVALUATION OF HYPERTENSION IN CHILDREN AND ADOLESCENTS

After establishing a diagnosis of elevated BP or hypertension, evaluation is important to help identify a possible underlying etiology and any comorbidities. Assessment should begin with a complete history, including maternal history of hypertension during pregnancy and low birth weight, both of which may be associated with elevated BP later in life.[53] Nutritional history should assess for intake of foods that are associated with high BP such as high salt and caffeine, and low potassium.[38,39] Level of physical activity should be assessed to help the clinician decide whether prescribing exercise is warranted because sufficient physical activity can lead to reductions in BP.[54] Last, a family history should be obtained on the initial visit and updated at regular intervals because the development of hypertension or comorbid conditions can develop in family members during the time the child is followed in the pediatric clinic.

Physical Examination

Although the physical examination is often normal in hypertensive children, the focus of the examination is to elicit clues to the etiology of the hypertension and to identify evidence of end-organ damage. Physical examination findings suggestive of secondary hypertension include heart murmur or diminished femoral pulses, decreased BP in lower extremities compared with upper extremities as seen in aortic coarctation, goiter in patients with hyperthyroidism, acne, hirsutism, and/or ambiguous or virialized genitalia in congenital adrenal hyperplasia or hypercortisolism, café-au-lait spots in patients with neurofibromatosis, and abdominal mass or palpable kidneys in the cases of renal tumors or polycystic kidney disease. Physical signs of hypertensive end-organ damage include retinal changes, apical heave with left ventricular hypertrophy, and the edema seen in advanced cardiac or renal disease.[1]

Diagnostic Studies

Follow-up and reassessment of BP relies on recording the BP measurement at well-child visits. A child with normal BP should have repeated measurements with scheduled well-child appointments. Children with elevated BP readings should return for a repeat check in 6 months, whereas those with hypertensive BP readings require more rapid reassessment. Time between visits depends on the degree of hypertension ranging from 1 week for stage II hypertension to 6 months for elevated BP.[1] The diagnostic workup for patients with elevated BP or stage I hypertension should be done when abnormal BP is confirmed on the third visit. For patients with stage II hypertension, diagnostic workup should be accomplished sooner, at the time of the second BP confirmed as stage II hypertension. All patients who are undergoing a diagnostic workup for hypertension should have a urinalysis, electrolyte panel, creatinine with an estimated glomerular filtration rate calculation (bedside CKiD Schwartz equation)[55] and lipid panel. For obese children, screening for diabetes, steatohepatitis, and dyslipidemia by obtaining hemoglobin A1c, alanine and aspartate aminotransferases, and a fasting lipid panel is also recommended. Other laboratory testing should be guided by specific clinical findings.[56]

Electrocardiogram and echocardiogram have been used to assess patients for left ventricular hypertrophy. However, the electrocardiogram has not been shown to be sensitive in the detection of left ventricular hypertrophy in children.[57,58] In a change from the 4th Working Group recommendations, the 2017 American Academy of Pediatrics guidelines do not recommend the use of an echocardiogram until the time that pharmacologic management is being contemplated.[1] Left ventricular hypertrophy is defined as greater than 51 $g/m^{2.7}$ (boys and girls) for children and adolescents older than 8 years and defined by a left ventricular mass of greater than 115 g/body surface area for boys and left ventricular mass greater than 95 g/body surface area for girls.[1,59,60] An echocardiogram can be repeated at 6- to 12-month intervals to monitor the progression or resolution of target organ damage in patients with an abnormal initial echocardiogram or those with uncontrolled hypertension.[1]

Renal ultrasound examination and renal vascular imaging are an important part of the evaluation of the hypertensive patient. Renal and renovascular disease are among the most common causes of secondary hypertension in pediatric patients. A renal ultrasound examination should be obtained in patients with a history of renal disease, who are less than 6 years of age, and who have an abnormal urinalysis or plasma creatinine. Patients who are suspected to have primary hypertension, such as adolescents, obese patients, or children with a family history of hypertension, do not require a renal ultrasound evaluation unless they are found to have an abnormal plasma creatinine or history suggestive of renal disease.

TREATMENT OF HYPERTENSION IN CHILDREN AND ADOLESCENTS

Patients with elevated BP and hypertension are at increased risk for target organ damage, including potentially accelerated cardiovascular disease. Left ventricular hypertrophy has been shown to be preventable or even reversible with appropriate treatment.[61,62] The goals of treatment include achieving a systolic and diastolic BP of less than the 90th percentile in younger children and less than 130/80 mm Hg for children greater than 13 years old.[1]

The first-line treatment for primary hypertension consists of nonpharmacologic therapy, such as nutritional intervention and exercise. Moderate decreases in sodium intake and a high potassium diet have been associated with improved BPs.[38] The DASH diet, which is a diet high in fruits and vegetables and low in fat and sodium, has been found to be associated with significantly lower BPs compared with the BP in those receiving usual care.[40] Additionally, at least 60 minutes of physical activity 3 times per week can confer modest reductions in BP.[54,63]

For patients who are still hypertensive despite a 6-month trial of lifestyle modification, who have symptomatic hypertension, who have stage II hypertension, or who have evidence end-organ disease, pharmacologic intervention is warranted. Although a specific recommendation is beyond the scope of this review, initiation of antihypertensive medication should begin with lowest dose as monotherapy and titrated upward or with a second agent added every 2 to 4 weeks until the goal BP is achieved (BP <90th percentile or <50th percentile if chronic kidney disease).[1] Preferred agents include ACE inhibitors, angiotensin receptor blockers, calcium channel blockers, and diuretics, although no specific class has been shown superior as a first-line agent.[64] Other classes of antihypertensives should be reserved for patients who remain hypertensive despite treatment with 2 or more of the preferred drugs.[1] Unless contraindicated, ACE inhibitors or ARBs should be first line in patients with diabetes or proteinuric chronic kidney disease. African American children may require higher doses of ACE inhibitors owing to racial differences in response to ACE inhibitors.[65,66] Last, ACE inhibitors and ARBs are teratogenic; if used in adolescent females, these classes of medications require counseling over the teratogenic effects and may require prescription of oral contraceptive medication as appropriate.

SUMMARY

Early identification and appropriate management of hypertension in children and adolescents is important to prevent the development of hypertensive end organ disease. The etiology of hypertension in children and adolescents is varied; however, the prevalence of pediatric primary hypertension is increasing. The 2017 American Academy of Pediatrics Clinical Practice Guidelines for the Screening and Management of High Blood Pressure in Children and Adolescents provide a comprehensive reference for evaluation and management of hypertension in this age group and should be used when assessing patients with elevated BP and hypertension.

REFERENCES

1. Flynn JT, Kaelber DC, Baker-Smith CM, et al. Clinical practice guideline for screening and management of high blood pressure in children and adolescents. Pediatrics 2017;140(3) [pii:e20171904].
2. Singh M, Mensah GA, Bakris G. Pathogenesis and clinical physiology of hypertension. Cardiol Clin 2010;28(4):545–59.
3. Suzuki H, Saruta T. An overview of blood pressure regulation associated with the kidney. Contrib Nephrol 2004;143:1–15.
4. Hiner LB, Gruskin AB. The physiology of blood pressure regulation–normal and abnormal. Pediatr Ann 1977;6(6):373–83.

5. Thompson M, Dana T, Bougatsos C, et al. Screening for hypertension in children and adolescents to prevent cardiovascular disease. Pediatrics 2013;131(3): 490–525.

6. Centers for Disease Control and Prevention (CDC). CDC high blood pressure fact sheet. Available at: https://www.cdc.gov/dhdsp/data_statistics/fact_sheets/fs_bloodpressure.htm. Accessed August 1, 2018.

7. Samuels JA, Bell C, Flynn JT. Screening children for high blood pressure: where the US Preventive Services Task Force went wrong. J Clin Hypertens (Greenwich) 2013;15(8):526–7.

8. Samuels J. Blood pressure measurement in pediatrics. J Clin Hypertens (Greenwich) 2016;18(12):1235–6.

9. Duncombe SL, Voss C, Harris KC. Oscillometric and auscultatory blood pressure measurement methods in children: a systematic review and meta-analysis. J Hypertens 2017;35(2):213–24.

10. Flynn J, Ingelfinger JR, editors. Pediatric hypertension, vol, 3rd edition. New York: Humana Press; 2013. p. 134, 160.

11. Savoca MR, MacKey ML, Evans CD, et al. Association of ambulatory blood pressure and dietary caffeine in adolescents. Am J Hypertens 2005;18(1):116–20.

12. Becton LJ, Egan BM, Hailpern SM, et al. Blood pressure reclassification in adolescents based on repeat clinic blood pressure measurements. J Clin Hypertens (Greenwich) 2013;15(10):717–22.

13. Samuels J, Bell C. Recognizing elevated blood pressure in pediatrics: the value of repeated measures. J Clin Hypertens (Greenwich) 2018;20(1):183–5.

14. Falkner B. Hypertension in children and adolescents: epidemiology and natural history. Pediatr Nephrol 2010;25(7):1219–24.

15. Dionne JM, Abitbol CL, Flynn JT. Hypertension in infancy: diagnosis, management and outcome. Pediatr Nephrol 2012;27(1):17–32.

16. National High Blood Pressure Education Program (NHBPEP). Report of the Second Task Force on Blood Pressure Control in Children–1987. Task Force on Blood Pressure Control in Children. National Heart, Lung, and Blood Institute, Bethesda, Maryland. Pediatrics 1987;79(1):1–25.

17. Whelton PK, Carey RM, Aronow WS, et al. 2017 ACC/AHA/AAPA/ABC/ACPM/AGS/APhA/ASH/ASPC/NMA/PCNA guideline for the prevention, detection, evaluation, and management of high blood pressure in adults: executive summary: a report of the American College of Cardiology/American Heart Association Task Force on Clinical Practice Guidelines. Hypertension 2017;71(6):1269–324.

18. Flynn JT, Daniels SR, Hayman LL, et al. Update: ambulatory blood pressure monitoring in children and adolescents: a scientific statement From the American Heart Association. Hypertension 2014;63(5):1116–35.

19. Soergel M, Kirschstein M, Busch C, et al. Oscillometric twenty-four-hour ambulatory blood pressure values in healthy children and adolescents: a multicenter trial including 1141 subjects. J Pediatr 1997;130(2):178–84.

20. Wühl E, Witte K, Soergel M, et al. Distribution of 24-h ambulatory blood pressure in children: normalized reference values and role of body dimensions. J Hypertens 2002;20(10):1995–2007.

21. Flynn JT, Urbina EM. Pediatric ambulatory blood pressure monitoring: indications and interpretations. J Clin Hypertens (Greenwich) 2012;14(6):372–82.

22. Hansen ML, Gunn PW, Kaelber DC. Underdiagnosis of hypertension in children and adolescents. JAMA 2007;298(8):874–9.

23. McNiece KL, Poffenbarger TS, Turner JL, et al. Prevalence of hypertension and pre-hypertension among adolescents. J Pediatr 2007;150(6):640–4, 644.e1.

24. Cheung EL, Bell CS, Samuel JP, et al. Race and obesity in adolescent hypertension. Pediatrics 2017;139(5) [pii:e20161433].

25. Steinthorsdottir SD, Eliasdottir SB, Indridason OS, et al. Prevalence of hypertension in 9- to 10-year-old Icelandic school children. J Clin Hypertens (Greenwich) 2011;13(10):774–9.

26. Meng L, Liang Y, Liu J, et al. Prevalence and risk factors of hypertension based on repeated measurements in Chinese children and adolescents. Blood Press 2013;22(1):59–64.

27. National High Blood Pressure Education Program Working Group on High Blood Pressure in Children and Adolescents. The fourth report on the diagnosis, evaluation, and treatment of high blood pressure in children and adolescents. Pediatrics 2004;114(2):555–76.

28. Chen X, Wang Y. Tracking of blood pressure from childhood to adulthood: a systematic review and meta-regression analysis. Circulation 2008;117(25):3171–80.

29. Kelly RK, Thomson R, Smith KJ, et al. Factors affecting tracking of blood pressure from childhood to adulthood: the childhood determinants of adult health study. J Pediatr 2015;167(6):1422–8.e2.

30. Schieken RM, Eaves LJ, Hewitt JK, et al. Univariate genetic analysis of blood pressure in children (the Medical College of Virginia Twin Study). Am J Cardiol 1989;64(19):1333–7.

31. Snieder H, Harshfield GA, Treiber FA. Heritability of blood pressure and hemodynamics in African- and European-American Youth. Hypertension 2003;41(6):1196–201.

32. McIlhany ML, Shaffer JW, Hines EA Jr. The heritability of blood pressure: an investigation of 200 pairs of twins using the cold pressor test. Johns Hopkins Med J 1975;136(2):57–64.

33. Baird J, Osmond C, MacGregor A, et al. Testing the fetal origins hypothesis in twins: the Birmingham twin study. Diabetologia 2001;44(1):33–9.

34. Hong Y, de Faire U, Heller DA, et al. Genetic and environmental influences on blood pressure in elderly twins. Hypertension 1994;24(6):663–70.

35. Wu T, Snieder H, Li L, et al. Genetic and environmental influences on blood pressure and body mass index in Han Chinese: a twin study. Hypertens Res 2010;34(2):173–9.

36. Yu MW, Chen CJ, Wang CJ, et al. Chronological changes in genetic variance and heritability of systolic and diastolic blood pressure among Chinese Twin Neonates. Acta Genet Med Gemellol (Roma) 1990;39(01):99–108.

37. Obarzanek E, Wu CO, Cutler JA, et al. Prevalence and incidence of hypertension in adolescent girls. J Pediatr 2010;157(3):461–7, 467.e1-5.

38. Simons-Morton DG, Obarzanek E. Diet and blood pressure in children and adolescents. Pediatr Nephrol 1997;11(2):244–9.

39. He FJ, MacGregor GA. Importance of salt in determining blood pressure in children: meta-analysis of controlled trials. Hypertension 2006;48(5):861–9.

40. Couch SC, Saelens BE, Levin L, et al. The efficacy of a clinic-based behavioral nutrition intervention emphasizing a DASH-type diet for adolescents with elevated blood pressure. J Pediatr 2008;152(4):494–501.

41. Flynn J. The changing face of pediatric hypertension in the era of the childhood obesity epidemic. Pediatr Nephrol 2013;28(7):1059–66.

42. Kapur G, Ahmed M, Pan C, et al. Secondary hypertension in overweight and stage 1 hypertensive children: a midwest pediatric nephrology consortium report. J Clin Hypertens 2010;12(1):34–9.

43. Gupta-Malhotra M, Banker A, Shete S, et al. Essential hypertension vs. secondary hypertension among children. Am J Hypertens 2014;28(1):73–80.

44. Baracco R, Kapur G, Mattoo T, et al. Prediction of primary vs secondary hypertension in children. The J Clin Hypertens 2012;14(5):316–21.

45. Hager A, Kanz S, Kaemmerer H, et al. Coarctation Long-term Assessment (COALA): significance of arterial hypertension in a cohort of 404 patients up to 27 years after surgical repair of isolated coarctation of the aorta, even in the absence of restenosis and prosthetic material. J Thorac Cardiovasc Surg 2007; 134(3):738–45.

46. Di Salvo G, Castaldi B, Baldini L, et al. Masked hypertension in young patients after successful aortic coarctation repair: impact on left ventricular geometry and function. J Hum Hypertens 2011;25(12):739–45.

47. Young W. Endocrine hypertension. In: Melmed S, Polonsky KS, Larsen R, et al, editors. Williams textbook of endocrinology. 13th edition. Philadelphia: Elsevier Inc; 2016. p. 556–88.

48. Lenders JWM, Duh Q-Y, Eisenhofer G, et al. Pheochromocytoma and paraganglioma: an endocrine society clinical practice guideline. J Clin Endocrinol Metab 2014;99(6):1915–42.

49. Aggarwal A, Rodriguez-Buritica D. Monogenic hypertension in children: a review with emphasis on genetics. Adv Chronic Kidney Dis 2017;24(6):372–9.

50. Baid S, Nieman LK. Glucocorticoid excess and hypertension. Curr Hypertens Rep 2004;6(6):493–9.

51. Samuels JA, Franco K, Wan F, et al. Effect of stimulants on 24-h ambulatory blood pressure in children with ADHD: a double-blind, randomized, cross-over trial. Pediatr Nephrol 2005;21(1):92–5.

52. Sharma S, Meyers KE, Vidi SR. Secondary forms of hypertension in children: overview. In: Flynn JT, Ingelfinger JR, Redwine KM, editors. Pediatric hypertension. Cham (Switzerland): Springer International Publishing; 2018. p. 431–49.

53. Staley JR, Bradley J, Silverwood RJ, et al. Associations of blood pressure in pregnancy with offspring blood pressure trajectories during childhood and adolescence: findings from a prospective study. J Am Heart Assoc 2015;4(5):e001422.

54. García-Hermoso A, Saavedra JM, Escalante Y. Effects of exercise on resting blood pressure in obese children: a meta-analysis of randomized controlled trials. Obes Rev 2013;14(11):919–28.

55. Schwartz GJ, Munoz A, Schneider MF, et al. New equations to estimate GFR in children with CKD. J Am Soc Nephrol 2009;20(3):629–37.

56. Wiesen J, Adkins M, Fortune S, et al. Evaluation of pediatric patients with mild-to-moderate hypertension: yield of diagnostic testing. Pediatrics 2008;122(5): e988–93.

57. Bratincsák A, Williams M, Kimata C, et al. The electrocardiogram is a poor diagnostic tool to detect left ventricular hypertrophy in children: a comparison with echocardiographic assessment of left ventricular mass. Congenit Heart Dis 2015;10(4):E164–71.

58. Rijnbeek PR, van Herpen G, Kapusta L, et al. Electrocardiographic criteria for left ventricular hypertrophy in children. Pediatr Cardiol 2008;29(5):923–8.

59. Lang RM, Badano LP, Mor-Avi V, et al. Recommendations for cardiac chamber quantification by echocardiography in adults: an update from the American Society of Echocardiography and the European Association of Cardiovascular Imaging. J Am Soc Echocardiogr 2015;28(1):1–39.e14.

60. Lopez L, Colan SD, Frommelt PC, et al. Recommendations for quantification methods during the performance of a pediatric echocardiogram: a report from

the Pediatric Measurements Writing Group of the American Society of Echocardiography Pediatric and Congenital Heart Disease Council. J Am Soc Echocardiogr 2010;23(5):465–95 [quiz: 576–7].

61. Litwin M, Niemirska A, Śladowska-Kozlowska J, et al. Regression of target organ damage in children and adolescents with primary hypertension. Pediatr Nephrol 2010;25(12):2489–99.

62. Kupferman JC, Paterno K, Mahgerefteh J, et al. Improvement of left ventricular mass with antihypertensive therapy in children with hypertension. Pediatr Nephrol 2010;25(8):1513–8.

63. Farpour-Lambert NJ, Aggoun Y, Marchand LM, et al. Physical activity reduces systemic blood pressure and improves early markers of atherosclerosis in prepubertal obese children. J Am Coll Cardiol 2009;54(25):2396–406.

64. Samuel JP, Samuels JA, Brooks LE, et al. Comparative effectiveness of antihypertensive treatment for older children with primary hypertension: study protocol for a series of n-of-1 randomized trials. Trials 2016;17:16.

65. Li JS, Baker-Smith CM, Smith PB, et al. Racial differences in blood pressure response to angiotensin-converting enzyme inhibitors in children: a meta-analysis. Clin Pharmacol Ther 2008;84(3):315–9.

66. Samuels J, Negroni-Balasquide X, Bell C. Ethnic differences in childhood blood pressure. In: Flynn JT, Ingelfinger JR, Redwine KM, editors. Pediatric hypertension. Cham (Switzerland): Springer International Publishing; 2018. p. 351–64.

Infection-Related Glomerulonephritis

Elizabeth A.K. Hunt, MD[a],*, Michael J.G. Somers, MD[b]

KEYWORDS

- Postinfectious • Glomerulonephritis • Poststreptococcal • Hepatitis • Shunt
- Endocarditis

KEY POINTS

- Although glomerulonephritis can follow illness with multiple infectious agents, poststreptococcal glomerulonephritis has been most extensively characterized and is used as a prototype for postinfectious glomerulonephritis.
- Most glomerulonephritis associated with infections present clinically after a latent phase during which the infection begins to resolve.
- Macroscopic hematuria, proteinuria, hypertension, and edema are the most common clinical features, with acute hypocomplementemia in the overwhelming majority.
- With supportive care only, most children begin to have resolution of concerning clinical features within 4 to 6 weeks. Hypocomplementemia usually resolves within 3 months.
- Glomerulonephritis associated with bacterial endocarditis or infected shunts tends to occur without a latent phase while the infection is still active and responds best to specific therapy for the underlying infection.

CLINICAL SPECTRUM OF POSTINFECTIOUS GLOMERULONEPHRITIS

The sudden appearance of tea- or cola-colored urine, often accompanied by edema and high blood pressure, frequently leads to a clinical concern for an acute nephritis. Unlike chronic nephritis that is often more insidious in onset and the result of an ongoing glomerular process, acute nephritis is most commonly associated with a recent infection.

Although acute postinfectious glomerulonephritis (APIGN) has been described after several viral or bacterial infections, group A beta-hemolytic streptococcal infection is the prototypical cause. Acute poststreptococcal glomerulonephritis (APSGN) affects

Disclosure Statement: Neither E.A.K. Hunt nor M.J.G. Somers has anything to disclose.
[a] Division of Pediatric Nephrology, University of Vermont Children's Hospital, Larner College of Medicine, UVM Medical Center, 111 Colchester Avenue, Smith 5, Burlington, VT 05405, USA;
[b] Division of Nephrology, Boston Children's Hospital, Harvard Medical School, 300 Longwood Avenue, Boston, MA 02115, USA
* Corresponding author.
E-mail address: Liz.hunt@uvmhealth.org

upwards of 500,000 children worldwide each year, accounting for 5000 deaths, generally in areas with limited medical resources. Seasonal and geographic variations in APSGN incidence generally parallel differences in overall streptococcal disease burden, though epidemics of APSGN have been described as a result of particularly nephritogenic strains of streptococcus.[1]

The clinical spectrum of APIGN can vary widely, from asymptomatic microscopic hematuria incidentally detected on routine urinalysis to a rapidly progressive glomerulonephritis (RPGN) with acute kidney injury requiring emergent dialysis. The changes in glomerular integrity that accompany APIGN often result in an acute nephritic syndrome with hematuria, hypertension, and a reduction in kidney function. In some cases, there can be a mixed nephritic-nephrotic picture, with additional heavy proteinuria mediating hypoalbuminemia and volume imbalance. Infrequently, APIGN can mediate widespread crescentic glomerular injury with rapid loss of kidney function and serious clinical consequences related to impairment of normal solute and volume homeostasis.

Although most children affected by APIGN require little more than monitoring for the development of significant initial sequelae and recover completely with no long-term renal residuals, the potential for serious or even life-threatening complications underscores the need for pediatric clinicians to be familiar with its clinical presentation, diagnostic evaluation, and management, including when involvement of a pediatric nephrologist may be useful.

CAUSE AND EPIDEMIOLOGY
Acute Postinfectious Glomerulonephritis

Clinical presentation
Because streptococcal disease is often easier to clinically diagnose and confirm, much of the literature that exists on postinfectious nephritis focuses on APSGN. The presentation, clinical course, and outcomes of nonstreptococcal cases of APIGN are generally similar to those of APSGN; many clinical reports do not differentiate between various causes in analyzing their data.

Although APIGN can be seen in children of all ages, it tends to be more commonly seen in school-aged children, with a mean age of presentation between 6 and 8 years of age.[2–6] The reason for a lower incidence in children younger than 3 years of age is thought to be less frequent streptococcal carriage[7] and lower colonization rates as well as potentially decreased immunogenicity in younger children.[8] Most studies report a male preponderance, ranging from 54% to 87%,[2,3] although the reason for this difference is not clear; rates of overall group A streptococcal infection do not vary between boys and girls.

As suggested by the name, there is usually a recent identifiable illness that precedes APIGN. A review of 474 patients with APIGN in Armenia over a 5-year period exemplifies the variability in presentation, with 51% experiencing a preceding upper respiratory tract infection, 23% with scarlet fever, 13% with impetigo, 5% with cervical adenitis, and only 8% with no recalled illness.[5]

In APSGN, although there is usually a preceding pharyngeal or skin infection, results from multiple case series show that preceding symptoms can also vary[9] (**Table 1**). Dagan and colleagues[10] reported that although 85% of their cohort had positive antistreptolysin O (ASO) titers, only 45% had a clinical episode of pharyngitis, with just 31% having had a positive streptococcal throat culture. Of the others, 25% had experienced typical upper respiratory tract infection symptoms and 11% gastroenteritis. Interestingly, even though these patients did not have classic streptococcal infection

Table 1
Presenting features of postinfectious glomerulonephritis

Clinical Features	Study, n (%)					
	Dagan et al,[10] 2016 n = 125	Ilyas & Tolaymat,[2] 2008 n = 45[b]	Becquet et al,[3] 2010 n = 50	Wong et al,[6] 2013 n = 176	Blyth & Robertson,[4] 2006 n = 37	Sarkissian et al,[5] 1997 n = 474
Study population	APIGN, Israel	APSGN, United States	APSGN	APSGN, New Zealand	APSGN, Australia	APIGN, Armenia
Male (%)	74.40%	87%	54%	65%	64.90%	65%
Macroscopic hematuria	21 of 125 (16.8%)	82%	32 of 50 (64%)	153 of 176 (87%)	28 (75.7%)	442 (93%)
Oliguria	42 of 125 (33.6%)	—	9 of 50 (18%)	86 of 167 (51%)	—	—
Hypertension	103 (82.4%)	—	32 of 50 (64%)	126 of 176 (72%)	25 (67.6%)	340 (72%)
Fever	49 of 125 (40.2%)	51%	—	—	—	—
Edema	74 of 125 (59.2%)	—	33 of 50 (66%)	109 of 176 (62%)	19 (51.4%)	397 of 474 (72%)
Azotemia/impaired renal function[a]	87 (70.2%)	40%	14 of 32 (43.7%)	120 of 176 (68%)	30 (81.1%)	134 of 474 (28%)
Proteinuria[a]	116 (92.8%)	—	49 of 50 (98%)	55 of 133 (44%)	14 of 14	134 of 474 (28%)
Nephrotic range proteinuria	40 (32.5%)	—	15 of 50 (25%)	4 of 58 (7%)	—	5 of 474 (1%)
Hypoalbuminemia	27 (22%)	33%	30 of 50 (60%)	—	—	5 of 474 (1%)
Low C3	110 (89%)	88%	45 of 50 90%	161 of 173 (93%)	—	149 of 157 (95%)
Low C4	29 (23.8%)	—	—	—	37 (100%)	—
Anemia	98 (79%)	51%	—	—	—	—
Hyperkalemia	36 (28.8%)	51%	—	—	—	—
Elevated ASO	109 (85%)	84%	73.60%	—	29 (78.4)	—
A Dnase B positive	—	—	97.30%	—	24 (64.9%)	—
Elevated ASO or DNase	—	—	—	138 of 176 (79%)	35 (94.6%)	—
Encephalopathy/seizure[a]	1 (0.8%)	6%	2 of 50 (4%)	16 of 176 (9%)	2 of 37 (5.6%)	16 (3%)
Pulmonary edema/CHF	—	50% of those with CXR	7 of 50, 14%	10 of 176 (6%)	2 (5.6%)	45 (10%)
Dialysis	1 (0.8%)	—	—	3 of 176	3 of 37 (8.3%)	3 of 474

[a] Definitions differ by study.
[b] n is not available, reported for current cohort.

symptoms, more than three-quarters had a positive ASO titer. In this series, impetigo was less common (6%) and 16% had no obvious preceding infection. Leung and colleagues[11] prospectively enrolled 74 children who presented with acute glomerulonephritis over a 2-year period. Half the children had a clear history of throat infection, and nearly 20% had a recent skin infection. Throat cultures, ASO titers, and serum C3 levels were obtained in all children. Group A hemolytic strep was isolated from 10 throat cultures from the study subjects and in 6 children from a control group of 60 otherwise healthy children hospitalized for acute illness. Seventy percent of the study cohort had positive ASO titers, compared with 18% of the control group. C3 was low at presentation in 73 of 74 children, all returning to normal levels within 6 weeks. Many patients had been treated with antibiotics for their preceding illness.

Although it has anecdotally been suggested that APSGN presents later after skin infections than with pharyngitis, several studies looking specifically at the latent phase report similar periods of time between acute illness and onset of nephritis, averaging 9 to 10 days with both pharyngitis and impetigo.[3,6] A seasonal variation with preceding illness has been seen, however, with pharyngitis-associated APSGN predominating in winter and spring and impetigo-associated APSGN seen more commonly in the summer and fall.[2]

The phenotypic spectrum of APIGN ranges from clinically insignificant involvement to a RPGN with loss of kidney function. Hematuria, either microscopic or macroscopic, is present in nearly all cases and most patients have some degree of proteinuria (see **Table 1**). In one retrospective review of 125 hospitalized children, 41% met the criteria for nephritic syndrome (some combination of hematuria, hypertension, oliguria, edema, and increased serum creatinine level) with 23% of these also demonstrating concomitant nephrotic range proteinuria and hypoalbuminemia. Just less than 10% had nephrotic syndrome without a nephritic component.[10] Some decrease in normal kidney function is fairly common at presentation, with rates ranging from 28% to 68%.[2,3,5,6] Most patients recover kidney function with supportive care; dialysis is relatively rarely needed, reported in only cases that manifested a rapidly progressive course.[5,6] Most clinical signs and symptoms resolve spontaneously within a few weeks of presentation, but microscopic hematuria can persist for up to 2 years. Gross hematuria can sometimes recur with new episodes of acute illness during early stages of APIGN recovery.[12] Recurrent episodes of frank APIGN are rare but have been reported.[13] One series documented recurrence in 12 out of 590 children followed over 15 years. The first episode was preceded by pyoderma in 9 of these patients. The second episode occurred 9 to 28 months after the initial episode and was preceded by pyoderma in 9 patients and sore throat in 3. Eleven of the 12 patients were followed long-term after their second episode of APSGN. Ten of these children had a complete recovery with no residual renal or urinary findings, whereas one had persistent proteinuria.[14]

Most case series focus on children ill enough to present for medical care, but family screening of identified index cases has shown that subclinical or unrecognized APIGN is possible. Tasic and Polenakovic[15] evaluated urine from families of 75 APSGN index cases and found no evidence of APSGN in parents. However, 22% of 170 siblings had an abnormal urinalysis. Further evaluation showed that 4% of siblings had clinical glomerulonephritis (gross hematuria, edema, hypertension) and 5% had hematuria and proteinuria but no edema, hypertension, or gross hematuria. Another study of 20 index patients and 91 sibling contacts found clinical or laboratory evidence of kidney disease in 19 children from 10 of 20 families. Sixteen had no recalled history of recent illness. Six underwent renal biopsy, which was consistent with APSGN in all.[12]

Diagnostic evaluation

- Urine and blood work
- Imaging findings
- Role of biopsy

APIGN is usually a diagnosis that arises from clinical signs and symptoms. Urinalysis is the first step in helping to confirm this diagnosis and shows hematuria with variable proteinuria. Microscopy almost always demonstrates dysmorphic urinary red blood cells and often red blood cell casts. Urine protein/creatinine ratios can range from modestly elevated to nephrotic range. Chemistries can demonstrate decreased renal function, especially in cases of more pronounced nephritic syndrome. A typical clinical course and laboratory values are illustrated in **Fig. 1**.

Often the most useful confirmatory test for APIGN is a complement C3 level. C3 levels are classically depressed early in the course and rebound to normal levels by 6 to 8 weeks.[3,11,16] There are some reports of C3 levels taking longer to normalize; but if recovery exceeds 3 months, an alternate diagnosis, such as membranoproliferative glomerulonephritis, must be considered.[5]

Patients with APSGN may have had a previously diagnosed streptococcal infection that facilitates the diagnosis. If not, antistreptolysin O (ASO) antibodies and anti-DNAse titers can be helpful. ASO typically begins to increase by 1 week after infection and peaks at 3 to 5 weeks after infection, and DNase B increases 2 weeks after infection and peaks at 6 to 8 weeks. In one series of poststreptococcal illness, the sensitivity of ASO for a preceding streptococcal illness was 73% and the specificity was 93% compared with a sensitivity of 71% and specificity of 93% for anti–DNase B. Combining the two resulted in an improved sensitivity of 96% but reduced specificity to 89%.[4] This study did not show a difference between pharyngeal and skin infections; but other studies have reported that ASO has decreased sensitivity after skin infections compared with DNase B.[16,17]

There is no clear role for renal imaging in diagnosing APIGN, though often in the setting of hematuria and decreased renal function it is prudent to obtain a screening renal ultrasound to document urinary tract anatomy. Imaging findings in APIGN range from normal to parenchymal echogenicity and renal enlargement secondary to tissue edema and inflammation.

Most children with a clear diagnosis of APIGN do not require an initial diagnostic renal biopsy. In more atypical cases or in the setting of a progressive loss of renal function, a biopsy helps to establish a definitive diagnosis and can rule out another cause that may require specific therapy for recovery. If children fail to recover as expected or exhibit persistent hypocomplementemia or ongoing high-grade proteinuria, then a biopsy should be done to help guide further management. Guidelines point to 3 months as a typical period to wait to see substantive recovery in complement levels.[18]

Management and treatment

- Indications for supportive care and monitoring
- Indication and types of specific therapies

There are no clear trials comparing treatment strategies in APIGN, and most treatment is supportive in nature. If an underlying bacterial infection is identified, it should be treated with appropriate antibiotics, although such therapy does not change the course of the glomerulonephritis once it is underway.

Monitoring for the development or exacerbation of hypertension or renal impairment is important, as is avoiding further kidney injury by exposure to nephrotoxic

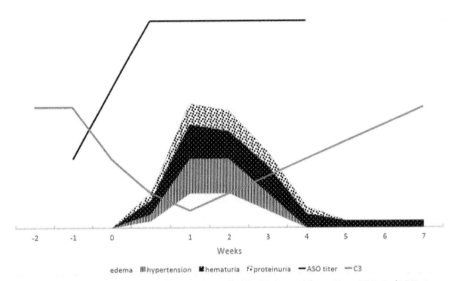

-2   -1   0   1   2   3   4   5   6   7

Weeks

edema ▥hypertension ▧hematuria ░proteinuria ━ASO titer ━C3

Fig. 1. Course of postinfectious glomerulonephritis. (*Adapted from* Eison TM, Ault BH, Jones DP, et al. Post-streptococcal acute glomerulonephritis in children: clinical features and pathogenesis. Pediatr Nephrol 2011;26(2):165–80 with additional data from Refs.[2–6,12,16])

medications or to periods of significant or prolonged effective volume depletion. Hospital admission is generally recommended for children who present with hypertension, significant generalized edema, or impaired renal function. Often diuretics or a combination of a diuretic and a vasodilator, such as a calcium channel blocker, can be helpful for hypertension, as the presumed cause is volume excess from sodium and water retention. Angiotensin-converting enzyme inhibitors or angiotensin receptor blockers are usually avoided in the acute phase because they may exacerbate any reduction in glomerular perfusion arising from the glomerulonephritis itself. Edematous or hypertensive patients should also be instructed in a reduced-sodium diet and may require fluid restriction.

Children with APIGN can on occasion develop pronounced hypertension, including hypertensive urgencies and emergencies. Hypertension-related seizures with documentation of posterior reversible encephalopathy syndrome can be seen. It is especially important in the early phases of a suspected case of APIGN for blood pressures to continue to be assessed at regular intervals, even in children who are normotensive at presentation and are being followed in an ambulatory care setting.

Dialysis is indicated in the setting of severe renal impairment leading to volume excess or electrolyte abnormalities that cannot otherwise be medically managed. With significant acute kidney injury, Kidney Disease: Improving Global Outcomes (KDIGO) guidelines recommend considering treating with intravenous (IV) methylprednisolone if there are extensive acute glomerular crescents on biopsy; but there are no randomized trials of steroid treatment of APIGN-associated RPGN.[18] There are some case reports using plasma exchange in RPGN associated with APIGN, but again the specific efficacy of this therapy in APIGN is unclear; it has generally been used along with steroids or other immunosuppression as empirical therapy in severe cases of APIGN-associated RPGN.[19]

Outcomes

Long-term outcomes are thought to be good with preserved renal function in most children and adults who have an uncomplicated case of APIGN. Kasahara and colleagues[20] reported on 138 patients with APSGN followed for 9 years. The most common initial complication was hypertension in 64%, with only 2 individuals manifesting a serum creatinine greater than 1 mg/dL, and no patients with a creatinine greater than 1.5 mg/dL or requiring dialysis. All had a normal C3 complement level within 3 months. Patients were followed every 1 to 3 months initially and then at less frequent intervals. By 3 years after diagnosis, no patients had residual proteinuria; by 4 years, no patients had hematuria. Although many patients would be expected to become normotensive over time, data were not provided as to the long-term rates of hypertension or the recurrence of either hypertension or proteinuria as long-term residuals for the acute kidney injury that accompanied their APIGN.

Sarkissian and colleagues[5] reported short-term and intermediate outcomes in their retrospective review of 474 patients with APIGN. Initial hypocomplementemia resolved in half of the patients in the first 3 weeks, and only one child continued to have hypocomplementemia after 3 months. Seventy-eight percent of 368 children had complete remission (normal renal function and urinalysis, no edema or hypertension) 3 months after diagnosis. Ninety-seven percent of 171 patients who followed up at 1 year had no evidence of such residual renal involvement. Of the 4 patients with an initial RPGN and crescentic changes on renal biopsy who were treated with steroids and cyclophosphamide, 3 had improvement in renal function; but the other patient developed ESRD within 7 months.

On the more severe end of the spectrum, Wong and colleagues[21] reviewed 27 patients in New Zealand with APSGN referred for renal biopsy. Acute dialysis was needed in 12 of the 27. In 11 patients, there were more than 50% crescents on biopsy. Six of these 11 patients presented with anuric renal failure, and 2 progressed to end-stage renal disease (ESRD) despite treatment with methylprednisolone and cyclophosphamide. Follow-up was available in 18 patients over a mean period of 3.2 years (range 1–8 years). Patients who needed dialysis tended to have residual proteinuria throughout the follow-up, and 2 patients never recovered function after their initial RPGN. Of the 12 patients who needed initial dialysis, 8 had developed ESRD, chronic kidney disease (CKD) with impaired glomerular filtration rate (GFR), or persistent proteinuria at the last follow-up. Of the 15 patients who did not need dialysis acutely, nearly half were lost to follow-up, which unfortunately limits conclusions about long-term outcomes.

More recently, residents in an Aboriginal community in Australia with a high incidence of kidney disease and APSGN have been studied longitudinally. A history of APSGN was associated with a higher level of albuminuria compared with those without such history. The odds ratio for long-term overt albuminuria after ASPGN was 4.96 in males and 3.3 in females when adjusted for age, body mass index, blood pressure, and diabetes status. The significance of this in the general population is unclear, but it suggests the need for long-term prospective follow-up of children with APSGN.[22]

Other Infectious Causes Associated with Glomerulonephritis

Although streptococcal infection is the prototypical cause of APIGN, multiple infectious causes have been associated with renal manifestations as listed in **Box 1**. In addition, there are several specific infectious conditions that have historically been linked to associated nephritis. The authors discuss these conditions in the following sections, with emphasis on their presentation and management.

Nephritis associated with endocarditis

- Clinical presentation
- Management and outcomes

Nephritis associated with infectious endocarditis (IE) is more common in adults due to higher baseline rates of endocarditis in an older patient population.[23–27] The frequency of an IE-associated nephritis and the specific clinical manifestations vary, likely related to the underlying infectious organism. The renal histology with IE-associated nephritis is classically either a focal or diffuse endocapillary proliferation.

Postmortem analysis of 107 patients with IE treated between 1965 and 1979 showed that 22% had histologic evidence of glomerulonephritis, 14% with diffuse disease and 8% with focal glomerulonephritis. Histologic changes were similar with either acute or subacute IE. *S aureus* endocarditis predisposed to glomerulonephritis more than nonstaphylococcal disease (31% vs 19%).[28]

A more recent case series reviewed 49 patients (2 children) between 2001 to 2011 with IE-associated nephritis who underwent renal biopsy. The cause of IE was *Staphylococcus aureus* in 53% of cases and *Streptococcus* species in 23%. The most common presenting feature was acute kidney injury in 79%, with a classic acute nephritic syndrome present in 9%, RPGN in 6%, and nephrotic syndrome in 6%. Hematuria was found in 97% and hypocomplementemia in 56%. Renal histology demonstrated crescentic changes in half, with diffuse proliferative glomerular changes in 33% and mild mesangial hypercellularity in 10%. Treatment provided for the renal disease included antibiotics in 67% and antibiotics with immunosuppression in 33%. After an average of 25 months follow-up, 21% had died, 10% had progressed to ESRD, 37% had CKD, and 32% had complete renal recovery. Because this report only looked at patients who were chosen to be biopsied because of clinical concern, it may overestimate the proportion of cases with more serious renal disease and subsequent adverse outcomes.[29]

In general, the mainstay of treatment is antibiotics to treat the IE. There are no randomized trials to evaluate the efficacy of additional treatment specifically for the associated nephritis. Some reports suggest using corticosteroids, although this is controversial because of the potential for worsening the underlying infection. With crescentic or rapidly progressive glomerulonephritis, more aggressive immunomodulatory therapy, including plasmapheresis, has been advocated; but this is based on typical clinical practice for these conditions with increased likelihood for adverse renal outcomes without aggressive therapy.[30–33]

Nephritis associated with shunt infection

- Clinical presentation
- Management and outcomes

When ventriculoatrial (VA) shunts were more commonly placed by neurosurgeons, nephritis associated with shunt infection was more frequent. Shunt nephritis is a prototypical immune complex-induced nephritis, although a key difference from a classic APIGN is that it occurs during an active infection as opposed to following a latent period. In a series from 1975 of pediatric patients with shunts, 48 of 205 (23%) VA shunts became infected and 4% of the patients were subsequently diagnosed with nephritis.[34] Another retrospective review of 138 VA shunts showed that 15% became infected, with nearly a third of those infected then developing nephritis.[35]

Two retrospective reviews encompassing 138 cases of shunt nephritis suggest that most patients have symptoms of a shunt malfunction or a systemic illness before onset of any renal manifestations. When renal disease presents, both gross and microscopic hematuria with varying levels of proteinuria were common as was a decrease from baseline GFR. Hypertension seemed to be a less prominent feature of shunt nephritis than other forms of APIGN. C3 hypocomplementemia is frequent with a

---

Box 1
Infections associated with renal manifestations

Bacterial
  Mycobacterium leprae, Mycobacterium tuberculosis
  Treponema pallidum
  Salmonella typhi, Salmonella paratyphi, Salmonella typhimurium
  Streptococcus pneumoniae, Streptococcus viridans, Streptococcus pyogenes, Staphylococcus aureus, Staphylococcus epidermidis, Streptomyces albus, Streptococcus equi[a]
  Leptospira species[a]
  Yersinia enterocolitica[a]
  Neisseria meningitidis, Neisseria gonorrhoeae[a]
  Corynebacterium diphtheriae[a]
  Coxiella burnetii[a]
  Brucella abortus[a]
  Listeria monocytogenes[a]
  Bartonella henselae[a]

Helminthic
  Schistosoma mansoni, Schistosoma japonicum
  Schistosoma haematobium
  Wuchereria bancrofti
  Brugia malayi
  Loa loa
  Onchocerca volvulus
  Trichinella spiralis[a]

Protozoal
  Plasmodium malariae, Plasmodium falciparum
  Leishmania donovani
  Toxoplasma gondii
  Trypanosoma cruzi, Trypanosoma brucei
  Toxocara canis[a]
  Strongyloides stercoralis[a]

Fungal
  Histoplasma capsulatum[a]
  Candida[a]
  Coccidioides immitis[a]

Viral
  Human immunodeficiency virus
  Hepatitis B and C
  Epstein-Barr virus
  Coxsackie B
  Cytomegalovirus
  Varicella zoster
  Mumps
  Rubella
  Influenza
  Echovirus
  Adenovirus[a]

[a] Case reports only.
Adapted from Kidney Disease: Improving Global Outcomes (KDIGO) Glomerulonephritis Work Group. KDIGO clinical practice guideline for glomerulonephritis. Kidney Int 2012;Suppl 2:201; with permission; and Additional information from Refs.[27,47–49]

---

rebound to normal with treatment of the infection that often also corresponded to clinical improvement in the glomerulonephritis. During active infection, cryoglobulins and antinuclear antibody were frequently positive, related to the immune complexes generated by the underlying infection.[36,37]

The most common renal biopsy finding with a shunt nephritis is diffuse proliferative disease in a membranoproliferative or mesangioproliferative pattern. Although extracapillary changes with crescent formation can be seen, it is much rarer than the nearly ubiquitous endocapillary proliferation.[36,37]

Management is aimed at treating the shunt infection, often necessitating shunt removal as well as antibiotic provision. Although historically about half of patients have complete resolution of their renal disease after successful treatment of the infection, there is significant morbidity and mortality with up to 10% in some series dying of their infection and related complications, up to 20% left with CKD, including progression to ESRD, and 20% showing persistent urinary abnormalities.[36,37]

Nephritis associated with hepatitis viruses

- Clinical presentation of Hepatitis B and C
- Management and outcomes

Although multiple viruses have been associated with renal complications, the hepatitis viruses are best known for their link to an infectious nephritis. Similar to shunt nephritis, hepatitis-linked nephritis occurs while the infection is ongoing. Nearly 260 million people worldwide have hepatitis B, with another 7 million with chronic hepatitis C infection.[38] In some parts of the world, nearly 10% of the population has an active hepatitis infection.

Renal involvement with hepatitis B has been associated with a spectrum of findings. One report from Turkey showed that both nephritic and nephrotic presentations were common, with just more than a quarter having reduced GFR at diagnosis. Renal biopsy generally demonstrates a membranous pattern in those with a more nephrotic presentation and a membranoproliferative pattern in those with more nephritic overtones. The clearing of hepatitis B e antigen and hepatitis B surface antigen was found to accompany clinical remission; in those who continued to have active renal disease, there were higher rates of CKD and progression to ESRD.[39,40]

In addition to usual supportive treatment, the KDIGO guidelines suggest that patients with hepatitis B–associated nephropathy be treated with interferon-α or nucleoside analogues with doses adjusted for renal function.[18]

With hepatitis C, renal involvement generally presents with proteinuria, with decreased renal function, hypocomplementemia, and, on occasion, detectable cryoglobulinemia.[41,42] A study of protocol renal biopsies in patients with cirrhosis secondary to hepatitis C who were undergoing liver transplant showed that 25 of 30 patients had immune complex glomerulonephritis with mesangial or mesangiocapillary proliferation.[43] Autopsy studies have shown that up to half of infected individuals can have renal histologic changes, with varying degrees of mesangial proliferation most commonly noted.[44] A frank membranoproliferative pattern can be seen in up to 11%, with a pure membranous pattern seen in 3%.[45]

In addition to symptomatic treatment, including blood pressure control most often with renin-angiotensin blockade and diuretics, specific treatment of hepatitis C nephritis is also indicated if available. KDIGO treatment guidelines recommend using combined antiviral treatment with pegylated interferon and ribavirin for patients with hepatitis C and CKD stage 1 or 2 and glomerulonephritis. For patients with more advanced CKD and active glomerulonephritis who are not on dialysis, KDIGO recommends monotherapy with pegylated interferon, with the dose adjusted for renal function. More aggressive therapy in addition to antiviral therapy, including plasmapheresis, rituximab, or cyclophosphamide with IV methylprednisolone, have been suggested for hepatitis C nephritis with mixed cryoglobulinemia and nephrotic range proteinuria or decreasing GFR.[18] Although there are limited data assessing the efficacy of these recommended approaches, treatment with interferon-α and ribavirin seems to decrease hepatitis C viral loads with ensuing reduction in proteinuria, improving serum albumin and complement levels, and stabilization of renal function.[46]

PATHOGENESIS AND PATHOLOGY

- Mechanisms of immune-mediated injury
- Histologic findings (light microscopy, immunofluorescence, electron microscopy)

The pathogenesis of APIGN is focused on immune complex disease prompted by the acute infection and ultimately resulting in disruption of normal glomerular integrity. In many types of APIGN, and certainly in the case of APSGN, complement activation and local inflammatory response play a key role in the ensuing renal injury.

With APIGN, there is the production of some sort of nephritogenic antigen that then plays a key role in triggering a damaging immune response. Certain strains of bacteria may inherently be more nephritogenic. For instance, there has been a great deal of research done on the bacterial cell wall proteins used to characterize the various subtypes of *Streptococcus*, with various M protein serotypes found to be more likely to cause nephritis.

A variety of host factors then likely underlies an individual's predisposition to respond to a specific antigen and also modulates the inflammatory reaction. In APSGN, there has been recent focus on streptococcal pyogenic exotoxin B (SPE B), with immunohistochemistry demonstrating its presence colocalized with complement factors in the subepithelial immune deposits that characterize APSGN. Specific immune testing has also found the widespread presence of SPE B antibodies in serum samples of convalescing patients with APSGN.

The nephritogenic factor is thought to help create an immune complex. Various mechanisms of glomerular injury have been proposed, including direct deposition of preformed antigen-antibody complexes, in situ immune complex formation from antibody binding to antigen that was filtered and trapped in the glomerular basement membrane, and in situ immune complex formation from antibodies to the antigen possessing an ability to cross-react with normal glomerular structures.

Regardless of the specific mechanism that does occur, the resulting interaction between immune complex and glomerular cells results in an inflammatory reaction that consumes complement, damages the glomerular endothelial cells and glomerular basement membrane (GBM), and results in the formation of subepithelial humps that further perturb GBM and epithelial foot process integrity. In addition to activation of the classic complement cascade, this process also involves activation of the coagulation cascade, recruitment of white cells to the area, and generation of numerous cytokines and proinflammatory factors.

Histologically, this is manifested on light microscopy by varying degrees of endocapillary proliferation with neutrophil infiltration of the glomerulus; on immunofluorescence by predominant C3 deposition along with immunoglobulin G in the mesangium and capillary wall; and on electron microscopy by electron-dense deposits gathered as humps in a subepithelial distribution and also found subendothelially.

Individuals who have more pronounced glomerular capillary subendothelial injury will have a more nephritic presentation than those with primary epithelial cell damage who are more disposed to nephrotic syndrome. Damage to both endothelial and epithelial cells of the capillary mediates a mixed nephritic-nephrotic picture.

The extent of the initial inflammatory reaction and ensuing local capillary damage and the host's ability to clear the deposits and repair any damage will account for variable clinical presentations and outcomes in APIGN.

REFERENCES

1. Carapetis JR, Steer AC, Mulholland EK, et al. The global burden of group A streptococcal diseases. Lancet Infect Dis 2005;5(11):685–94.
2. Ilyas M, Tolaymat A. Changing epidemiology of acute post-streptococcal glomerulonephritis in Northeast Florida: a comparative study. Pediatr Nephrol 2008; 23(7):1101–6.
3. Becquet O, Pasche J, Gatti H, et al. Acute post-streptococcal glomerulonephritis in children of French Polynesia: a 3-year retrospective study. Pediatr Nephrol 2010;25(2):275–80.
4. Blyth CC, Robertson PW. Anti-streptococcal antibodies in the diagnosis of acute and post-streptococcal disease: streptokinase versus streptolysin O and deoxyribonuclease B. Pathology 2006;38(2):152–6.
5. Sarkissian A, Papazian M, Azatian G, et al. An epidemic of acute postinfectious glomerulonephritis in Armenia. Arch Dis Child 1997;77(4):342–4.
6. Wong W, Lennon DR, Crone S, et al. Prospective population-based study on the burden of disease from post-streptococcal glomerulonephritis of hospitalised children in New Zealand: epidemiology, clinical features and complications. J Paediatr Child Health 2013;49(10):850–5.
7. Alpert JJ, Pickering MR, Warren RJ. Failure to isolate streptococci from children under the age of 3 years with exudative tonsillitis. Pediatrics 1966;38(4):663–6.
8. Bingler MA, Ellis D, Moritz ML. Acute post-streptococcal glomerulonephritis in a 14-month-old boy: why is this uncommon? Pediatr Nephrol 2007;22(3):448–50.
9. Eison TM, Ault BH, Jones DP, et al. Post-streptococcal acute glomerulonephritis in children: clinical features and pathogenesis. Pediatr Nephrol 2011;26(2): 165–80.
10. Dagan R, Cleper R, Davidovits M, et al. Post-infectious glomerulonephritis in pediatric patients over two decades: severity-associated features. Isr Med Assoc J 2016;18(6):336–40.
11. Leung DT, Tseng RY, Go SH, et al. Post-streptococcal glomerulonephritis in Hong Kong. Arch Dis Child 1987;62(10):1075–6.
12. Dodge WF, Spargo BH, Bass JA, et al. The relationship between the clinical and pathologic features of poststreptococcal glomerulonephritis. A study of the early natural history. Medicine (Baltimore) 1968;47(3):227–67.
13. Watanabe T, Yoshizawa N. Recurrence of acute poststreptococcal glomerulonephritis. Pediatr Nephrol 2001;16(7):598–600.
14. Roy S 3rd, Wall HP, Etteldorf JN. Second attacks of acute glomerulonephritis. J Pediatr 1969;75(5):758–67.
15. Tasic V, Polenakovic M. Occurrence of subclinical post-streptococcal glomerulonephritis in family contacts. J Paediatr Child Health 2003;39(3):177–9.
16. Derrick CW, Reeves MS, Dillon HC Jr. Complement in overt and asymptomatic nephritis after skin infection. J Clin Invest 1970;49(6):1178–87.
17. Kaplan EL, Anthony BF, Chapman SS, et al. The influence of the site of infection on the immune response to group A streptococci. J Clin Invest 1970;49(7): 1405–14.
18. Kidney Disease: Improving Global Outcomes Work Group. KDIGO Clinical Practice Guideline for Glomerulonephritis. Kidney Int 2012;(Supplement 2):139–274.

19. D'Amico G, Sinico R, Fornasieri A, et al. Effect of intensive plasma exchange (PE) in rapidly progressive crescentic glomerulonephritis (RPCGN). Int J Artif Organs 1983;6(Suppl 1):3–9.
20. Kasahara T, Hayakawa H, Okubo S, et al. Prognosis of acute poststreptococcal glomerulonephritis (APSGN) is excellent in children, when adequately diagnosed. Pediatr Int 2001;43(4):364–7.
21. Wong W, Morris MC, Zwi J. Outcome of severe acute post-streptococcal glomerulonephritis in New Zealand children. Pediatr Nephrol 2009;24(5):1021–6.
22. Hoy WE, White AV, Dowling A, et al. Post-streptococcal glomerulonephritis is a strong risk factor for chronic kidney disease in later life. Kidney Int 2012; 81(10):1026–32.
23. Elzouki AY, Akthar M, Mirza K. Brucella endocarditis associated with glomerulonephritis and renal vasculitis. Pediatr Nephrol 1996;10(6):748–51.
24. Sadikoglu B, Bilge I, Kilicaslan I, et al. Crescentic glomerulonephritis in a child with infective endocarditis. Pediatr Nephrol 2006;21(6):867–9.
25. Itoh M, Kann DC, Schwenk HT, et al. Fever and renal failure in a child with Di-George syndrome and tetralogy of fallot. J Pediatric Infect Dis Soc 2015;4(4): 373–5.
26. Krishnamurthy S, Chandrasekaran V, Mahadevan S, et al. Severe acute kidney injury in children owing to infective endocarditis-associated immune complex glomerulonephritis: a report of two cases. Paediatr Int Child Health 2017;37(2): 144–7.
27. Ouellette CP, Joshi S, Texter K, et al. Multiorgan involvement confounding the diagnosis of bartonella henselae infective endocarditis in children with congenital heart disease. Pediatr Infect Dis J 2017;36(5):516–20.
28. Neugarten J, Baldwin DS. Glomerulonephritis in bacterial endocarditis. Am J Med 1984;77(2):297–304.
29. Boils CL, Nasr SH, Walker PD, et al. Update on endocarditis-associated glomerulonephritis. Kidney Int 2015;87(6):1241–9.
30. Couzi L, Morel D, Deminiere C, et al. An unusual endocarditis-induced crescentic glomerulonephritis treated by plasmapheresis. Clin Nephrol 2004;62(6):461–4.
31. Daimon S, Mizuno Y, Fujii S, et al. Infective endocarditis-induced crescentic glomerulonephritis dramatically improved by plasmapheresis. Am J Kidney Dis 1998;32(2):309–13.
32. Kannan S, Mattoo TK. Diffuse crescentic glomerulonephritis in bacterial endocarditis. Pediatr Nephrol 2001;16(5):423–8.
33. Rovzar MA, Logan JL, Ogden DA, et al. Immunosuppressive therapy and plasmapheresis in rapidly progressive glomerulonephritis associated with bacterial endocarditis. Am J Kidney Dis 1986;7(5):428–33.
34. Schoenbaum SC, Gardner P, Shillito J. Infections of cerebrospinal fluid shunts: epidemiology, clinical manifestations, and therapy. J Infect Dis 1975;131(5): 543–52.
35. Samtleben W, Bauriedel G, Bosch T, et al. Renal complications of infected ventriculoatrial shunts. Artif Organs 1993;17(8):695–701.
36. Arze RS, Rashid H, Morley R, et al. Shunt nephritis: report of two cases and review of the literature. Clin Nephrol 1983;19(1):48–53.
37. Haffner D, Schindera F, Aschoff A, et al. The clinical spectrum of shunt nephritis. Nephrol Dial Transplant 1997;12(6):1143–8.
38. World Health Organization Global hepatitis report. Hepatitis C. Global hepatitis report 2017. 2018. Available at: http://www.who.int/mediacentre/factsheets/fs164/en/. Accessed January 22, 2018.

39. Bhimma R, Coovadia HM, Adhikari M. Hepatitis B virus-associated nephropathy in black South African children. Pediatr Nephrol 1998;12(6):479–84.

40. Ozdamar SO, Gucer S, Tinaztepe K. Hepatitis-B virus associated nephropathies: a clinicopathological study in 14 children. Pediatr Nephrol 2003;18(1):23–8.

41. Burstein DM, Rodby RA. Membranoproliferative glomerulonephritis associated with hepatitis C virus infection. J Am Soc Nephrol 1993;4(6):1288–93.

42. Johnson RJ, Gretch DR, Yamabe H, et al. Membranoproliferative glomerulonephritis associated with hepatitis C virus infection. N Engl J Med 1993;328(7): 465–70.

43. McGuire BM, Julian BA, Bynon JS Jr, et al. Brief communication: glomerulonephritis in patients with hepatitis C cirrhosis undergoing liver transplantation. Ann Intern Med 2006;144(10):735–41.

44. Gopalani A, Ahuja TS. Prevalence of glomerulopathies in autopsies of patients infected with the hepatitis C virus. Am J Med Sci 2001;322(2):57–60.

45. Arase Y, Ikeda K, Murashima N, et al. Glomerulonephritis in autopsy cases with hepatitis C virus infection. Intern Med 1998;37(10):836–40.

46. Kamar N, Rostaing L, Alric L. Treatment of hepatitis C-virus-related glomerulonephritis. Kidney Int 2006;69(3):436–9.

47. Khalighi MA, Nguyen S, Wiedeman JA, et al. Bartonella endocarditis-associated glomerulonephritis: a case report and review of the literature. Am J Kidney Dis 2014;63(6):1060–5.

48. Thorley AM, Campbell D, Moghal NE, et al. Post streptococcal acute glomerulonephritis secondary to sporadic Streptococcus equi infection. Pediatr Nephrol 2007;22(4):597–9.

49. Garty BZ, Amir A, Scheuerman O, et al. Post-infectious glomerulonephritis associated with adenovirus infection. Isr Med Assoc J 2009;11(12):758–9.

Nephrotic Syndrome

Chia-shi Wang, MD, MSc*, Larry A. Greenbaum, MD, PhD

KEYWORDS

- Nephrotic syndrome • Edema • Peritonitis • Thrombosis • Minimal change disease
- Focal segmental glomerulosclerosis

KEY POINTS

- The classic features of nephrotic syndrome are edema, proteinuria, hypoalbuminemia, and hyperlipidemia.
- Minimal change disease, the most common cause of nephrotic syndrome in childhood, usually goes into remission within 4 weeks after starting corticosteroids, but there is a high risk of relapse after corticosteroids are stopped.
- Focal segmental glomerulosclerosis is the most common diagnosis in children who do not respond to corticosteroids, and it is an important cause of kidney failure in childhood.
- Complications of nephrotic syndrome include infections, including spontaneous bacterial peritonitis and cellulitis, and blood clots due to hypercoagulability.
- Nephrotic syndrome may be secondary to gene mutations, especially in infants, or systemic diseases, such as hepatitis or systemic lupus erythematosus.

INTRODUCTION

There are 4 classic features of nephrotic syndrome (**Box 1**).[1] There are many different causes of nephrotic syndrome (**Table 1**), but they share a common pathophysiology: massive loss of protein in the urine due to a defect in the glomerular filtration barrier.[2]

The most common causes of nephrotic syndrome in childhood are idiopathic minimal change disease (MCD) and focal segmental glomerulosclerosis (FSGS). The excellent response to corticosteroids in most patients with MCD has led to the empiric use of corticosteroids in most children with nephrotic syndrome, unless there are clinical features or laboratory findings suggesting a different cause.[3]

Disclosure: C. Wang and L.A. Greenbaum have received funding from Mallinckrodt Pharmaceuticals for an investigator-initiated clinical trial of H.P. Acthar Gel in childhood nephrotic syndrome. L.A. Greenbaum serves on the Data and Safety Monitoring Board for a clinical trial sponsored by Retrophin in patients with nephrotic syndrome. L.A. Greenbaum is a co-investigator of CureGN, an observational study of nephrotic syndrome patients sponsored by the National Institutes of Health.
Division of Pediatric Nephrology, Department of Pediatrics, Emory University School of Medicine and Children's Healthcare of Atlanta, 2015 Uppergate Drive Northeast, Atlanta, GA 30322-1015, USA
* Corresponding author.
E-mail address: chia-shi.wang@emory.edu

Pediatr Clin N Am 66 (2019) 73–85
https://doi.org/10.1016/j.pcl.2018.08.006
0031-3955/19/© 2018 Elsevier Inc. All rights reserved.

Box 1
Classic features of nephrotic syndrome
Proteinuria
Hypoalbuminemia
Edema
Hyperlipidemia

There are a variety of ways of classifying nephrotic syndrome (**Box 2**), and a patient's classification may change over time. For example, new knowledge may reveal a genetic cause or a pathogenic pathway. The histology does not determine other classifications: a patient with FSGS may have primary or secondary disease; genetic or nongenetic cause; or steroid-sensitive or steroid-resistant disease.

Some patients with nephrotic syndrome may have nephritic features (hypertension, hematuria, and decreased kidney function). Similarly, patients with a nephritic disease may have nephrotic features. This article does not discuss diseases that rarely present with nephrotic syndrome (eg, IgA nephropathy) or diseases that typically present with nephritic syndrome, but may have nephrotic features (eg, postinfectious glomerulonephritis).

For idiopathic nephrotic syndrome, response to corticosteroids is currently the best predictor of disease outcome. Ongoing research attempts to integrate genetic, epigenetic, molecular, and clinical data to determine a more precise disease taxonomy and improve outcome prediction.[4]

CLINICAL EVALUATION

The evaluation of a child with nephrotic syndrome includes a history and physical examination targeted at identifying secondary causes and complications of the disease. Diagnostic evaluation is dictated by the findings on history and physical examination and the response to corticosteroids.

History

The age of the child with nephrotic syndrome dictates the most likely causes. Congenital nephrotic syndrome (CNS; presentation during the first 3 months of life) most commonly has a genetic cause (see later discussion), but may be secondary to a congenital infection. Infantile nephrotic syndrome (3–12 months of age at presentation) is also likely to be genetic.[5–7] Idiopathic nephrotic syndrome most commonly presents between ages 2 and 7 years, and there is a male predominance (up to 3.8:1 male-to-female ratio).[8] Most of these children have MCD that is responsive to corticosteroids, although steroid-resistant disease, typically idiopathic FSGS, can also occur. In older children, and especially in adolescents, MCD becomes less common, and primary FSGS, membranous nephropathy (MN), and membranoproliferative glomerulonephritis (MPGN) are more common than in younger children.[2] Older children and adolescents are also at increased risk for secondary causes (eg, systemic lupus erythematosus [SLE], hepatitis B and C, human immunodeficiency virus [HIV]).[9]

A family history of nephrotic syndrome, FSGS, chronic kidney disease, or consanguinity should prompt consideration of a genetic cause. Autosomal recessive and autosomal dominant disease typically present in younger children and adolescents, respectively. A genetic cause should also be considered if there are congenital anomalies, such as occur in a variety of syndromic disorders (see **Table 1**).[10]

Table 1
Classification and causes of nephrotic syndrome in childhood

Examples of genetic disorders (associated gene)	Common age at presentation
Finnish-type congenital nephrotic syndrome (*NPHS1*)	Infancy
Diffuse mesangial sclerosis (eg, *PLCE1*, *WT1*)	Infancy
Early-onset autosomal recessive SRNS (eg, *NPHS2*, *PLCE1*)	Infancy and early childhood
Late-onset SRNS (eg, *ACTN4*, *TRPC6*)	Late childhood and adolescence
Examples of syndromic genetic disorders (associated gene)	
Denys-Drash and WAGR (*WT1*)	Infancy
Schimke immuno-osseus dysplasia (*SMARCAL1*)	Childhood
Pierson syndrome (*LAMB2*)	Infancy
Galloway-Mowat syndrome (eg, *WDR73* and *LAGE3*)	Infancy
Frasier syndrome (*WT1*)	Childhood or adolescence
Idiopathic (histologic classification)	
MCD	Early childhood to adolescence
FSGS	Early childhood to adolescence
MN	Late childhood and adolescence
MPGN	Late childhood and adolescence
Rheumatologic	
SLE	Late childhood and adolescence
Infections	
Hepatitis B, C	Variable; infancy for congenital exposure
HIV-1	Variable
Malaria	Variable
Congenital syphilis, toxoplasmosis	Infancy
Drugs/toxins	
Penicillamine	Variable
Gold	Variable
Nonsteroidal anti-inflammatory drugs	Variable
Pamidronate	Variable
Interferon	Variable
Mercury	Variable
Heroin	Variable
Lithium	Variable
Malignancy	
Lymphoma	Variable
Leukemia	Variable
Glomerular hyperfiltration	
Sickle-cell disease	Adolescence
Oligomeganephronia	Adolescence
Morbid obesity	Adolescence

Abbreviations: FSGS, focal segmental glomerulosclerosis; HIV-1, human immunodeficiency virus type 1; MCD, minimal change disease; MN, membranous nephropathy; MPGN, membranoproliferative glomerulonephritis; SLE, systemic lupus erythematosus; SRNS, steroid-resistant nephrotic syndrome; WAGR, Wilms tumor, aniridia, genitourinary abnormalities, and intellectual disability.
    Data from Refs.[2,5,45]

Box 2
Classifications of nephrotic syndrome

Age of presentation
  Congenital (first 3 months of life)
  Infantile (4–12 months)
  Childhood (>12 months)

Idiopathic versus secondary

Genetic versus acquired

Histology (eg, MCD, FSGS)

Steroid-sensitive versus steroid-resistant

The history should include questions about symptoms of lupus (joint pain, stiffness, and swelling; rash; photosensitivity; mouth ulcers; hair loss; fevers; and malaise), medication exposures (see **Table 1**); risk factors for or symptoms suggestive of infections that may cause nephrotic syndrome (ie, hepatitis B or C, HIV). Lymphadenopathy, pallor, fevers, and fatigue may suggest malignancy, which is a very rare cause of nephrotic syndrome in childhood.[2]

Patients typically present with insidious onset of edema, which may not be detected until significant fluid accumulation has occurred (**Fig. 1**). The edema is gravity dependent, and thus periorbital edema, occasionally misdiagnosed as allergies, is more prominent in the morning. After daytime ambulation, edema becomes more noticeable in the feet and legs. Scrotal, penile, and labial edema can be particularly distressing.

Although the chief complaint in nephrotic syndrome is usually edema, other clinical presentations may occur:

- Incidental finding on urinalysis or when screening due to a positive family history
- Complication of nephrotic syndrome (see later discussion)
  - Blood clot (pulmonary embolus [**Fig. 2**], deep venous thrombosis, arterial thrombosis)
  - Spontaneous bacterial peritonitis
  - Cellulitis
  - Abdominal pain due to bowel wall edema or hypoperfusion[11]

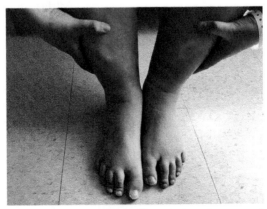

Fig. 1. Bilateral lower extremity edema in a patient with nephrotic syndrome with indentations visible bilaterally after applying pressure with a thumb.

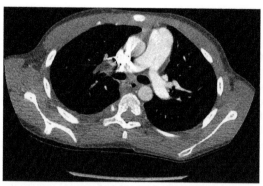

Fig. 2. Computed tomography angiography of the chest showing a right main pulmonary artery embolus (*red arrow*) in a child with nephrotic syndrome. (*Courtesy of* Stephen Simoneaux, MD, Emory University and Children's Healthcare of Atlanta, Atlanta, GA.)

Physical Examination

Edema is the dominant finding; the location of the most prominent edema can be quite variable between children. Rarely, the edema may be subtle despite massive proteinuria. The examination should include looking for findings suggestive of a syndromic condition, malignancy, or SLE (see earlier discussion) or complications of nephrotic syndrome (blood clot, peritonitis, or cellulitis). Hypertension may be present, especially in patients with FSGS or MPGN.[2]

Diagnostic Evaluation

The initial evaluation of a child with suspected nephrotic syndrome should establish the diagnosis of nephrotic syndrome (**Box 3**). Additional testing should screen for the most likely causes and complications.

Evaluations Done in All Patients

- Complete blood count: Elevated hemoglobin may occur due to hemoconcentration from intravascular volume contraction from fluid moving into the interstitial space.[12] Anemia may be present if there is chronic kidney disease or a secondary cause (SLE or malignancy). Depression of white cells or platelets also raises concerns of SLE or malignancy.
- Chemistries: Hyponatremia, typically mild, is a common finding due to secretion of antidiuretic hormone secondary to intravascular volume depletion.[12] Serum

---

Box 3
Laboratory testing to establish the diagnosis of nephrotic syndrome

Serum albumin ≤2.5 mg/L

Proteinuria
Random UPCR ≥2 mg/mg
24-h urine with greater than 50 mg/kg/day or greater than 40 mg/h/m² protein

Hyperlipidemia (elevated cholesterol and/or triglycerides)

Abbreviation: UPCR, urine protein to creatinine ratio.
Data from Lombel RM, Gipson DS, Hodson EM. Kidney disease: improving global outcomes. Treatment of steroid-sensitive nephrotic syndrome: new guidelines from KDIGO. Pediatr Nephrol 2013;28(3):415–26.

total calcium is low due to the low serum albumin since ~50% of calcium normally binds to albumin. The ionized calcium is typically normal, but may be low, possibly due to urinary loss of 25-hydroxyvitamin D.[13]

- Creatinine: Kidney function is usually normal in idiopathic nephrotic syndrome, although it may be diminished if there is significant intravascular volume depletion. Elevated serum creatinine not related to intravascular volume depletion is more common with FSGS and in secondary nephrotic syndrome.[14]
- Complement levels: Low C3 is common in MPGN; C3 and C4 are typically low in lupus nephritis. A low C3 is also consistent with postinfectious glomerulonephritis, which may occasionally be confused with idiopathic nephrotic syndrome.[15]
- Chest radiograph: This may rarely detect evidence of malignancy. Small pleural effusions are almost universally present and do not require intervention.[16]

Evaluations Done in Select Patients

- Antinuclear antibody: Screens for SLE in older children and adolescents or if there are signs and symptoms suggestive of SLE. Additional serologies for SLE may be indicated if suspicion is high.
- Viral testing (HIV, hepatitis B and C): Screen in children with CNS, older children, and adolescents or if biopsy findings suggest infection as a possible cause.[7]
- Kidney biopsy: A kidney biopsy is done in patients with steroid-resistant disease, older adolescents, or patients with other findings suggestive of a cause other than MCD. Although previously done in CNS, rapid genetic testing may make this unnecessary.[1]
- Genetic testing: This is most useful in congenital and infantile nephrotic syndrome, syndromic disease, familial disease, or if there is a history of consanguinity. Genetic testing is increasingly used in children with steroid-resistant disease.[10]
- Histology-specific testing: There are specific additional tests that should be considered in patients diagnosed with MN and MPGN (see later discussion).

COMPLICATIONS
Infections

Infections are common in children with nephrotic syndrome. Infections are due to urinary loss of immunoglobulins and complement factors, impaired lymphocytic function, treatment with immunosuppressive agents, ascites, and edema. Infections include pneumonia, bacteremia, spontaneous bacterial peritonitis, and cellulitis, with increased susceptibility to encapsulated organisms such as *Streptococcus pneumoniae*.[2,17,18]

Acute Kidney Injury

Acute kidney injury (AKI) is commonly due to intravascular volume depletion, which may be exacerbated by diuretics if concurrent intravenous replacement of albumin is not performed. AKI is more likely in children with steroid-resistant disease, concomitant infections, and nephrotoxic medication exposure.[19]

Thromboembolism

Thromboembolism is estimated to occur in approximately 3% of childhood nephrotic syndrome patients, with venous clots accounting for 97% of the cases.[20] The hypercoagulability in nephrotic syndrome is multifactorial: increased platelet aggregability, increased synthesis of prothrombotic factors, and urinary loss and decreased levels of antithrombin III, protein C, and protein S.[21] Traditional risk factors, such as heritable thrombophilia, intravascular volume depletion, and use of central venous catheters further increase the risk. Presenting complaints include asymmetric limb swelling, central venous catheter malfunction, gross hematuria (renal vein thrombosis), superior vena cava syndrome, and respiratory compromise (pulmonary embolism).[20]

CAUSES
Minimal Change Disease and Primary Focal Segmental Glomerulosclerosis

Epidemiology and clinical presentation
MCD and FSGS are the causes of more than 80% of idiopathic nephrotic syndrome cases in childhood, with MCD occurring more frequently than FSGS.[22] The prevalence of FSGS increases with age; the median age of onset is 6 years for FSGS and 3 years for MCD.[8] FSGS is present in 20% to 30% of adolescents presenting with nephrotic syndrome and is more common in Hispanic and black patients.[2]

On initial presentation, it is not possible to distinguish between MCD and FSGS, although microscopic hematuria, hypertension, and elevated serum creatinine occur more frequently with FSGS.[8] Approximately 80% of patients with suspected idiopathic childhood nephrotic syndrome have resolution of proteinuria within 8 weeks when treated with high-dose oral corticosteroids.[1] Failure to respond to corticosteroids is predictive of non-MCD histology; approximately 92% of MCD patients respond to corticosteroids and half of non-responders have FSGS. Approximately 70% of FSGS patients do not respond to corticosteroid therapy.[22] Thus, a biopsy is recommended for those who fail to respond to an adequate course of corticosteroid therapy.[3]

Pathophysiology
By definition, the cause of idiopathic MCD and FSGS is unknown. There is ongoing debate whether MCD and FSGS represent a spectrum of the same disease or are separate diseases.[23] There is convincing evidence that the podocyte is the target cell in these diseases. Based on the clinical response to corticosteroids and other immunosuppressive agents, it is hypothesized that there is an underlying immune mechanism leading to podocyte dysfunction, but proof of this hypothesis remains elusive.[2] However, there is also evidence for a direct effect of some medications on the podocyte.[24,25]

Disease course and prognosis
Steroid response is the most important predictor of prognosis. Long-term prognosis is good for patients who are responsive to corticosteroid therapy, with greater than 80% of patients no longer experiencing disease relapses at 8 years following disease onset.[26] Frequent disease relapses occur in approximately 60% of patients, causing morbidity from disease complications and treatment side effects.[2] Prognosis among steroid-resistant patients—the minority of MCD and majority of FSGS patients—is much less promising. Those who are refractory to treatment have a greater than 50% risk of progression to end-stage renal disease (ESRD) within 5 years of diagnosis.[3] In fact, FSGS is the second leading diagnosis among pediatric dialysis patients in North America.[27]

Treatment
The treatment of the initial episode of nephrotic syndrome is oral prednisone at 60 mg/m^2/day or 2 mg/kg/day (maximum 60 mg/day) for 4 to 6 weeks, followed by 40 mg/m^2 or 1.5 mg/kg (maximum 40 mg/day) on alternate days for 1 to 2 months. Daily prednisone is given for relapses and is reduced to alternate day dosing once the urine is

negative or trace for protein for 3 days.[1,3] For patients with frequent relapses, especially if there are significant steroid side effects, a variety of agents are used to prevent relapses: alkylating agents, calcineurin inhibitors, mycophenolate mofetil, and rituximab.[28] Home urine monitoring for relapses is a critical component of management.[29] The recommended treatment of steroid-resistant patients is a minimum 6-month course of a calcineurin inhibitor and an angiotensin converting enzyme inhibitor (ACEi) or angiotensin II receptor blocker (ARB). Evidence for other therapeutic approaches is limited.[28]

Membranous Nephropathy

Epidemiology and clinical presentation
MN is uncommon in childhood. Secondary causes include SLE, hepatitis B, drugs, and toxins. Idiopathic MN causes approximately 1.5% of childhood nephrotic syndrome.[8] In MN secondary to SLE, typical age of onset is around 13 years, with female predominance; AKI, hematuria, and hypertension can be seen on presentation.[30,31] The mean age at presentation for idiopathic MN in childhood is around 10 years with a slight male predominance. Microscopic hematuria is common, and gross hematuria may also occur. Hypertension is less common.[32]

Pathophysiology
A major advancement in the understanding of the pathogenesis was the discovery of antiphospholipase A_2 receptor (PLA_2R) antibodies in patients with MN. PLA_2R is a transmembrane glycoprotein expressed by the podocyte. Circulating anti-PLA_2R autoantibodies are found in 70% of primary adult MN patients and levels correlate with disease activity; screening for autoantibodies has thus become an important component of management.[32] Autoantibodies against other glomerular antigens may also cause primary MN.[33,34]

Disease course and prognosis
The degree of proteinuria is an important prognostic indicator in idiopathic MN. Patients with proteinuria without complete features of nephrotic syndrome often achieve disease remission spontaneously, although relapses can occur. Those with nephrotic syndrome have a 50% remission rate, with renal dysfunction developing in approximately one-third of the patients.[32] In addition, age greater than 10 years, hypertension on presentation, and presence of renal venous thrombosis are poor prognostic indicators.[35,36] Prognosis in secondary MN depends on the cause.

Treatment
Treatment of secondary MN depends on the cause and will not be reviewed here. Data on treatment of idiopathic MN in children are limited given its low incidence. Children without nephrotic syndrome are generally given ACEis/ARBs and other supportive therapy without immunosuppressants. Those with nephrotic syndrome, especially if decreased kidney function or fibrosis on biopsy, may be treated with alkylating agents, calcineurin inhibitors, or rituximab, with limited evidence on the optimal approach in children.[32]

Membranoproliferative Glomerulonephritis, C3 Glomerulopathy, and Immune-Complex–Mediated Membranoproliferative Glomerulonephritis

Epidemiology and clinical presentation
MPGN is a clinically diverse group of diseases traditionally grouped together based on common histologic findings. A key serologic feature is low C3, seen in 80% to 95% of the patients.[37] MPGN is further subdivided based on the location of immune deposits:

type 1 (subendothelial), type 2 (also called dense deposit disease [DDD]; intramembranous deposits), and type 3 (subendothelial and subepithelial). This histologic classification offers limited information on the underlying disease process due to extensive overlap. Thus, a new classification is based on whether the immune complexes are predominantly composed of C3 (C3 glomerulopathy [C3G]) or immunoglobulins (immune-complex-mediated MPGN [IC-MPGN]). C3G is further subdivided based on the location and quality of deposits into DDD or C3 glomerulonephritis (C3GN). The new classification improves diagnostic precision, but is imperfect.[38]

The incidence of MPGN or C3G/IC-MPGN is estimated to be 2 cases per 10^6 children, comprising approximately 7.5% of nephrotic syndrome cases in pediatrics. Onset is typically in late childhood or adolescence, with a slight male predominance.[8,37] Nearly half of patients present with isolated hematuria and proteinuria that is found on routine evaluation. About one-third of patients present with nephrotic syndrome, usually accompanied by microscopic hematuria. Others present with gross hematuria with acute nephritic syndrome, often associated with rapidly progressive glomerulonephritis. Hypertension and renal insufficiency can be seen on presentation.[39]

Pathophysiology

Table 2 summarizes causes of C3G and IC-MPGN and the associated traditional histologic classification. IC-MPGN is most commonly secondary to chronic infections, autoimmune disorders, or malignancies. In chronic infections and autoimmune disorders, antigen-antibody immune complexes trigger classical complement pathway-medicated injury. The monoclonal immunoglobulins formed in malignancies, which are rare in childhood, also trigger the classical complement pathway, resulting in IC-MPGN. C3G is generally thought to be caused by abnormalities in the alternative complement pathway, due to either mutations in genes for complement or complement regulatory proteins or autoantibodies against complement system components, leading to uncontrolled activity and complement-mediated damage of glomeruli.

Table 2
Causes and traditional histologic classification of immune-complex-mediated membranoproliferative glomerulonephritis and C3 glomerulopathy

Causes	Traditional Classification
IC-MPGN	
Infections: hepatitis B, hepatitis C, staphylococcus, *Mycobacterium tuberculosis*, *Propionibacterium acnes*, brucella, *Coxiella burnetii*, streptococci, nocardia, meningococcus, malaria, schistosomiasis, HIV	Type 1
Autoimmune: SLE, mixed cryoglobulinemia, Sjögren syndrome, scleroderma	Type 1
Malignancy: monoclonal gammopathy, chronic lymphocytic leukemia, low-grade B-cell lymphoma, multiple myeloma	Type 1
C3G	
Dysregulation of the alternative complement pathway: mutations in complement-regulating proteins (CFH, CFI, CFHR5), autoantibodies to complement-regulating proteins (anti-C3bBb, anti-CFH, anti-CFI, anti-CFB), C3 mutations	Type I, II, and III

Abbreviations: C3G, C3 glomerulopathy; IC-MPGN, immune-complex-mediated membranoproliferative glomerulonephritis; SLE, systemic lupus erythematosus.
Data from Refs.[38,40,47,48]

There is, however, some overlap between IC-MPGN and C3G, and the association of IC-MPGN with the classical complement system and C3G with the alternative complement system may not be absolute.[38,40]

Disease course and prognosis

Long-term outcome for MPGN (C3G and IC-MPGN) is poor. Fifty percent and 90% develop ESRD by 10 years and 20 years, respectively. Outcome is worse in those presenting with nephrotic syndrome, renal insufficiency, and crescents on initial biopsy. C3G may be more refractory to treatment than IC-MPGN.[37,41]

Treatment

There is limited evidence to guide therapy in C3G and IC-MPGN. Corticosteroids, mycophenolate mofetil, and rituximab have been used, along with ACEis/ARBs, without consistent efficacy. More recently, targeted complement pathway inhibitors have been evaluated in patients with C3G, but benefit still needs to be established.[42,43]

Congenital Nephrotic Syndrome

Cause and clinical presentation

CNS, defined as nephrotic syndrome presenting in the first 3 months of life, is rare. Secondary causes include congenital infections (syphilis, toxoplasmosis, cytomegalovirus, rubella, HIV), infantile SLE, and fetomaternal alloimmunization. Screening for congenital infections is an important component of the evaluation of the infant with CNS. CNS is most commonly caused by mutations in genes encoding proteins that are essential for proper function of the glomerular filtration barrier. CNS of the Finnish type is caused by mutations in the gene (NPHS1) encoding nephrin, a protein that is a critical component of the slit diaphragm between glomerular podocytes. Mutations in multiple other genes may cause CNS (**Box 4**).[44]

Presentation differs depending on the mutation involved. Patients with NPHS1 mutations typically present with nephrotic syndrome in the first weeks of life, with massive proteinuria that is associated with worse outcomes, although milder forms exist. An enlarged placenta is classically observed at birth (>25% of the infant's birth weight). NPHS2 mutations typically present after 1 month of life, with many cases presenting in early childhood. Children with syndromic causes of CNS have extrarenal manifestations:

- Urogenital abnormalities with WT1 mutations in Denys-Drash syndrome
- Eye defects with LAMB2 mutations in Pierson syndrome
- Neurologic findings in Galloway-Mowat syndrome[10,45]

Box 4
Examples of genes and associated proteins where mutations may cause congenital nephrotic syndrome

NPHS1 (nephrin)

NPHS2 (podocin)

WT1 (Wilms tumor protein)

LAMB2 (laminin)

PLCε1 (phospholipase C epsilon 1)

Data from Machuca E, Benoit G, Nevo F, et al. Genotype-phenotype correlations in non-Finnish congenital nephrotic syndrome. J Am Soc Nephrol 2010;21(7):1209–17.

Prognosis

Secondary CNS generally resolves with treatment of the underlying cause or after disappearance of maternal autoantibodies. Primary CNS is generally not responsive to treatment and progresses to ESRD. Classic Finnish-type CNS patients frequently reach ESRD by 2 to 3 years. In contrast, patients with mutations in podocin generally develop ESRD between 6 and 9 years.[44] CNS is complicated by failure to thrive, infections, and thrombosis.[6,46]

Treatment

Goals of treatment are to control edema with a combination of albumin infusions and diuretics and to prevent and treat complications such as infections and thromboembolism. Nutritional support and thyroxine and cholecalciferol to replace urinary losses are important to promote growth and development. Children eventually need kidney transplantation, which is commonly preceded by nephrectomies to address hypercoagulability and hyperlipidemia if the patient remains nephrotic.[11]

REFERENCES

1. Lombel RM, Gipson DS, Hodson EM, Kidney Disease: Improving Global Outcomes. Treatment of steroid-sensitive nephrotic syndrome: new guidelines from KDIGO. Pediatr Nephrol 2013;28(3):415–26.
2. Eddy AA, Symons JM. Nephrotic syndrome in childhood. Lancet 2003;362(9384): 629–39.
3. Lombel RM, Hodson EM, Gipson DS, et al. Treatment of steroid-resistant nephrotic syndrome in children: new guidelines from KDIGO. Pediatr Nephrol 2013;28(3):409–14.
4. Mariani LH, Pendergraft WF 3rd, Kretzler M. Defining glomerular disease in mechanistic terms: implementing an integrative biology approach in nephrology. Clin J Am Soc Nephrol 2016;11(11):2054–60.
5. Warejko JK, Tan W, Daga A, et al. Whole exome sequencing of patients with steroid-resistant nephrotic syndrome. Clin J Am Soc Nephrol 2018;13(1):53–62.
6. Kari JA, Montini G, Bockenhauer D, et al. Clinico-pathological correlations of congenital and infantile nephrotic syndrome over twenty years. Pediatr Nephrol 2014;29(11):2173–80.
7. Soares SF, Donatti TL, Souto FJ. Serological markers of viral, syphilitic and toxoplasmic infection in children and teenagers with nephrotic syndrome: case series from Mato Grosso State, Brazil. Rev Inst Med Trop Sao Paulo 2014;56(6): 499–504.
8. Nephrotic syndrome in children: prediction of histopathology from clinical and laboratory characteristics at time of diagnosis. A report of the International Study of Kidney Disease in Children. Kidney Int 1978;13(2):159–65.
9. Jiang M, Xiao Z, Rong L, et al. Twenty-eight-year review of childhood renal diseases from renal biopsy data: a single centre in China. Nephrology (Carlton) 2016;21(12):1003–9.
10. Preston R, Stuart HM, Lennon R. Genetic testing in steroid-resistant nephrotic syndrome: why, who, when and how? Pediatr Nephrol 2017. [Epub ahead of print].
11. McCaffrey J, Lennon R, Webb NJ. The non-immunosuppressive management of childhood nephrotic syndrome. Pediatr Nephrol 2016;31(9):1383–402.
12. Siddall EC, Radhakrishnan J. The pathophysiology of edema formation in the nephrotic syndrome. Kidney Int 2012;82(6):635–42.

13. Sato KA, Gray RW, Lemann J Jr. Urinary excretion of 25-hydroxyvitamin D in health and the nephrotic syndrome. J Lab Clin Med 1982;99(3):325–30.

14. Primary nephrotic syndrome in children: clinical significance of histopathologic variants of minimal change and of diffuse mesangial hypercellularity. A Report of the International Study of Kidney Disease in Children. Kidney Int 1981;20(6): 765–71.

15. Thurman JM, Nester CM. All things complement. Clin J Am Soc Nephrol 2016; 11(10):1856–66.

16. Niaudet P, Boyer O. Idiopathic nephrotic syndrome in children: clinical aspects. In: Avner ED, Harmon WE, Niaudet P, et al, editors. Pediatric nephrology. 7th edition. Berlin (Germany): Springer; 2016. p. 839–82.

17. Wei CC, Yu IW, Lin HW, et al. Occurrence of infection among children with nephrotic syndrome during hospitalizations. Nephrology (Carlton) 2012;17(8): 681–8.

18. Gipson DS, Messer KL, Tran CL, et al. Inpatient health care utilization in the United States among children, adolescents, and young adults with nephrotic syndrome. Am J Kidney Dis 2013;61(6):910–7.

19. Rheault MN, Wei CC, Hains DS, et al. Increasing frequency of acute kidney injury amongst children hospitalized with nephrotic syndrome. Pediatr Nephrol 2014; 29(1):139–47.

20. Kerlin BA, Haworth K, Smoyer WE. Venous thromboembolism in pediatric nephrotic syndrome. Pediatr Nephrol 2014;29(6):989–97.

21. Loscalzo J. Venous thrombosis in the nephrotic syndrome. N Engl J Med 2013; 368(10):956–8.

22. The primary nephrotic syndrome in children. Identification of patients with minimal change nephrotic syndrome from initial response to prednisone. A report of the International Study of Kidney Disease in Children. J Pediatr 1981;98(4): 561–4.

23. Maas RJ, Deegens JK, Smeets B, et al. Minimal change disease and idiopathic FSGS: manifestations of the same disease. Nat Rev Nephrol 2016;12(12):768–76.

24. Ransom RF, Lam NG, Hallett MA, et al. Glucocorticoids protect and enhance recovery of cultured murine podocytes via actin filament stabilization. Kidney Int 2005;68(6):2473–83.

25. Faul C, Donnelly M, Merscher-Gomez S, et al. The actin cytoskeleton of kidney podocytes is a direct target of the antiproteinuric effect of cyclosporine A. Nat Med 2008;14(9):931–8.

26. Tarshish P, Tobin JN, Bernstein J, et al. Prognostic significance of the early course of minimal change nephrotic syndrome: report of the International Study of Kidney Disease in Children. J Am Soc Nephrol 1997;8(5):769–76.

27. Leonard MB, Donaldson LA, Ho M, et al. A prospective cohort study of incident maintenance dialysis in children: an NAPRTC study. Kidney Int 2003;63(2): 744–55.

28. Greenbaum LA, Benndorf R, Smoyer WE. Childhood nephrotic syndrome–current and future therapies. Nat Rev Nephrol 2012;8(8):445–58.

29. Wang CS, Yan J, Palmer R, et al. Childhood nephrotic syndrome management and outcome: a single center retrospective analysis. Int J Nephrol 2017;2017: 2029583.

30. Boneparth A, Wenderfer SE, Moorthy LN, et al. Clinical characteristics of children with membranous lupus nephritis: the Childhood Arthritis and Rheumatology Research Alliance Legacy Registry. Lupus 2017;26(3):299–306.

31. Pereira M, Muscal E, Eldin K, et al. Clinical presentation and outcomes of childhood-onset membranous lupus nephritis. Pediatr Nephrol 2017;32(12): 2283–91.
32. Ayalon R, Beck LH Jr. Membranous nephropathy: not just a disease for adults. Pediatr Nephrol 2015;30(1):31–9.
33. Tomas NM, Beck LH Jr, Meyer-Schwesinger C, et al. Thrombospondin type-1 domain-containing 7A in idiopathic membranous nephropathy. N Engl J Med 2014;371(24):2277–87.
34. Bullich G, Ballarin J, Oliver A, et al. HLA-DQA1 and PLA2R1 polymorphisms and risk of idiopathic membranous nephropathy. Clin J Am Soc Nephrol 2014;9(2): 335–43.
35. Tsukahara H, Takahashi Y, Yoshimoto M, et al. Clinical course and outcome of idiopathic membranous nephropathy in Japanese children. Pediatr Nephrol 1993;7(4):387–91.
36. Lee BH, Cho HY, Kang HG, et al. Idiopathic membranous nephropathy in children. Pediatr Nephrol 2006;21(11):1707–15.
37. Medjeral-Thomas NR, O'Shaughnessy MM, O'Regan JA, et al. C3 glomerulopathy: clinicopathologic features and predictors of outcome. Clin J Am Soc Nephrol 2014;9(1):46–53.
38. Noris M, Remuzzi G. Genetics of immune-mediated glomerular diseases: focus on complement. Semin Nephrol 2017;37(5):447–63.
39. Licht C, Riedl M, Pickering MC, et al. Membranoproliferative and C3-Mediated GN in Children. In: Avner ED, Harmon WE, Niaudet P, et al, editors. Pediatric nephrology. 7th edition. Berlin (Germany): Springer; 2016. p. 1036–55.
40. Noris M, Remuzzi G. Glomerular diseases dependent on complement activation, including atypical hemolytic uremic syndrome, membranoproliferative glomerulonephritis, and C3 glomerulopathy: core curriculum 2015. Am J Kidney Dis 2015; 66(2):359–75.
41. Okuda Y, Ishikura K, Hamada R, et al. Membranoproliferative glomerulonephritis and C3 glomerulonephritis: frequency, clinical features, and outcome in children. Nephrology (Carlton) 2015;20(4):286–92.
42. Bomback AS, Smith RJ, Barile GR, et al. Eculizumab for dense deposit disease and C3 glomerulonephritis. Clin J Am Soc Nephrol 2012;7(5):748–56.
43. Sanghera P, Ghanta M, Ozay F, et al. Kidney diseases associated with alternative complement pathway dysregulation and potential treatment options. Am J Med Sci 2017;354(6):533–8.
44. Machuca E, Benoit G, Nevo F, et al. Genotype-phenotype correlations in non-Finnish congenital nephrotic syndrome. J Am Soc Nephrol 2010;21(7):1209–17.
45. Braun DA, Rao J, Mollet G, et al. Mutations in KEOPS-complex genes cause nephrotic syndrome with primary microcephaly. Nat Genet 2017;49(10):1529–38.
46. Lau KK, Chan HH, Massicotte P, et al. Thrombotic complications of neonates and children with congenital nephrotic syndrome. Curr Pediatr Rev 2014;10(3): 169–76.
47. Fervenza FC, Sethi S, Glassock RJ. Idiopathic membranoproliferative glomerulonephritis: does it exist? Nephrol Dial Transplant 2012;27(12):4288–94.
48. Sethi S, Fervenza FC. Membranoproliferative glomerulonephritis–a new look at an old entity. N Engl J Med 2012;366(12):1119–31.

Lupus Nephritis

Scott E. Wenderfer, MD, PhD[a],*, Karen W. Eldin, MD[b]

KEYWORDS

- Lupus • Nephritis • Glomerulopathy • Complement • Autoantibody • Proteinuria
- Hematuria • Biopsy

KEY POINTS

- Lupus nephritis is a cause of hypocomplementemic glomerulonephritis.
- Kidney involvement in lupus often warrants immunosuppression beyond that required for extrarenal manifestations.
- Biopsy is the gold standard for classification of kidney involvement in lupus and primarily drives treatment decisions.
- Frequent monitoring is required for assessing the therapeutic response, relapse of active disease, and renal scarring.
- The dramatic improvements in renal and patient outcomes from 1950 to 1990 have slowed substantially.

INTRODUCTION

Pediatric lupus nephritis (LN) is a common cause of glomerular disease in children. The prevalence of systemic lupus erythematosus (SLE) is 70 to 90 per 100,000 individuals, with 20% diagnosed before 18 years of age.[1,2]

The prevalence is approximately 2-fold higher in Asians and Hispanics and up to 4-fold higher in blacks of African descent.[3] Between 40% and 70% of children with SLE develop LN, 10% to 30% higher than in adult-onset SLE.[4,5] Genetic polymorphisms are more common in childhood-onset SLE (cSLE), such as signal transducer and activator of transcription 4 (STAT4)[6,7] and integrin alpha M (ITGAM)-integrin alpha X (ITGAX)[8] polymorphisms and reduced Fc-receptor gene copy number.[9] However,

Disclosure Statement: Neither Dr S.E Wenderfer nor Dr K.W. Eldin have any relationships to disclose with commercial companies that have direct financial interest in the subject matter or materials discussed in this article or with any company making a competing product.
[a] Pediatric Nephrology, Department of Pediatrics, Baylor College of Medicine, Texas Children's Hospital, 1102 Bates Avenue, Suite 245, Houston, TX 77030, USA; [b] Department of Pathology and Immunology, Baylor College of Medicine, Texas Children's Hospital, 6621 Fannin Street, Suite AB195, Houston, TX 77030, USA
* Corresponding author.
E-mail address: wenderfe@bcm.edu

the numerous genes identified so far explain only 20% of disease heritability.[10] The missing heritability likely comes from complex interactions between genes and the environment (ultraviolet light, heavy metals, viral infections) and disrupted epigenetic regulation of gene expression.

PATHOPHYSIOLOGY

Systemic autoimmunity in SLE begins with the loss of tolerance to intracellular self-antigens (chromatin, nucleosomes, DNA, RNA, ribonuclear proteins).[11] Defects in the classic pathway of complement (such as C1q deficiency), DNase enzymes, and phagocyte receptors all contribute to autoantibody generation.[12] Type-I interferon and nuclear factor kappa-B pathways, neutrophil extracellular traps, and perturbations in B-cell signaling and B-cell cytokines (such as B-cell activating factor [BAFF][13]) all predispose to LN development. Ultimately, immune complexes form and localize to glomeruli, driving proliferation of resident kidney cells and inflammation by macrophage, dendritic cells, basophils,[14] and B and T lymphocytes.

CLINICAL PRESENTATION

Presenting features of LN are nonspecific for acute glomerulonephritis[2]:

- Hematuria (microscopic or gross)
- Proteinuria (± nephrotic syndrome)
- Urinary casts (red blood cell [RBC], granular, hyaline)
- Hypertension
- Peripheral edema
- Acute/chronic kidney injury

Laboratory Evaluation

Testing for antinuclear antibodies (ANAs) has a low false-negative rate but is nonspecific. An extractable nuclear antigen (ENA) panel or ANA profile can provide data on specificity of ANA and help confirm an SLE diagnosis. Anti–double-stranded DNA antibody titers loosely correlate with LN activity. Anti-C1q antibodies are also more specific for LN.[15,16] Low levels of complement components C3 and C4 help in the diagnosis; however, normal complement levels do not exclude LN.

Kidney biopsy remains the gold standard for diagnosis. Immunofluorescent antibody staining of glomeruli is typically positive for C1q, C3, immunoglobulin A (IgA), IgG, and IgM (full house pattern). Kidney injury is classified by the International Society of Nephrology/Renal Pathology Society (ISN/RPS).[17] The prevalence for each LN class is similar in children and adults.[18] The utility of distinguishing nonproliferative (Fig. 1) from proliferative classes (Fig. 2) is supported by pediatric studies.[19–23] The ISN/RPS's revised 2018 classification includes scoring for both disease activity and chronicity, based on the National Institutes of Health's (NIH) indices that are valid in pediatric LN.[24,25]

PATHOLOGY
Proliferative Lupus Nephritis

- Prevalence (class III/IV): 50% to 80%[2]
- Segmental or global glomerular hypercellularity lesions, in a mesangial, endocapillary, or mesangiocapillary pattern

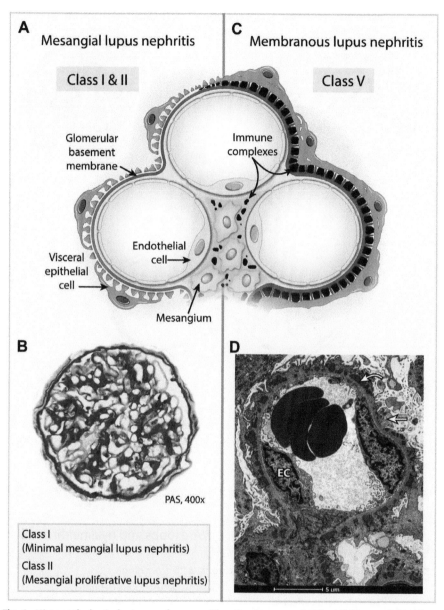

Fig. 1. Histopathologic features of nonproliferative lupus nephritis. (*A*) Mesangial LN (ISN/RPS class I and class II). In class I, glomeruli are histologically normal with immune complex deposition by ancillary immunofluorescence or electron microscopy studies. (*B*) Glomerulus with mildly increased mesangial hypercellularity by light microscopy, class II (periodic acid–Schiff, original magnification × 400). (*C*) Membranous LN (ISN/RPS class V). Glomeruli have immune complex deposition along the glomerular basement membranes with visceral epithelial cell (podocyte) injury, ± mesangial alternations. (*D*) Electron microscopy imaging demonstrates epi-membranous to intramembranous electron-dense deposits (*curved arrow*) with podocyte foot process effacement (*straight arrow*). EC, endothelial cell.

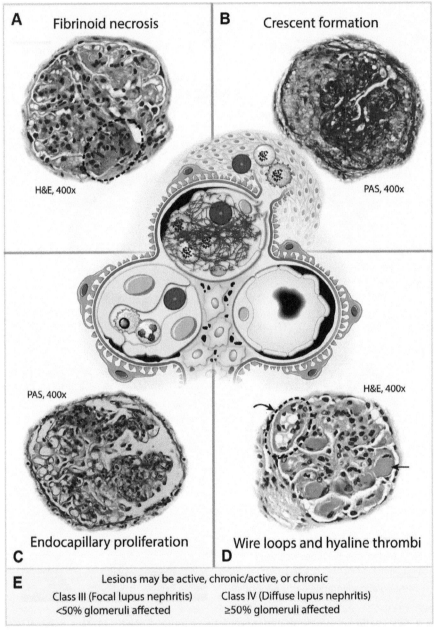

A Fibrinoid necrosis

H&E, 400x

B Crescent formation

PAS, 400x

PAS, 400x

H&E, 400x

C Endocapillary proliferation

D Wire loops and hyaline thrombi

E Lesions may be active, chronic/active, or chronic

Class III (Focal lupus nephritis)
<50% glomeruli affected

Class IV (Diffuse lupus nephritis)
≥50% glomeruli affected

Fig. 2. Histopathologic features of proliferative LN (*central schematic*). Subendothelial immune complex mediated injury compromises the intracapillary circulation. (*A*) Luminal inflammatory cells with fibrinoid necrosis of glomerular capillary loop (*dashed circle*) (hematoxylin-eosin, original magnification ×400). (*B*) Glomerular capillary loop rupture may incite extracapillary hypercellularity (crescent) (periodic acid–Schiff, original magnification × 400). (*C*) Endocapillary hypercellularity with swollen endothelium and intraluminal inflammatory cells (periodic acid–Schiff, original magnification × 400). (*D*) Massive subendothelial immune complexes, wire loops (*curved arrow, dashed circle*), focally bulging into capillary lumen as hyaline thrombi (*straight arrow*) (hematoxylin-eosin, original magnification ×400). (*E*) The proportion of affected glomeruli characterizes ISN/RPS class III or class IV disease.

- Usually accompanied by positive immunostaining of capillary loops for immuno-globulins and complement components and extensive subendothelial electron dense deposits
- Untreated, has high rate of morbidity, mortality, and end-stage kidney disease (ESKD)

Membranous Lupus Nephritis

- Prevalence (pure class V LN): 10% to 25%[2]
- Segmental or global thickening of glomerular basement membranes, often with spikes noted on silver stain
- Positive immunostaining of capillary loops for immunoglobulins and complement
- Electron-dense deposits in epi-membranous or subepithelial locations
- Resemble idiopathic membranous nephropathy on biopsy but distinguishable by presence of tubuloreticular inclusions and/or C1q immunostaining

Membranous and proliferative lesions can coexist (mixed-class LN).

Nonclassifiable Lupus Nephritis

- Lupus vasculitis: pauci-immune, necrotizing glomerulonephritis (often segmental with crescents)[26]
- Thrombotic microangiopathy: intraglomerular fibrin staining in association with thrombocytopenia and microangiopathic hemolytic anemia; often associated with antiphospholipid syndrome (anticardiolipin/beta2 glycoprotein I antibodies or positive lupus anticoagulant)[27]
- Lupus podocytopathy: isolated proteinuria and greater than 50% podocyte foot process effacement, with minimal change, mesangial, or focal segmental glo-merulosclerosis histopathology, without significant electron dense deposits[28]

MANAGEMENT
Proliferative Lupus Nephritis

Initial therapy

- The NIH's regimen of cyclophosphamide (CYC) and high-dose IV solumedrol[29] or
- The Euro-Lupus protocol of low-dose CYC[30] (remains unstudied in children) or
- Mycophenolate mofetil (MMF) alone[31–33] or in combination with tacrolimus (TAC)[34]
- Azathioprine (AZA), cyclosporine (CsA),[35] and TAC (one study includes adoles-cents)[36] are effective second-line agents

To standardize approaches for future comparative effectiveness research in chil-dren, consensus treatment plans (CTPs) have been developed for initial episodes of proliferative LN (**Table 1**).[37] CTPs use either MMF or CYC for an initial 6-month induc-tion, combined with one of 3 corticosteroid strategies: primarily oral, primarily intrave-nous (IV), and mixed oral/IV.

Maintenance therapy

- Clinical trials support either MMF or AZA for long-term maintenance.[38–41]
- Hydroxychloroquine reduces rates of disease flare, allows tapering of corticoste-roids, and improves renal outcomes.[42]
- Renin angiotensin blockade reduces proteinuria in patients with or without renal scarring.[43]

Table 1
Approach toward therapy for lupus nephritis in children

Proliferative LN (Class III or IV) or Mixed Proliferative/Membranous (Classes III + V, IV + V)	
Initial therapy	• CYC or MMF for 6 mo • Oral steroids ± IV steroid pulses, with tapering
Maintenance therapy	• MMF or AZA, duration undefined • Oral steroids as needed to control extrarenal disease • Hydroxychloroquine (can be started with initial therapy) • Renin angiotensin blockade (for persistent HTN or proteinuria, if not already started with initial therapy)
Nonproliferative LN (class I, II, V)	
Initial therapy (low risk)[a]	• Oral ± IV steroids, as dictated by extrarenal manifestations • No additional immunosuppression recommended
Initial therapy (high risk)[a]	• MMF (most common), AZA, CsA, TAC, or CYC (no strong evidence to support any as first line) until complete response • Oral steroids, with tapering after resolution of risk factors[a]
Maintenance therapy	• Same as proliferative LN
LN relapses	
Proteinuric flares	• Encourage medication adherence • Restart or increase steroid ± maintenance immunosuppression
Nephritic flares	• Encourage medication adherence • Consider repeat biopsy • Restart initial therapy, based on prior responsiveness
AKI	• Encourage medication adherence • Consider repeat biopsy, consider nonclassifiable causes • Restart initial therapy, including IV steroids
End-stage LN (class VI)	
Conservative therapy	• Avoid additional immunosuppression • Low-dose oral steroids and hydroxychloroquine • Consider renin angiotensin blockade

Abbreviations: AKI, acute kidney injury; HTN, hypertension; IV, intravenous.
[a] Risk factors for ESKD nonproliferative LN include proteinuria greater than 3.5 g/d, nephrotic syndrome, or acute kidney injury.

Definitions for response
Pediatric CTPs also define outcome measures for assessing the response to induction therapy (**Table 2**).[37] Patients with mild to moderate responses can continue to show improvement for months after completion of induction therapy.

Refractory therapy
One-third of patients are refractory to conventional therapy, with active urine sediment and deterioration of renal function. Medication nonadherence is a common contributor. Repeat kidney biopsy can be highly informative:

- Increased activity index may justify more aggressive immunosuppression.
- Improvements in histopathology may be reassuring.

Table 2
Definitions of renal outcomes in patients with childhood-onset systemic lupus erythematosus and lupus nephritis

	Definition
Outcome Measure	
Core renal parameters	Proteinuria (spot uPCR) Renal function (creatinine clearance or serum creatinine) Urine sediment (urine WBC, RBC, or casts)
Renal Response	
Complete	• Inactive urine sediment (<5 WBCs and <5 RBCs per high-power field, no casts) • uPCR <0.2 • Normal renal function (estimated GFR >90 mL/min/1.73 m^2)
Moderate	• At least 50% improvement in 2 of 3 core renal parameters (uPCR $\leq$1.0) without worsening of remaining parameter
Mild	• 30%–50% improvement in 2 of 3 core renal parameters without clinically relevant worsening of the remaining core parameter
No response	• Patients who do not improve

Abbreviations: GFR, glomerular filtration rate; uPCR, urine protein/creatinine ratio; WBC, white blood cell.

- Increased chronicity index suggests poor prognosis; with lower activity, the index predicts a decline in renal function regardless of therapy.
- A nonclassifiable disease, such as pauci-immune vasculitis or thrombotic microangiopathy, may guide alternative therapies.

Management of refractory LN with a persistently high activity index starts with switching from MMF to CYC or vice versa, switching from oral to IV therapies, or adding a B-cell depletion agent like rituximab.[44,45]

Membranous Lupus Nephritis

Initial therapy

- For patients with normal renal function, non–nephrotic-range proteinuria, antiproteinuric therapy, and corticosteroids $\pm$ immunosuppressive therapy as dictated by extrarenal manifestations (see **Table 1**).[46]
- For proteinuria greater than 3.5 g/d $\pm$ nephrotic syndrome, steroids and additional immunosuppression are more effective than steroids alone.[47] MMF is most commonly used[48,49]; but favorable data exist for the use of AZA, CsA, TAC, or CYC.[47]

Oral corticosteroid dosing is similar to the treatment of proliferative LN,[37] but IV pulse steroids are often unnecessary.[48,49] The optimal approach to mixed membranous and proliferative LN is uncertain, but most treat similarly to pure proliferative LN.[18]

Maintenance therapy

Similar to proliferative LN, steroid-sparing strategies have been used (antimalarials with either MMF or AZA and RAS blockade for persistent proteinuria or hypertension).[40]

Refractory therapy

It can take 2 to 3 years to fully respond to therapy.[48,49] Refractory therapy is reserved for children who develop progressive renal failure or persistent edema from nephrotic syndrome for greater than 3 to 6 months. Options include switching immunosuppressive agents or add-on therapy with rituximab, IV immunoglobulin, or IV corticosteroids.[44–46]

Definitions for response

Five core renal parameters are typically considered: (1) proteinuria, (2) hypoalbuminemia, (3) edema, (4) renal function, and (5) urine sediment. Complete resolution of membranous lesions is rarely seen on repeat biopsy.[48–50]

Lupus Nephritis Relapses

The rate of renal flares due to SLE is 25% to 50% on therapy.[48–52] Three types have been defined[37]:

- Proteinuric flare: abnormal proteinuria after complete remission or doubling of proteinuria after mild/moderate response
- Nephritic flare: increase or recurrence of active urinary sediment (increased hematuria ± reappearance of cellular casts) ± increased proteinuria
- Acute kidney injury (AKI) with worsening serologies

Management

Treatment of flares is not evidence based and must be individualized (see **Table 1**). Determination of patients' adherence to their medication regimen is crucial. Proteinuric renal flares are usually manageable without repeat biopsy with increased dose corticosteroids or maintenance immunosuppression. Coexistence of extrarenal involvement must also be considered. For flares on weaning immunosuppression, returning to the dose that last controlled the disease may be the best initial strategy.

Repeat biopsy is often helpful for nephritic flares, which often require a change in immunosuppressive agent or more induction therapy.

OUTCOMES
Patient Survival

Outcomes in pediatric LN have improved since the 1980s,[2] with improvement in 5-year patient survival from 83% to 91% over 3 decades.[41]

Disease Complications

Patients with cSLE carry an increased burden of both traditional and nontraditional cardiovascular risk factors.[2] Hypertension persists in 20% of patients often with left ventricular hypertrophy, increased arterial stiffness, and carotid intima media hyperplasia.[53]

Renal Survival

ESKD rates in children with SLE have greatly improved from 50% in the 1970s to less than 10% in 1990.[2] The addition of maintenance immunosuppression is credited with the largest improvement.[41] Further improvements since 1990 have not been appreciated.

The risk factors for progressive chronic kidney disease in SLE are well defined[21–23,51]:

- APOL1 risk alleles[54]
- Male sex
- Hypertension or nephrotic range proteinuria at time of diagnosis
- Antiphospholipid antibodies
- Proliferative LN
- High chronicity index on biopsy
- No response to treatment in the first 6 months
- Occurrence of nephritic renal flare

CONTROVERSIES
Weaning Immunosuppression

Evidence guiding discontinuation of immunosuppression after complete response is lacking. A study on withdrawing MMF in patients with quiescent adult SLE is underway (ClinicalTrials.gov NCT01946880). Many centers prioritize weaning steroids before other immunosuppression. Unless contraindicated, hydroxychloroquine is rarely discontinued.

Management of End-Stage Kidney Disease in Childhood-Onset Systemic Lupus Erythematosus

The mortality rate on dialysis (22% at 5 years) is similar to that reported for other causes of ESKD[55] regardless of dialysis modality. Because of concerns for peritonitis in chronic peritoneal dialysis patients on immunosuppression, some centers prefer hemodialysis. Because of the thrombosis risk, peritoneal dialysis may be preferable in patients with antiphospholipid antibodies. Survival is better for those taking prednisone and hydroxychloroquine than corticosteroids alone and worse for patients off immunosuppression.[56]

Management of Patients with Childhood-Onset Systemic Lupus Erythematosus Post Kidney Transplantation

Graft survival and infection rates are comparable between transplantation patients with LN and ESKD from other causes.[55,57] However, mortality from SLE with ESKD is double among the black versus white race.[55] Persistent antiphospholipid antibodies present a risk for early graft failure, not reduced by anticoagulation.[58] Markers of disease activity (complement C3 and C4, double-stranded–DNA antibodies) are less accurate after the transplant. Although glomerular immune complex deposition is common, recurrent LN is rare. Graft failures from rejection are far more common than from recurrent LN.[57]

SUMMARY

LN is a common cause of hypocomplementemic glomerulonephritis that warrants aggressive therapy with immunosuppression. Variability in cause and pathogenic mechanisms is reflected in several classes of kidney involvement. Kidney biopsy remains the diagnostic test of choice for guiding therapy. Frequent monitoring is required to assess the therapeutic response, flare, and disease damage.

ACKNOWLEDGMENTS

The authors would like to thank Karen Prince (graphics designer, Department of Pathology, Texas Children's Hospital) for the artwork included in Figures **1** and **2**.

REFERENCES

1. Silva CA, Avcin T, Brunner HI. Taxonomy for systemic lupus erythematosus with onset before adulthood. Arthritis Care Res 2012;64:1787–93.
2. Wenderfer SE, Ruth NM, Brunner HI. Advances in the care of children with lupus nephritis. Pediatr Res 2016;81:406–14.
3. Stojan G, Petri M. Epidemiology of systemic lupus erythematosus: an update. Curr Opin Rheumatol 2018;30:144–50.
4. Hiraki LT, Feldman CH, Liu J, et al. Prevalence, incidence, and demographics of systemic lupus erythematosus and lupus nephritis from 2000 to 2004 among children in the US Medicaid beneficiary population. Arthritis Rheum 2012;64: 2669–76.
5. Ambrose N, Morgan TA, Galloway J, et al. Differences in disease phenotype and severity in SLE across age groups. Lupus 2016;25:1542–50.
6. Dagna L, Frontino G, Praderio L. Rheumatoid arthritis, systemic lupus erythematosus, and STAT4. N Engl J Med 2007;357:2517–8 [author reply: 8].
7. Remmers EF, Plenge RM, Lee AT, et al. STAT4 and the risk of rheumatoid arthritis and systemic lupus erythematosus. N Engl J Med 2007;357:977–86.
8. Hom G, Graham RR, Modrek B, et al. Association of systemic lupus erythematosus with C8orf13-BLK and ITGAM-ITGAX. N Engl J Med 2008;358: 900–9.
9. Yuan J, Zhao D, Wu L, et al. FCGR3B copy number loss rather than gain is a risk factor for systemic lupus erythematous and lupus nephritis: a meta-analysis. Int J Rheum Dis 2015;18:392–7.
10. So HC, Gui AH, Cherny SS, et al. Evaluating the heritability explained by known susceptibility variants: a survey of ten complex diseases. Genet Epidemiol 2011; 35:310–7.
11. Tsokos GC. Systemic lupus erythematosus. N Engl J Med 2011;365:2110–21.
12. Arbuckle MR, McClain MT, Rubertone MV, et al. Development of autoantibodies before the clinical onset of systemic lupus erythematosus. N Engl J Med 2003; 349:1526–33.
13. Steri M, Orru V, Idda ML, et al. Overexpression of the cytokine BAFF and autoimmunity risk. N Engl J Med 2017;376:1615–26.
14. Kaveri SV, Mouthon L, Bayry J. Basophils and nephritis in lupus. N Engl J Med 2010;363:1080–2.
15. Moroni G, Trendelenburg M, Del Papa N, et al. Anti-C1q antibodies may help in diagnosing a renal flare in lupus nephritis. Am J Kidney Dis 2001;37: 490–8.
16. Trouw LA, Groeneveld TW, Seelen MA, et al. Anti-C1q autoantibodies deposit in glomeruli but are only pathogenic in combination with glomerular C1q-containing immune complexes. J Clin Invest 2004;114:679–88.
17. Bajema IM, Wilhelmus S, Alpers CE, et al. Revision of the International Society of Nephrology/Renal Pathology Society classification for lupus nephritis: clarification of definitions, and modified National Institutes of Health activity and chronicity indices. Kidney Int Suppl 2018;93(4):789–96.
18. Boneparth A, Ilowite N. Comparison of renal response parameters for juvenile membranous plus proliferative lupus nephritis versus isolated proliferative lupus nephritis: a cross-sectional analysis of the CARRA Registry. Lupus 2014;23: 898–904.
19. Hagelberg S, Lee Y, Bargman J, et al. Longterm followup of childhood lupus nephritis. J Rheumatol 2002;29:2635–42.

20. Zappitelli M, Duffy C, Bernard C, et al. Clinicopathological study of the WHO classification in childhood lupus nephritis. Pediatr Nephrol 2004;19:503–10.

21. Marks SD, Sebire NJ, Pilkington C, et al. Clinicopathological correlations of paediatric lupus nephritis. Pediatr Nephrol 2007;22:77–83.

22. Rianthavorn P, Buddhasri A. Long-term renal outcomes of childhood-onset global and segmental diffuse proliferative lupus nephritis. Pediatr Nephrol 2015;30:1969–76.

23. Lee BS, Cho HY, Kim EJ, et al. Clinical outcomes of childhood lupus nephritis: a single center's experience. Pediatr Nephrol 2007;22:222–31.

24. Zappitelli M, Duffy CM, Bernard C, et al. Evaluation of activity, chronicity and tubulointerstitial indices for childhood lupus nephritis. Pediatr Nephrol 2008;23:83–91.

25. Brunner HI, Bennett M, Abulaban K, et al. Development of a novel renal activity index of lupus nephritis in children & young adults. Arthritis Care Res 2016;68:1003–11.

26. Anders HJ, Weening JJ. Kidney disease in lupus is not always 'lupus nephritis. Arthritis Res Ther 2013;15:108.

27. Giannakopoulos B, Krilis SA. The pathogenesis of the antiphospholipid syndrome. N Engl J Med 2013;368:1033–44.

28. Hu W, Chen Y, Wang S, et al. Clinical–morphological features and outcomes of lupus podocytopathy. Clin J Am Soc Nephrol 2016;11:585–92.

29. Austin HA 3rd, Klippel JH, Balow JE, et al. Therapy of lupus nephritis. Controlled trial of prednisone and cytotoxic drugs. N Engl J Med 1986;314:614–9.

30. Houssiau FA, Vasconcelos C, D'Cruz D, et al. The 10-year follow-up data of the Euro-Lupus Nephritis Trial comparing low-dose and high-dose intravenous cyclophosphamide. Ann Rheum Dis 2010;69:61–4.

31. Appel GB, Contreras G, Dooley MA, et al. Mycophenolate mofetil versus cyclophosphamide for induction treatment of lupus nephritis. J Am Soc Nephrol 2009;20:1103–12.

32. Lau KK, Ault BH, Jones DP, et al. Induction therapy for pediatric focal proliferative lupus nephritis: cyclophosphamide versus mycophenolate mofetil. J Pediatr Health Care 2008;22:282–8.

33. Buratti S, Szer IS, Spencer CH, et al. Mycophenolate mofetil treatment of severe renal disease in pediatric onset systemic lupus erythematosus. J Rheumatol 2001;28:2103–8.

34. Liu Z, Zhang H, Liu Z, et al. Multitarget therapy for induction treatment of lupus nephritis: a randomized, controlled trial. Ann Intern Med 2015;162:18–26.

35. Fu LW, Yang LY, Chen WP, et al. Clinical efficacy of cyclosporin a neoral in the treatment of paediatric lupus nephritis with heavy proteinuria. Br J Rheumatol 1998;37:217–21.

36. Chen W, Tang X, Liu Q, et al. Short-term outcomes of induction therapy with tacrolimus versus cyclophosphamide for active lupus nephritis: a multicenter randomized clinical trial. Am J Kidney Dis 2011;57:235–44.

37. Mina R, von Scheven E, Ardoin SP, et al. Consensus treatment plans for induction therapy of newly diagnosed proliferative lupus nephritis in juvenile systemic lupus erythematosus. Arthritis Care Res 2012;64:375–83.

38. Contreras G, Pardo V, Leclercq B, et al. Sequential therapies for proliferative lupus nephritis. N Engl J Med 2004;350:971–80.

39. Kizawa T, Nozawa T, Kikuchi M, et al. Mycophenolate mofetil as maintenance therapy for childhood-onset systemic lupus erythematosus patients with severe lupus nephritis. Mod Rheumatol 2014;25:210–4.

40. Tamirou F, D'Cruz D, Sangle S, et al. Long-term follow-up of the MAINTAIN Nephritis Trial, comparing azathioprine and mycophenolate mofetil as maintenance therapy of lupus nephritis. Ann Rheum Dis 2015;75:526–31.

41. Pereira T, Abitbol CL, Seeherunvong W, et al. Three decades of progress in treating childhood-onset lupus nephritis. Clin J Am Soc Nephrol 2011;6:2192–9.

42. Fessler BJ, Alarcon GS, McGwin G Jr, et al. Systemic lupus erythematosus in three ethnic groups: XVI. Association of hydroxychloroquine use with reduced risk of damage accrual. Arthritis Rheum 2005;52:1473–80.

43. Tse KC, Li FK, Tang S, et al. Angiotensin inhibition or blockade for the treatment of patients with quiescent lupus nephritis and persistent proteinuria. Lupus 2005;14:947–52.

44. Watson L, Beresford MW, Maynes C, et al. The indications, efficacy and adverse events of rituximab in a large cohort of patients with juvenile-onset SLE. Lupus 2015;24:10–7.

45. Tambralli A, Beukelman T, Cron RQ, et al. Safety and efficacy of rituximab in childhood-onset systemic lupus erythematosus and other rheumatic diseases. J Rheumatol 2015;42:541–6.

46. Kidney Disease: Improving Global Outcomes (KDIGO) Glomerulonephritis Work Group t. KDIGO clinical practice guideline for glomerulonephritis. Kidney Inter Suppl 2012;2:221–32.

47. Swan JT, Riche DM, Riche KD, et al. Systematic review and meta-analysis of immunosuppressant therapy clinical trials in membranous lupus nephritis. J Investig Med 2011;59:246–58.

48. Hugle B, Silverman E, Tyrrell P, et al. Presentation and outcome of paediatric membranous non-proliferative lupus nephritis. Pediatr Nephrol 2014;30:113–21.

49. Pereira M, Muscal E, Eldin K, et al. Clinical presentation and outcomes of childhood-onset membranous lupus nephritis. Pediatr Nephrol 2017;32:2283–91.

50. Donadio JV Jr, Burgess JH, Holley KE. Membranous lupus nephropathy: a clinicopathologic study. Medicine (Baltimore) 1977;56:527–36.

51. Gibson KL, Gipson DS, Massengill SA, et al. Predictors of relapse and end stage kidney disease in proliferative lupus nephritis: focus on children, adolescents, and young adults. Clin J Am Soc Nephrol 2009;4:1962–7.

52. Aragon E, Resontoc LP, Chan YH, et al. Long-term outcomes with multi-targeted immunosuppressive protocol in children with severe proliferative lupus nephritis. Lupus 2016;25:399–406.

53. Sozeri B, Deveci M, Dincel N, et al. The early cardiovascular changes in pediatric patients with systemic lupus erythematosus. Pediatr Nephrol 2013;28(3):471–6.

54. Freedman BI, Langefeld CD, Andringa KK, et al. End-stage kidney disease in African Americans with lupus nephritis associates with APOL1. Arthritis Rheum 2014;66:390–6.

55. Hiraki LT, Lu B, Alexander SR, et al. End-stage renal disease due to lupus nephritis among children in the US, 1995-2006. Arthritis Rheum 2011;63:1988–97.

56. Broder A, Khattri S, Patel R, et al. Undertreatment of disease activity in systemic lupus erythematosus patients with end stage renal failure is associated with increased all-cause mortality. J Rheumatol 2011;38:2382–9.

57. Bartosh SM, Fine RN, Sullivan EK. Outcome after transplantation of young patients with systemic lupus erythematosus: a report of the North American pediatric renal transplant cooperative study. Transplantation 2001;72:973–8.

58. Vaidya S. Ten-yr renal allograft survival of patients with antiphospholipid antibody syndrome. Clin Transplant 2012;26:853–6.

Immunoglobulin A Nephropathy and Immunoglobulin A Vasculitis

Oana Nicoara, MD, Katherine Twombley, MD*

KEYWORDS

- Henoch- Schönlein purpura nephritis (HSPN)
- Immunoglobulin A (IgA) nephropathy (IgAN)
- Immunoglobulin A vasculitis (IgAV) or anaphylactoid purpura nephropathy

KEY POINTS

- Immunoglobulin (Ig)A nephropathy and IgA vasculitis share many similarities.
- Monitoring for renal disease is crucial.
- Patients with renal symptoms need referral to pediatric nephrology.

CAUSE, EPIDEMIOLOGY, AND PATHOGENESIS

Henoch-Schönlein purpura (HSP) nephritis (HSPN), sometimes referred to as immunoglobulin (Ig)A vasculitis (IgAV) or anaphylactoid purpura nephropathy, and IgA nephropathy (IgAN) are 2 common glomerulopathies in the pediatric population that are thought to be related for several reasons: both have been described consecutively in the same patient[1] and in identical twins,[2] and both have similar pathologic and biological abnormalities.[3] Yet there are also some unique differences. What is truly interesting is that HSP is typically a self-resolving vasculitis but its prognosis depends on the extent of renal involvement. A useful review of this topic outlining the major similarities and differences was published by Davin and colleagues,[4] and the major ones are highlighted in **Table 1**.

Both HSPN and IgAN result from the glomerular deposition of an abnormally glycosylated IgA1 with resulting mesangial proliferative changes; however, just having elevated abnormally glycosylated IgA1 is not enough to cause nephritis. In fact, Kiryluk and colleagues[5] showed that children with IgAN or HSPN frequently have a parent with a similar

O. Nicoara, no conflicts of interest; K. Twombley, grant funding from: Alexion, Novartis, Kaneka Pharma of America, Takeda Pharmaceuticals, Arbor Pharmaceuticals, LLC.
Department of Pediatrics, Medical University of South Carolina, 96 Jonathan Lucas Street, 428 CSB, MSC 608, Charleston, SC 29425, USA
* Corresponding author.
E-mail address: twombley@musc.edu

Table 1
Similarities and differences in immunoglobulin-A nephropathy and Henoch-Schönlein purpura nephritis

	HSPN	IgAN
Description	Most common vasculitis in children[5]	Most common form of chronic glomerulonephritis[6]
Peak age or sex	<15 y or male	15–30 y or male
Organ systems involved	Skin (palpable purpura), gastrointestinal, joints, renal (~40%), neurologic, pulmonary, urologic	Renal only
Pathophysiology	Large (>19 S) circulating IgA1 O-glycoform-containing immune complexes (IgA-IC) Higher IgG content Greater incidence of increased plasma IgE levels Small-vessel leukocytoclastic vasculitis Associated with hypersensitivity type 1	Small (7 S-19 S) IgA-CC Deposit only in the glomeruli
Presenting symptoms	Macro or microscopic hematuria associated with a purpuric rash, colicky pain, bloody stools, edema and arthralgia	Macroscopic hematuria at the same time of a respiratory infection
Nephrotic	+	+/−
Nephritic	+	+/−
Renal Pathology		
IgA mesangial deposition	+	+
Increased lambda or kappa	−	−
IgA along capillary walls	+	−
Crescents	+	+/−
Neutrophil infiltration	+	+/−
Subendothelial deposits	+	+/−

Abbreviation: S, secretory.

serum IgA1 O-glycoform profile but without kidney disease. This suggests that a second hit is needed to manifest renal disease **Fig. 1**. The mechanisms responsible for the differences in clinical presentation and symptoms among patients are poorly understood; however, possible mechanisms, including differences in the duration of production, amount, composition, and localization of IgA circulating immune complexes, as well as differences in the intensity of the local interactions between cells, are capably reviewed by Davin and Coppo.[6] Taking all of this into consideration, it is important to remember that measuring IgA levels is rarely useful in making these diagnoses and should only be done in consultation with a subspecialist.

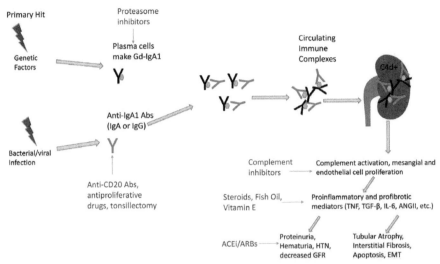

Fig. 1. Suggested pathogenesis of IgA-mediated renal disease (*thick yellow arrows*) and potential treatment targets (*thin blue arrows*). ABS, antibodies; ACEi, angiotensin converting enzyme inhibitor; ANGII, angiotensin II; ARB, angiotensin II receptor blockers; CD20, cluster of differention 20; EMT, epithelial-mesenchymal transition; gd, glycosalated; GFR, glomerular filtration rate; HTN, hypertension; IL-6, interleukin-6; TGF, transforming growth factor-beta; TNF, tumor necrosis factor.

Familial clustering, ethnic differences, and regional discrepancies suggest a genetic component to IgAN. Genome-wide association studies (GWASs) have identified several susceptibility genes and loci that have been associated with IgAN, including pathways involving the major histocompatibility complex, complement system, mucosal innate immunity, and mucosal IgA production regulation. Not only are some of these pathways implicated in immune regulation but also they are shared with other autoimmune diseases such as lupus erythematosus, rheumatoid arthritis, and multiple sclerosis. Zhang and colleagues[7] recently published a detailed review of these GWASs and the role of the immune function in IgAN. Although there are investigations taking place on the genotypic and phenotypic correlations of IgA, this work is in the early stages. Future work will likely focus on predictive or prognostic genetic factors as well as on potential targets for therapy.

DIAGNOSIS

HSP is a cutaneous small-vessel vasculitis (also known as leukocytoclastic vasculitis) and the hallmark lesion that should clue a practitioner into making the clinical diagnosis is the palpable purpura that predominate on the ankles and lower legs (ie, dependent areas). It can have other concurrent clinical manifestations such as arthritis, abdominal pain, pancreatitis, nephritis, pulmonary involvement, and neurologic involvement. HSPN is a clinical diagnosis, whereas IgAN is a pathologic diagnosis. HSPN tends to present as acute glomerular inflammatory lesions, whereas IgAN tends to develop slow but progressive mesangial lesions.[6] The Oxford Classification of IgAN originally included 4 parameters called the MEST scores: mesangial hypercellularity (M), segmental glomerulosclerosis (S), tubular atrophy or interstitial fibrosis (T), and endocapillary hypercellularity (E).[8,9] Crescents were not included in the original classification because they were not found to be an independent predictor of renal outcomes. Unfortunately, subjects with a glomerular filtration rate (GFR) of less than 30 mL/min per 1.73 m^2 were excluded from these studies.[10–13] When further analysis was done to include subjects with severe renal impairment, crescents were found to be potential predictors of renal outcomes.[8,14,15] More recently, in 2017, the Oxford classification was updated to MEST-C score, with the C representing crescents.[16] It is currently only recommended for use in IgAN; however, some investigators have begun to also look at the validity of the Oxford scores in HSPN.[17] The most updated information on the Oxford classification and the relevant studies validating this work can be found in a useful review by Trimarchi and colleagues.[16] Both of these disorders typically present at the same time or within a few days of an upper respiratory infection. This is a distinct difference from postinfectious glomerulonephritis, which presents at least 7 days after.

NATURAL HISTORY

IgAN typically presents as a slowly progressive disease in children but is known to progress to end-stage renal disease (ESRD). Yoshikawa and colleagues[18] showed that 10% of children with IgAN had ESRD 20 years after diagnosis; however, Wyatt and colleagues[19] showed that the predicted kidney survival from the time of apparent disease onset was only 70% at 20 years. HSP is typically a self-limiting vasculitis but the prognosis is worse when patients develop renal symptoms. As many as 20% of children can progress to ESRD 20 years after diagnosis.[20] According to the most recent United States Renal Data System report, 2.5% of the pediatric ESRD population is children with either IgAN or HSPN.[21]

Because both diseases can have variable outcomes, considerable attention has been focused on defining the predictors of outcomes so practitioners can provide more targeted treatments. Some have focused on clinical predictors such as blood pressure (BP), proteinuria, and GFR, whereas others have focused on the pathologic predictors. The most promising work has been the combination of clinical and pathologic predictors as was done in the VALIGA study.[15] The VALIGA (Validation of the Oxford classification of IgA nephropathy) study showed that when M, S, and T scores are evaluated in combination with known clinical variables, the ability to predict renal outcomes was significantly increased. The addition of C to the Oxford classification has also proved to be a valuable clinical predictive tool, and greater than 25% crescents have been shown to be associated with poorer renal outcomes.[22] Most of the IgAN work has been done is adult patients; however, a recent review by Rosanna Coppo[23] details what is known about these predictors in pediatric IgAN patients. More is known about pediatric HSPN and a review by Martin Pohl[24] reviews these data.

There are no accepted guidelines on recommended follow-up or screening for children who develop HSP with minimal or no renal involvement; however, it is clear that they warrant some type of close monitoring.[25] The authors have developed a pathway for suggested primary care follow-up called the rule of 4 (**Fig. 2**). If there is a normal BP, no significant proteinuria (negative first morning dip or protein/creatinine ratio <0.2), and only microscopic hematuria, the patient can be checked weekly for 4 weeks, then every 2 weeks for 4 checks, then once in 4 months, and then yearly.

There is a definite need to answer many questions about IgAN and HSPN. Cure Glomerulonephropathy (CureGN) is a multicenter study. The National Institute of Diabetes and Digestive and Kidney Diseases (NIDDK)-funded consortium is working collaboratively to address these challenges by recruiting a large cohort of subjects, including those with IgAN and HSPN, and following them prospectively. This study has the potential to address this and many more questions surrounding all aspects of these diseases. There is still a lot that is not known regarding the pathogenesis of

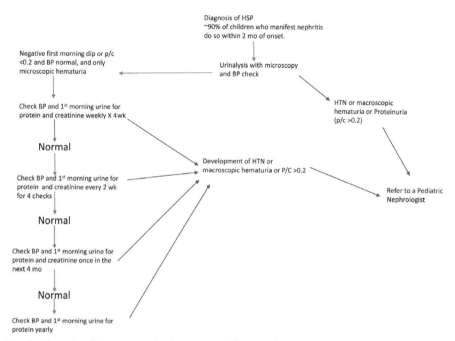

Diagnosis of HSP
~90% of children who manifest nephritis
do so within 2 mo of onset.

Urinalysis with microscopy
and BP check

Negative first morning dip or p/c
<0.2 and BP normal, and only
microscopic hematuria

Check BP and 1st morning urine for
protein and creatinine weekly X 4 wk

Normal

Check BP and 1st morning urine for
protein and creatinine every 2 wk
for 4 checks

Normal

Check BP and 1st morning urine for
protein and creatinine once in the
next 4 mo

Normal

Check BP and 1st morning urine for
protein yearly

HTN or macroscopic
hematuria or Proteinuria
(p/c >0.2)

Development of HTN or
macroscopic hematuria or P/C >0.2

Refer to a Pediatric
Nephrologist

Fig. 2. The rule of 4: suggested primary care follow-up for children with HSPN. p/c, protein/creatinine ratio.

IgAN and HSPN that will undoubtedly change how the diagnosis and treatment is approached in the future. Within IgAN and HSPN, there are wide variations in presentations and outcomes, suggesting the potential need for different treatments based on the class of the disease. More recently, efforts have focused on the genetic and epigenetic factors that play a part in the pathogenesis of these diseases. These exciting developments have and will continue to lead to a better understanding of the underlying pathways that can help differentiate distinct disease subtypes and, it is hoped, lead to the ultimate goal of patient-specific treatments.

TREATMENT

The Kidney Disease Improving Global Outcomes (KDIGO) working group on glomerulonephritis compiled the first evidence-based guidelines for the treatment of IgAN and HSPN[26] but it should be noted that the evidence for these guidelines closed in 2011. These treatment guidelines are based on the severity of disease and both IgAN and HSPN are treated the same. **Fig. 3** outlines the guidelines and the authors have taken the liberty to add what they think are reasonable proteinuria targets for children. There is still debate on the ideal urine protein target in children and some would argue that the target should be less than 0.5 g/d/1.73 m². Furthermore, goals for BP management in adults are given but no BP goals are specified for children. Both of these are areas that require further clarification in future trials.

Second-line treatment per KDIGO guidelines in children who have a GFR of greater than 50 mL/min/1.7 3m² is the addition of corticosteroids. Not all patients respond to corticosteroids and they have many potential dangerous side effects. In fact, the Therapeutic Evaluation of Steroids in IgA Nephropathy Global (TESTING) study was a multi-center, double-blind, randomized clinical trial that was subject to early termination

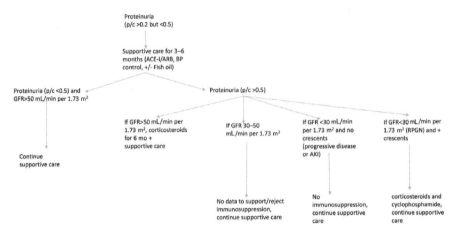

Fig. 3. Modified KDIGO guidelines for pediatric IgAN or HSPN. ACE, angiotensin converting enzyme inhibitor; AKI, acute kidney injury; ARB, angiotensin II receptor blocker; BP, blood pressure; p/c, protein/creatinine ratio; RPGN, rapidly progressive glomerulonephritis. (*From* Coppo R, Troyanov S, Bellur S, et al. Validation of the Oxford classification of IgA nephropathy in cohorts with different presentations and treatments. Kidney Int 2014;86(4):828–36; with permission.)

secondary to the high incidence of infections.[27] The STOP-IgAN (Supportive Versus Immunosuppressive Therapy of Progressive IgA Nephropathy) Trial was another more recent trial that compared supportive care or additional immunosuppression (GFR $\geq$60 mL/min per 1.73 m^2: 6-month corticosteroid monotherapy; GFR = 30–59 mL/min per 1.73 m^2: cyclophosphamide for 3 months followed by azathioprine plus oral prednisolone). Corticosteroid monotherapy induced disease remission in only a few patients but neither of the immunosuppressive regimens was able to prevent GFR loss. Again, both immunosuppressive groups were associated with substantial adverse events.[28] Other, more potent immunosuppressive agents are not recommended unless there is crescentic IgAN or HSPN as evidenced by more than 50% of the glomeruli being involved with rapidly deteriorating kidney function. In this situation, cyclophosphamide and corticosteroids are recommended. Because children have more naïve immune systems than adults, this is of particular concern and practitioners should be vigilant in monitoring for infections when treating with immunosuppression, especially in children. Future studies should consider examining infection prophylaxis.

Not only have corticosteroids been used to treat disease but there has been some controversy about using corticosteroids with HSP to prevent HSPN. Although earlier studies showed some benefit of corticosteroids in preventing disease[29–32] these studies were small and poorly designed. More recent randomized controlled trials have not shown this benefit.[33–36] Currently, corticosteroids are not recommended to prevent the development of renal disease in IgA or HSPN.

Another second-line treatment option that KDIGO recommends is fish oil because it was found to suppress interleukin-6–induced abnormal IgA production and deposition of IgA immune complexes in the mesangial region of the kidneys.[37,38] Although the initial evidence involving fish oil was conflicting,[39–42] a meta-analysis by Chou and colleagues[43] reviews the more recent clinical data available on fish oil quite satisfactorily. Considering the low-risk profile of fish oil and the potential added benefits on the cardiovascular system, such as lowering lipid levels and BP, it is typically started early in the disease process. **Fig. 1** and **Table 2** highlight some other potential targets for treatment, including vitamin E,[44] rituximab,[45–47] and tonsillectomy.[48,49]

Table 2 Alternatives to treatment			
Treatment	Pro	Con	Recommendation
Tonsillectomy	1. Reduce the number of infective events in the upper airways, therefore reducing the lymphatic tissue production of glycosylated-IgA1	1. Hard to draw conclusions because (1) patients received other immunosuppression such as steroids, (2) patients received renin angiotensin system-blocking drugs, (3) most studies were retrospective	Routine tonsillectomy is not indicated in IgAN per KDIGO
Vitamin E	1. Decreased proteinuria by decreasing transforming growth factor-beta1	No long-term trials	No formal recommendations
Fish oil rich in w-3 polyunsaturated fatty acids	1. Suppress interleukin -6–induced abnormal IgA production and deposition of IgA immune complexes in the mesangial region 2. Cardiovascular benefits	No long-term trials	Recommend

There is much left to be learned about both of these diseases. Continued research is critical to define better treatments with the goal of better long-term outcomes. Until that time, it is imperative that primary care providers accurately and promptly diagnose children with renal involvement and refer them to a pediatric nephrologist.

REFERENCES

1. Ravelli A, Carnevale-Maffe G, Ruperto N, et al. IgA nephropathy and Henoch-Schonlein syndrome occurring in the same patient. Nephron 1996;72(1):111–2.
2. Meadow SR, Scott DG. Berger disease: Henoch-Schonlein syndrome without the rash. J Pediatr 1985;106(1):27–32.
3. Knight JF. The rheumatic poison: a survey of some published investigations of the immunopathogenesis of Henoch-Schonlein purpura. Pediatr Nephrol 1990;4(5): 533–41.
4. Davin JC, Ten Berge IJ, Weening JJ. What is the difference between IgA nephropathy and Henoch-Schonlein purpura nephritis? Kidney Int 2001;59(3): 823–34.
5. Kiryluk K, Moldoveanu Z, Sanders JT, et al. Aberrant glycosylation of IgA1 is inherited in both pediatric IgA nephropathy and Henoch-Schonlein purpura nephritis. Kidney Int 2011;80(1):79–87.
6. Davin JC, Coppo R. Henoch-Schonlein purpura nephritis in children. Nat Rev Nephrol 2014;10(10):563–73.
7. Zhang YM, Zhou XJ, Zhang H. What genetics tells us about the pathogenesis of IgA nephropathy: the role of immune factors and infection. Kidney Int Rep 2017; 2(3):318–31.

8. Working Group of the International Ig ANN, the Renal Pathology Society, Cattran DC, Coppo R, Cook HT, et al. The Oxford classification of IgA nephropathy: rationale, clinicopathological correlations, and classification. Kidney Int 2009;76(5):534–45.

9. Working Group of the International Ig ANN, the Renal Pathology Society, Roberts IS, Cook HT, Troyanov S, et al. The Oxford classification of IgA nephropathy: pathology definitions, correlations, and reproducibility. Kidney Int 2009; 76(5):546–56.

10. Herzenberg AM, Fogo AB, Reich HN, et al. Validation of the Oxford classification of IgA nephropathy. Kidney Int 2011;80(3):310–7.

11. Shi SF, Wang SX, Jiang L, et al. Pathologic predictors of renal outcome and therapeutic efficacy in IgA nephropathy: validation of the oxford classification. Clin J Am Soc Nephrol 2011;6(9):2175–84.

12. Le W, Zeng CH, Liu Z, et al. Validation of the Oxford classification of IgA nephropathy for pediatric patients from China. BMC Nephrol 2012;13:158.

13. Lee H, Yi SH, Seo MS, et al. Validation of the Oxford classification of IgA nephropathy: a single-center study in Korean adults. Korean J Intern Med 2012;27(3): 293–300.

14. Working Group of the International Ig ANN, the Renal Pathology Society, Coppo R, Troyanov S, Camilla R, et al. The Oxford IgA nephropathy clinicopathological classification is valid for children as well as adults. Kidney Int 2010; 77(10):921–7.

15. Coppo R, Troyanov S, Bellur S, et al. Validation of the Oxford classification of IgA nephropathy in cohorts with different presentations and treatments. Kidney Int 2014;86(4):828–36.

16. Trimarchi H, Barratt J, Cattran DC, et al. Oxford Classification of IgA nephropathy 2016: an update from the IgA Nephropathy Classification Working Group. Kidney Int 2017;91(5):1014–21.

17. Xu K, Zhang L, Ding J, et al. Value of the Oxford classification of IgA nephropathy in children with Henoch-Schonlein purpura nephritis. J Nephrol 2018;31(2): 279–86.

18. Yoshikawa N, Ito H, Nakamura H. IgAN nephropathy in children from Japan. Child Nephrol Urol 1989;9:191–9.

19. Wyatt RJ, Kritchevsky SB, Woodford SY, et al. IgA nephropathy: long-term prognosis for pediatric patients. J Pediatr 1995;127(6):913–9.

20. White RHR, Yoshikawa N. Henoch- Schonlein nephritis. In: Barratt TM, Holiday M, editors. Pediatric nephrology. Baltimore (MD): Williams & Wilkins; 1993. p. 729–38.

21. United States Renal Data System. 2017 USRDS annual data report: epidemiology of kidney disease in the United States. Bethesda (MD): National Institutes of Health, National Institute of Diabetes and Digestive and Kidney Diseases; 2017. The data reported here have been supplied by the United States Renal Data System. The interpretation and reporting of these data are the responsibility of the authors and in no way should be seen as an official policy or interpretation of the US government.

22. Haas M, Verhave JC, Liu ZH, et al. A multicenter study of the predictive value of crescents in IgA nephropathy. J Am Soc Nephrol 2017;28(2):691–701.

23. Coppo R. Clinical and histological risk factors for progression of IgA nephropathy: an update in children, young and adult patients. J Nephrol 2017;30(3): 339–46.

24. Pohl M. Henoch-Schonlein purpura nephritis. Pediatr Nephrol 2015;30(2):245–52.

25. Narchi H. Risk of long term renal impairment and duration of follow up recommended for Henoch-Schonlein purpura with normal or minimal urinary findings: a systematic review. Arch Dis Child 2005;90(9):916–20.

26. Kidney Disease: Improving Global Outcomes (KDIGO) Glomerulonephritis Work Group. KDIGO clinical practice guideline for glomerulonephritis. Kidney Int Suppl 2012;2(2):139–274.

27. Lv J, Zhang H, Wong MG, et al. Effect of oral methylprednisolone on clinical outcomes in patients with IgA nephropathy: the TESTING randomized clinical trial. JAMA 2017;318(5):432–42.

28. Rauen T, Fitzner C, Eitner F, et al. Effects of two immunosuppressive treatment protocols for IgA nephropathy. J Am Soc Nephrol 2018;29(1):317–25.

29. Mollica F, Li Volti S, Garozzo R, et al. Effectiveness of early prednisone treatment in preventing the development of nephropathy in anaphylactoid purpura. Eur J Pediatr 1992;151(2):140–4.

30. Huber AM, King J, McLaine P, et al. A randomized, placebo-controlled trial of prednisone in early Henoch Schonlein Purpura [ISRCTN85109383]. BMC Med 2004;2:7.

31. Ronkainen J, Koskimies O, Ala-Houhala M, et al. Early prednisone therapy in Henoch-Schonlein purpura: a randomized, double-blind, placebo-controlled trial. J Pediatr 2006;149(2):241–7.

32. Weiss PF, Klink AJ, Localio R, et al. Corticosteroids may improve clinical outcomes during hospitalization for Henoch-Schonlein purpura. Pediatrics 2010; 126(4):674–81.

33. Chartapisak W, Opastiraku S, Willis NS, et al. Prevention and treatment of renal disease in Henoch-Schonlein purpura: a systematic review. Arch Dis Child 2009;94(2):132–7.

34. Jauhola O, Ronkainen J, Koskimies O, et al. Outcome of Henoch-Schonlein purpura 8 years after treatment with a placebo or prednisone at disease onset. Pediatr Nephrol 2012;27(6):933–9.

35. Jauhola O, Ronkainen J, Koskimies O, et al. Renal manifestations of Henoch-Schonlein purpura in a 6-month prospective study of 223 children. Arch Dis Child 2010;95(11):877–82.

36. Dudley J, Smith G, Llewelyn-Edwards A, et al. Randomised, double-blind, placebo-controlled trial to determine whether steroids reduce the incidence and severity of nephropathy in Henoch-Schonlein Purpura (HSP). Arch Dis Child 2013;98(10):756–63.

37. Dong W, Sell JE, Pestka JJ. Quantitative assessment of mesangial immunoglobulin A (IgA) accumulation, elevated circulating IgA immune complexes, and hematuria during vomitoxin-induced IgA nephropathy. Fundam Appl Toxicol 1991; 17(1):197–207.

38. Pestka JJ, Zhou HR. Interleukin-6-deficient mice refractory to IgA dysregulation but not anorexia induction by vomitoxin (deoxynivalenol) ingestion. Food Chem Toxicol 2000;38(7):565–75.

39. Donadio JV Jr, Grande JP, Bergstralh EJ, et al. The long-term outcome of patients with IgA nephropathy treated with fish oil in a controlled trial. Mayo Nephrology Collaborative Group. J Am Soc Nephrol 1999;10(8):1772–7.

40. Ferraro PM, Ferraccioli GF, Gambaro G, et al. Combined treatment with renin-angiotensin system blockers and polyunsaturated fatty acids in proteinuric IgA nephropathy: a randomized controlled trial. Nephrol Dial Transplant 2009;24(1): 156–60.

41. Bennett WM, Walker RG, Kincaid-Smith P. Treatment of IgA nephropathy with eicosapentanoic acid (EPA): a two-year prospective trial. Clin Nephrol 1989;31(3): 128–31.
42. Pettersson EE, Rekola S, Berglund L, et al. Treatment of IgA nephropathy with omega-3-polyunsaturated fatty acids: a prospective, double-blind, randomized study. Clin Nephrol 1994;41(4):183–90.
43. Chou HH, Chiou YY, Hung PH, et al. Omega-3 fatty acids ameliorate proteinuria but not renal function in IgA nephropathy: a meta-analysis of randomized controlled trials. Nephron Clin Pract 2012;121(1–2):c30–5.
44. Trachtman H, Chan JC, Chan W, et al. Vitamin E ameliorates renal injury in an experimental model of immunoglobulin A nephropathy. Pediatr Res 1996;40(4): 620–6.
45. Floege J. Glomerular disease: rituximab therapy for IgA nephropathy. Nat Rev Nephrol 2017;13(3):138–40.
46. Lafayette RA, Canetta PA, Rovin BH, et al. A randomized, controlled trial of rituximab in IgA nephropathy with proteinuria and renal dysfunction. J Am Soc Nephrol 2017;28(4):1306–13.
47. Lundberg S, Westergren E, Smolander J, et al. B cell-depleting therapy with rituximab or ofatumumab in immunoglobulin A nephropathy or vasculitis with nephritis. Clin Kidney J 2017;10(1):20–6.
48. Feehally J, Coppo R, Troyanov S, et al. Tonsillectomy in a European cohort of 1,147 patients with IgA nephropathy. Nephron 2016;132(1):15–24.
49. Birk PE. Surveillance biopsies in children post-kidney transplant. Pediatr Nephrol 2012;27(5):753–60.

Tubulointerstitial Nephritis

Rebecca L. Ruebner, MD, MSCE*, Jeffrey J. Fadrowski, MD, MHS

KEYWORDS

- Tubulointerstitial nephritis • Acute interstitial nephritis • Acute kidney injury
- Tubulointerstitial nephritis with uveitis

KEY POINTS

- Tubulointerstitial nephritis (TIN) is a cause of acute kidney injury characterized by an inflammatory cell infiltrate in the kidney interstitium.
- Common causes of TIN in children include medications, infections, rheumatologic diseases, inflammatory bowel disease, tubulointerstitial nephritis with uveitis, and genetic conditions.
- TIN typically presents with nonoliguric acute kidney injury due to impaired urinary concentrating ability. Systemic symptoms are common, including fever, rash, arthralgia, and flank pain.
- Urinalysis may show sterile pyuria, microscopic hematuria, and low-grade proteinuria; additional laboratory findings may include eosinophiluria, eosinophilia, elevated inflammatory markers, and anemia.
- The role of corticosteroids in managing children with TIN remains controversial; immunosuppressive therapy should be considered in patients with severe or prolonged disease.

DEFINITION

Tubulointerstitial nephritis (TIN) is a cause of acute kidney injury (AKI) that is characterized histologically by an inflammatory cell infiltrate in the kidney interstitium.[1] TIN accounts for 5% to 15% of cases of AKI in children and adults.[1,2] TIN may be associated with systemic symptoms, including the classic triad of fever, rash, and eosinophilia.[1,2] TIN can be caused by medications, infections, autoimmune disorders, and genetic conditions. The long-term prognosis is generally favorable with full kidney recovery but some patients with TIN may develop chronic kidney disease (CKD).[2]

CAUSES OF TUBULOINTERSTITIAL NEPHRITIS IN CHILDREN
Medications

Medications are the most common cause of TIN in adults and children.[3] Studies of TIN have reported that up to 90% of cases are medication-related.[1–5] The most commonly

Disclosure Statement: The authors have no disclosures to report.
Department of Pediatrics, Division of Nephrology, Johns Hopkins University School of Medicine, 200 North Wolfe Street, Room 3055, Baltimore, MD 21287, USA
* Corresponding author.
E-mail address: Rruebne1@jhmi.edu

Pediatr Clin N Am 66 (2019) 111–119
https://doi.org/10.1016/j.pcl.2018.08.009
pediatric.theclinics.com
0031-3955/19/© 2018 Elsevier Inc. All rights reserved.

associated medications include nonsteroidal antiinflammatory drugs (NSAIDs), antibiotics (eg, beta-lactam antibiotics, cephalosporins, sulfonamides), antivirals, antacids (proton pump inhibitors and H2 receptor antagonists), antiepileptics, and others (**Box 1**). Drug-induced TIN is thought to be an immune or allergic reaction in the kidney and can be associated with systemic signs of a hypersensitivity reaction, including fever, rash, arthritis, and eosinophilia.[6] NSAID-induced TIN may have fewer extrarenal symptoms compared with other medications.[6] TIN typically develops within a few weeks of exposure to a medication, with mean onset of symptoms of 10 days.[6] The severity of kidney injury is not necessarily dose-dependent, and the reaction may recur if there is reexposure to the same class of medications.[3,6]

Infections

Viral infections have been associated with TIN in children, including cytomegalovirus, Epstein-Barr virus, hepatitis, human immunodeficiency virus, and BK polyoma virus.[7–9] Bacterial infections that have been associated with TIN include brucellosis, campylobacter, legionella, salmonella, and streptococcus.[9,10] Other infectious causes include *Mycoplasma pneumoniae*, *Mycobacterium tuberculosis*, other mycobacterial infections, histoplasmosis, leptospirosis, candidiasis, and toxoplasmosis.[11,12] Although the pathogenesis of infection-associated TIN is not entirely clear, potential mechanisms include direct cytopathic effects by the organism or circulating immune complexes.[7,12]

Rheumatologic Diseases

Rheumatologic diseases such as systemic lupus erythematosus (SLE) are most commonly associated with glomerular disease in the kidney. However, TIN is also a common finding. TIN can occur in association with glomerular disease, and the degree of interstitial inflammation tends to correlate with the severity of the glomerular lesions.[13] However, TIN can be the predominant kidney finding in SLE without

---

Box 1
Drugs associated with tubulointerstitial nephritis

Analgesics

NSAIDs, selective cyclooxygenase-2 inhibitors

Antibiotics

Beta-lactams, cephalosporins, sulfonamides, fluoroquinolones, rifampin, doxycycline, erythromycin, vancomycin, minocycline, ethambutol, chloramphenicol, ciprofloxacin

Antivirals

Acyclovir, abacavir, indinavir

Antiepileptics

Phenytoin, carbamazepine, phenobarbital, lamotrigine, levetiracetam

Antacids

Proton pump inhibitors, histamine receptor antagonists

Other

Diuretics, allopurinol, cyclosporine, azathioprine, sulfasalazine

Adapted from Refs.[3,6,9]

significant glomerular involvement.[13,14] In patients with SLE, the degree of tubulointerstitial inflammation and interstitial fibrosis is an independent risk factor for long-term kidney prognosis.[13] TIN is also seen in patients with sarcoidosis, Sjögren syndrome, and granulomatosis with polyangiitis (GPA).[11,15–18]

Inflammatory Bowel Disease

Inflammatory bowel disease (IBD) is associated with several kidney abnormalities, including AKI, proteinuria, glomerulonephritis, nephrolithiasis, and CKD.[19,20] The most common histologic findings among patients with IBD undergoing kidney biopsy include IgA nephropathy and TIN.[19] Some cases of TIN in patients with IBD are related to exposure to aminosalicylates, which is thought to be a delayed-type hypersensitivity reaction independent of dose, similar to other forms of drug-induced TIN.[19] However, TIN has also been reported in patients with IBD before initiation of treatment with aminosalicylates, indicating that there may be an immune-mediated form of TIN unrelated to medication exposure in these patients.[19,21–25] TIN in patients with IBD can have a granulomatous pattern on kidney biopsy.[19,20]

Tubulointerstitial Nephritis and Uveitis Syndrome

TIN and uveitis (TINU) syndrome was first described in 1975 by Dobrin and colleagues[26] in 2 adolescent girls with interstitial nephritis and anterior uveitis. Since that time, TINU has become a well-recognized cause of TIN. TINU syndrome is most commonly seen among female patients, with median age of onset around 15 years.[27,28] The pathogenesis of TINU syndrome is unknown but seems to involve cell-mediated immunity.[28] TINU syndrome has been associated with certain HLA types, including HLA-A2, HLA-A24, HLA-DR4, HLA-DQA1, HLA-DQB1, and HLA-DRB1, although the role of these HLA antigens in the pathogenesis of TINU syndrome is unclear.[28,29] The combination of TIN and uveitis can also be seen in other conditions, including sarcoidosis, tuberculosis, IBD, SLE, and Sjögren syndrome.[18]

TINU syndrome can be associated with systemic symptoms, similar to other forms of TIN. These include fever, weight loss, fatigue, nausea, anorexia, flank pain, arthralgia, and myalgia. Rash is less common compared with other forms of TIN.[18,28] Laboratory findings may include elevated erythrocyte sedimentation rate (ESR), elevated immunoglobulin G (IgG), anemia, and eosinophilia. Urinalysis findings include dilute urine, pyuria, microscopic hematuria, low-grade proteinuria, aminoaciduria, and phosphaturia.[18] Kidney biopsy typically shows acute interstitial inflammation consisting of lymphocytes, plasma cells, and histiocytes. Eosinophils and neutrophils can also be present. Immunofluorescence is typically negative for immunoglobulins or complement. Noncaseating granulomas can be present.[18,28]

The uveitis associated with TINU syndrome is usually anterior, bilateral, and sudden in onset.[18,27,30] Uveitis can present at any time in relation to the kidney manifestations. Most commonly, the ocular manifestations occur after the onset of kidney disease, with a median onset of 1 month after TIN presentation, and most cases occurring within 6 months.[28] However, uveitis can also precede or occur concurrently with the kidney disease.[18,27,29,30] The clinical course of the uveitis is independent of the kidney disease.[28] The uveitis can have a chronic or relapsing-remitting course.[18,28,29] Uveitis can present with eye pain, redness, decreased visual acuity, or photophobia.[18,28] However, some patients have no ocular symptoms, so uveitis may be underdiagnosed.[29] Therefore, all patients with TIN of unknown cause should have an ophthalmologic examination at the time of diagnosis and again within approximately 6 months because the onset of uveitis may be delayed.

The role of immunosuppressive therapies in treating TINU syndrome is not well-understood. In a series of 26 children with TINU syndrome, 23 subjects were treated with oral corticosteroids for 4 to 7 weeks, followed by a tapering course. The remaining 3 subjects received intravenous corticosteroids due to rapidly rising creatinine. The median length of steroid treatment was 10 months. Most subjects had normalization of serum creatinine within a mean of 90 days, although 4 subjects did not have improvement in kidney function during follow-up.[29] Although the role for steroids in TINU syndrome is unclear, the uveitis should be treated with topical or systemic corticosteroids.[18] Refractory cases of uveitis may be treated with azathioprine, methotrexate, cyclosporine, or mycophenolate mofetil.[28]

Other Causes of Tubulointerstitial Nephritis in Children

Chronic environmental exposures have been associated with TIN, including heavy metals such as lead, cadmium, and mercury.[31] Exposure to aristolochic acid has been implicated in TIN related to traditional Chinese medicine herbs and Balkan endemic nephropathy, a condition found among residents of the Danube River plain in southeast Europe in which up to 5% of the population develops chronic TIN after living in the region for more than 15 years.[31,32]

IgG4-related TIN is a rare form of TIN. It is a multisystem disease associated with elevated serum IgG4 and tissue infiltration by IgG4. In addition to TIN, symptoms include pancreatitis, sclerosing cholangitis, sialadenitis, lymphadenopathy, retroperitoneal fibrosis, and interstitial pneumonitis. The disorder is more common in adults.[33,34]

TIN may also be secondary to a genetic mutation. TIN is seen with inherited diseases such as medullary cystic kidney disease and familial juvenile hyperuricemic nephropathy. Recently, the Kidney Disease: Improving Global Outcomes (KDIGO) group had a consensus conference and developed a new classification for inherited tubulointerstitial kidney diseases, now called autosomal dominant tubulointerstitial kidney disease (ADTKD).[35] ADTKD is characterized by an autosomal dominant pattern of inheritance, bland urinary sediment, nocturia or enuresis, absent or mild proteinuria, absence of severe hypertension, normal or small kidneys on kidney ultrasound, and no known drug exposures. These disorders are associated with progressive CKD, with renal replacement therapy often required by age 30 to 50 years.[35] Kidney biopsy may show tubulointerstitial inflammation, interstitial fibrosis, and tubular atrophy with negative immunofluorescence for complement or immunoglobulins.[35] Mutations of several genes have been associated with ADTKD including uromodulin (UMOD), renin (REN), hepatocyte nuclear factor (HNF1β), and mucin (MUC1), all of which are expressed in kidney tubular cells.[35–41] These genetic syndromes can be associated with extrarenal manifestations. For example, UMOD mutations are associated with hyperuricemia and gout.[35,37] HNF1β mutations can be associated with kidney cysts, kidney hypoplasia or agenesis, and maturity onset diabetes of youth type 5 (MODY5).[35,38,41] ADTKD should be suspected in a child with TIN which has a progressive course, particularly if there is a known family history of kidney disease or extrarenal findings suggestive of a genetic mutation.

PATHOGENESIS AND HISTOPATHOLOGY

TIN is characterized histologically by inflammation in the kidney interstitium. The inflammation is primarily related to cell-mediated immunity because immune deposits are rarely seen on kidney biopsy.[6,42] Drug-induced TIN is thought to be a delayed type hypersensitivity reaction mediated through T cells or, more rarely through humoral immunity.[3] Regardless of the underlying cause, the characteristic finding of TIN on kidney biopsy is tubulointerstitial inflammatory cell infiltrate with associated edema within the interstitium. The infiltrate in nondrug-associated TIN is composed primarily of lymphocytes and monocytes. Eosinophils, neutrophils, and plasma cells may also be present. An eosinophil dominant infiltrate is more suggestive of a drug-induced TIN. The glomeruli and blood vessels are typically normal.[3] With chronic cases of TIN, the biopsy may show interstitial fibrosis.[1] Immunofluorescence is negative in most cases.

Granulomatous TIN is a pathologic finding seen in a subset of patients with TIN. Granulomatous TIN is most commonly associated with medications, rheumatologic diseases, and infections.[15,17,43–45] Medications associated with granulomatous TIN include NSAIDs, antiepileptics, antibiotics, allopurinol, and diuretics.[16] Rheumatologic or inflammatory conditions can include sarcoidosis, GPA, and IBD.[11] Infectious causes include *Mycobacterium tuberculosis*, histoplasmosis, candidiasis, and toxoplasmosis.[11] Granulomatous TIN is thought to be a delayed hypersensitivity reaction, similar to other forms of TIN.[17] The histology on kidney biopsy is characterized by an interstitial infiltrate consisting of lymphocytes, monocytes, and eosinophils with aggregates of epithelioid cells with or without multinucleated giant cells.[3,16] The granulomas are typically noncaseating; however, caseating granulomas can be seen with tuberculosis or GPA.[16]

CLINICAL PRESENTATION

TIN classically presents as nonoliguric AKI.[3] In fact, patients can present with polyuria and polydipsia related to impaired urinary concentrating ability secondary to tubulointerstitial inflammation.[3] Patients typically do not have hypertension or edema.[6] In the case of drug-induced TIN, the creatinine typically starts to increase 7 to 10 days after drug exposure.[6] Some patients with severe disease can present with rapidly rising serum creatinine.[3]

TIN often presents with systemic symptoms in addition to the kidney manifestations. The classic triad of extrarenal symptoms includes fever, eosinophilia, and rash; however, this combination occurs in a small percentage of patients with TIN.[1,2,6] The rash is typically morbilliform or maculopapular.[3] Other systemic manifestations may include arthralgia, myalgias, flank pain, anorexia, nausea, vomiting, malaise, and lymphadenopathy.[2,3] Flank pain is thought to be a result of stretching of the kidney capsule in the setting of tubulointerstitial inflammation.[3,6] In a series of 60 adults with TIN, 45% had arthralgia, 30% had fever, and 21% had rash.[1] In another report of 27 children with biopsy-proven TIN, 81% had anorexia, 70% had malaise, 59% had vomiting, 41% had fever, 22% had arthralgia, and 15% had rash.[2]

Urinalysis may show pyuria, microscopic hematuria, and glucosuria, indicating kidney tubular injury. Additional findings of proximal tubular injury can include potassium and phosphate wasting.[2] With distal tubular injury, hyperkalemia can be present.[3] Low-grade proteinuria may occur but nephrotic-range proteinuria is rare.[2] Low-molecular-weight proteinuria may also be seen in the setting of tubular injury.[2] Eosinophiluria may be present; however, this finding has a low sensitivity and specificity for the diagnosis of TIN.[3] Additional laboratory findings can include eosinophilia, elevated ESR, and anemia.[3] Kidney ultrasound may show enlarged kidneys and/or increased cortical echogenicity; however, these findings are not specific to TIN.[2,3]

Although TIN may be suspected based on clinical features, the diagnosis is confirmed by kidney biopsy. Kidney biopsy is generally indicated when AKI is severe and/or does not improve after a period of conservative therapy. Kidney biopsy can confirm the diagnosis of TIN, as well as guide therapy.

PROGNOSIS AND TREATMENT

The long-term prognosis of TIN in children is generally thought to be favorable with complete kidney recovery in most patients. However, some patients with TIN may have progressive CKD. The literature on outcomes of TIN is limited because many patients with TIN are diagnosed clinically, and only those patients with severe or prolonged courses may undergo kidney biopsy. The risk of chronicity likely depends on the underlying cause, with progressive disease more likely in patients with systemic inflammatory conditions, genetic disorders, or delayed removal of the offending agent in medication-induced TIN.[9] In a series of 27 children with TIN, 60% had an estimated glomerular filtration rate less than 80 mL/min/1.73 m^2 after a median follow-up of 21 months, indicating CKD. However, all children in this study underwent kidney biopsy, likely indicating a selection bias of children with more severe disease.[2] In a study of 64 adult subjects with TIN, 31% had permanent kidney dysfunction. Subjects with TIN related to infection or idiopathic causes were more likely to have complete recovery. In cases of drug-induced TIN, prolonged intake of the offending agent for more than 1 month before diagnosis was associated with a worse long-term prognosis.[4] Factors associated with poor long-term kidney prognosis may include duration of AKI, more severe interstitial fibrosis on biopsy, and presence of granulomas.[3,6]

The treatment of TIN in children includes supportive management and removal of the offending agent in the case of drug-induced TIN.[3] The role of corticosteroids in managing TIN in children remains controversial, with the current literature limited by observational data or small randomized clinical trials. Some studies have shown no significant effect on kidney recovery among those treated with steroids compared with those managed with supportive care, with most subjects having good long-term prognosis regardless of therapy.[1] Jahnukainen and colleagues[46] published a small, randomized clinical trial of prednisone versus placebo in 17 children with newly diagnosed biopsy-proven TIN. Exclusion criteria included suspected self-limiting drug-induced TIN and underlying diseases such as sarcoidosis, connective tissue disorders, or lymphoma. The treatment group received prednisone 2 mg/kg/d to a maximum of 60 mg daily for 1 month, followed by a prednisone taper. Creatinine started to normalize earlier in the prednisone-treated group. However, creatinine was normal in all subjects at the end of the study. Low-molecular-weight proteinuria did not differ between the 2 groups at any point during follow-up. The investigators concluded that because many cases of TIN are self-limited it would be reasonable to observe for 2 weeks in uncomplicated cases before initiation of corticosteroids. However, other studies have reported a more beneficial effect of corticosteroids. Gonzalez and colleagues[5] reported an observational study of 61 subjects with drug-induced TIN, 52 of whom were treated with steroids. The 2 groups had similar baseline creatinine and proteinuria. Almost half (44%) of the untreated subjects developed end-stage kidney disease requiring dialysis (4 of 9 subjects) compared with only 4% (2 of 52 subjects) in the steroid group, $P<.001$. Among subjects who received steroids, more than half had complete recovery of kidney function. Prognosis was worse if steroids were delayed beyond 2 weeks after removal of the offending agent. In subjects who have refractory disease or significant steroid toxicity, other immunosuppressive agents, such as mycophenolate mofetil, have been reported to have benefit.[47]

Although the role of corticosteroids remains unclear, some experts suggest that corticosteroids should be considered for subjects who have minimal interstitial fibrosis on biopsy and no improvement in kidney function after 5 to 7 days of conservative therapy.[3] Optimal duration of corticosteroid therapy is also unclear, with some investigators suggesting a 4 to 6 week course followed by a taper, with discontinuation of steroids if there is no improvement after 3 to 4 weeks.[3]

SUMMARY

TIN is a cause of AKI in children. The most common causes of TIN in children include medications, infections, rheumatologic disorders, IBD, TINU, and genetic disorders. TIN is typically a nonoliguric form of AKI. Patients may present with polyuria and polydipsia related to impaired urinary concentrating ability. Systemic symptoms are common with TIN, including fever, rash, arthralgia, and flank pain. Urinalysis typically shows a dilute urine and may include sterile pyuria, microscopic hematuria, and low-grade proteinuria. Additional laboratory findings may include eosinophiluria, eosinophilia, elevated ESR, and anemia. Gross hematuria, high-grade proteinuria, hypertension, and edema are rare; these features would be more suggestive of a primary glomerular disease. The diagnosis of TIN is confirmed by kidney biopsy showing an inflammatory cell infiltrate and edema of the renal interstitium, with interstitial fibrosis seen in chronic cases. Most cases of TIN in children have a favorable prognosis; however, some patients may have progressive CKD. The role of corticosteroids in managing children with TIN remains controversial because cases may often be self-limited. Immunosuppressive therapy should be considered in patients with severe disease or in patients who have persistent elevation in serum creatinine after a period of conservative management.

REFERENCES

1. Clarkson MR, Giblin L, O'Connell FP, et al. Acute interstitial nephritis: clinical features and response to corticosteroid therapy. Nephrol Dial Transplant 2004; 19(11):2778–83.
2. Howell M, Sebire NJ, Marks SD, et al. Biopsy-proven paediatric tubulointerstitial nephritis. Pediatr Nephrol 2016;31(10):1625–30.
3. Perazella MA, Markowitz GS. Drug-induced acute interstitial nephritis. Nat Rev Nephrol 2010;6(8):461–70.
4. Schwarz A, Krause PH, Kunzendorf U, et al. The outcome of acute interstitial nephritis: risk factors for the transition from acute to chronic interstitial nephritis. Clin Nephrol 2000;54(3):179–90.
5. Gonzalez E, Gutierrez E, Galeano C, et al. Early steroid treatment improves the recovery of renal function in patients with drug-induced acute interstitial nephritis. Kidney Int 2008;73(8):940–6.
6. Rossert J. Drug-induced acute interstitial nephritis. Kidney Int 2001;60(2): 804–17.
7. Platt JL, Sibley RK, Michael AF. Interstitial nephritis associated with cytomegalovirus infection. Kidney Int 1985;28(3):550–2.
8. Rosen S, Harmon W, Krensky AM, et al. Tubulo-interstitial nephritis associated with polyomavirus (BK type) infection. N Engl J Med 1983;308(20):1192–6.
9. Joyce E, Glasner P, Ranganathan S, et al. Tubulointerstitial nephritis: diagnosis, treatment, and monitoring. Pediatr Nephrol 2017;32(4):577–87.
10. Praga M, Gonzalez E. Acute interstitial nephritis. Kidney Int 2010;77(11):956–61.
11. Shah S, Carter-Monroe N, Atta MG. Granulomatous interstitial nephritis. Clin Kidney J 2015;8(5):516–23.
12. Said MH, Layani MP, Colon S, et al. Mycoplasma pneumoniae-associated nephritis in children. Pediatr Nephrol 1999;13(1):39–44.

13. Yu F, Wu LH, Tan Y, et al. Tubulointerstitial lesions of patients with lupus nephritis classified by the 2003 International Society of Nephrology and Renal Pathology Society system. Kidney Int 2010;77(9):820–9.

14. Mori Y, Kishimoto N, Yamahara H, et al. Predominant tubulointerstitial nephritis in a patient with systemic lupus nephritis. Clin Exp Nephrol 2005;9(1):79–84.

15. Bijol V, Mendez GP, Nose V, et al. Granulomatous interstitial nephritis: a clinicopathologic study of 46 cases from a single institution. Int J Surg Pathol 2006; 14(1):57–63.

16. Joss N, Morris S, Young B, et al. Granulomatous interstitial nephritis. Clin J Am Soc Nephrol 2007;2(2):222–30.

17. Tong JE, Howell DN, Foreman JW. Drug-induced granulomatous interstitial nephritis in a pediatric patient. Pediatr Nephrol 2007;22(2):306–9.

18. Vohra S, Eddy A, Levin AV, et al. Tubulointerstitial nephritis and uveitis in children and adolescents. Four new cases and a review of the literature. Pediatr Nephrol 1999;13(5):426–32.

19. Ambruzs JM, Walker PD, Larsen CP. The histopathologic spectrum of kidney biopsies in patients with inflammatory bowel disease. Clin J Am Soc Nephrol 2014; 9(2):265–70.

20. Oikonomou K, Kapsoritakis A, Eleftheriadis T, et al. Renal manifestations and complications of inflammatory bowel disease. Inflamm Bowel Dis 2011;17(4): 1034–45.

21. Fraser JS, Muller AF, Smith DJ, et al. Renal tubular injury is present in acute inflammatory bowel disease prior to the introduction of drug therapy. Aliment Pharmacol Ther 2001;15(8):1131–7.

22. Herrlinger KR, Noftz MK, Fellermann K, et al. Minimal renal dysfunction in inflammatory bowel disease is related to disease activity but not to 5-ASA use. Aliment Pharmacol Ther 2001;15(3):363–9.

23. Kreisel W, Wolf LM, Grotz W, et al. Renal tubular damage: an extraintestinal manifestation of chronic inflammatory bowel disease. Eur J Gastroenterol Hepatol 1996;8(5):461–8.

24. Marcus SB, Brown JB, Melin-Aldana H, et al. Tubulointerstitial nephritis: an extraintestinal manifestation of Crohn disease in children. J Pediatr Gastroenterol Nutr 2008;46(3):338–41.

25. Tokuyama H, Wakino S, Konishi K, et al. Acute interstitial nephritis associated with ulcerative colitis. Clin Exp Nephrol 2010;14(5):483–6.

26. Dobrin RS, Vernier RL, Fish AL. Acute eosinophilic interstitial nephritis and renal failure with bone marrow-lymph node granulomas and anterior uveitis. A new syndrome. Am J Med 1975;59(3):325–33.

27. Mackensen F, Smith JR, Rosenbaum JT. Enhanced recognition, treatment, and prognosis of tubulointerstitial nephritis and uveitis syndrome. Ophthalmology 2007;114(5):995–9.

28. Mandeville JT, Levinson RD, Holland GN. The tubulointerstitial nephritis and uveitis syndrome. Surv Ophthalmol 2001;46(3):195–208.

29. Jahnukainen T, Ala-Houhala M, Karikoski R, et al. Clinical outcome and occurrence of uveitis in children with idiopathic tubulointerstitial nephritis. Pediatr Nephrol 2011;26(2):291–9.

30. Saarela V, Nuutinen M, Ala-Houhala M, et al. Tubulointerstitial nephritis and uveitis syndrome in children: a prospective multicenter study. Ophthalmology 2013; 120(7):1476–81.

31. Chan J. Environmental injury to the kidney: interstitial nephritis. Hong Kong J Nephrol 2014;16:23–8.

32. De Broe ME. Chinese herbs nephropathy and Balkan endemic nephropathy: toward a single entity, aristolochic acid nephropathy. Kidney Int 2012;81(6):513–5.
33. Saeki T, Nishi S, Imai N, et al. Clinicopathological characteristics of patients with IgG4-related tubulointerstitial nephritis. Kidney Int 2010;78(10):1016–23.
34. Zhang P, Cornell LD. IgG4-related tubulointerstitial nephritis. Adv Chronic Kidney Dis 2017;24(2):94–100.
35. Eckardt KU, Alper SL, Antignac C, et al. Autosomal dominant tubulointerstitial kidney disease: diagnosis, classification, and management–A KDIGO consensus report. Kidney Int 2015;88(4):676–83.
36. Bleyer AJ, Kmoch S, Antignac C, et al. Variable clinical presentation of an MUC1 mutation causing medullary cystic kidney disease type 1. Clin J Am Soc Nephrol 2014;9(3):527–35.
37. Dahan K, Devuyst O, Smaers M, et al. A cluster of mutations in the UMOD gene causes familial juvenile hyperuricemic nephropathy with abnormal expression of uromodulin. J Am Soc Nephrol 2003;14(11):2883–93.
38. Heidet L, Decramer S, Pawtowski A, et al. Spectrum of HNF1B mutations in a large cohort of patients who harbor renal diseases. Clin J Am Soc Nephrol 2010;5(6):1079–90.
39. Zivna M, Hulkova H, Matignon M, et al. Dominant renin gene mutations associated with early-onset hyperuricemia, anemia, and chronic kidney failure. Am J Hum Genet 2009;85(2):204–13.
40. Bollee G, Dahan K, Flamant M, et al. Phenotype and outcome in hereditary tubulointerstitial nephritis secondary to UMOD mutations. Clin J Am Soc Nephrol 2011;6(10):2429–38.
41. Kolatsi-Joannou M, Bingham C, Ellard S, et al. Hepatocyte nuclear factor-1beta: a new kindred with renal cysts and diabetes and gene expression in normal human development. J Am Soc Nephrol 2001;12(10):2175–80.
42. Ooi BS, Jao W, First MR, et al. Acute interstitial nephritis. A clinical and pathologic study based on renal biopsies. Am J Med 1975;59(5):614–28.
43. Javaud N, Belenfant X, Stirnemann J, et al. Renal granulomatoses: a retrospective study of 40 cases and review of the literature. Medicine (Baltimore) 2007;86(3):170–80.
44. Mignon F, Mery JP, Mougenot B, et al. Granulomatous interstitial nephritis. Adv Nephrol Necker Hosp 1984;13:219–45.
45. Viero RM, Cavallo T. Granulomatous interstitial nephritis. Hum Pathol 1995;26(12):1347–53.
46. Jahnukainen T, Saarela V, Arikoski P, et al. Prednisone in the treatment of tubulointerstitial nephritis in children. Pediatr Nephrol 2013;28(8):1253–60.
47. Preddie DC, Markowitz GS, Radhakrishnan J, et al. Mycophenolate mofetil for the treatment of interstitial nephritis. Clin J Am Soc Nephrol 2006;1(4):718–22.

Bartter Syndrome and Gitelman Syndrome

Rosanna Fulchiero, DO[a], Patricia Seo-Mayer, MD[a,b,c],*

KEYWORDS

- Salt-losing tubulopathy • Bartter syndrome (BS) • Gitelman syndrome (GS)
- Hypokalemic hypochloremic metabolic alkalosis • Polyuria • Failure to thrive

KEY POINTS

- The salt-losing tubulopathies are rare diseases that can present in infancy or later in childhood with renal salt wasting, hypokalemic hypochloremic metabolic alkalosis, and normal blood pressure despite hyperreninemia and hyperaldosteronism; Treatment varies by type but may include ample fluid delivery, electrolyte replacement, nutritional support, prostaglandin inhibition, and disruption of renin-angiotensin-aldosterone axis.
- Antenatal Bartter/hyperprostaglandin E syndrome presents with fetal polyhydramnios and life-threatening salt and water loss, with or without nephrocalcinosis, and is caused by several distinct gene mutations.
- Classic Bartter syndrome, caused by *CLCNKB* mutation, presents in a clinically heterogenous manner, with failure to thrive, polyuria, salt-wasting, and hypokalemic metabolic alkalosis; and may mimic antenatal Bartter syndrome or Gitelman-like syndrome.
- Gitelman syndrome patients have a mild or even incidental presentation, with hypokalemic metabolic alkalosis, hypomagnesemia, hypocalciuria, and normal blood pressure.
- Treatment varies by type but may include ample fluid delivery, electrolyte replacement, nutritional support, prostaglandin inhibition, and disruption of renin-angiotensin-aldosterone axis.
- Inclusion of patients in national and international registries may improve classification and treatment of these rare conditions, and could provide a framework for future clinical trials.

INTRODUCTION

The kidney is often considered to be an organ designed primarily to promote excretion of metabolic wastes. Though clearance is a vital function, this viewpoint overlooks the elegant and critical role of the kidneys in orchestrating acid-base balance, salt, and water

Disclosures: No relevant disclosures.
[a] Department of Pediatrics, Inova Children's Hospital, 3300 Gallows Road, Falls Church, VA 22042, USA; [b] Division of Nephrology and Hypertension, Pediatric Specialists of Virginia, 3023 Hamaker Court, Suite 600, Fairfax, VA 22031, USA; [c] Virginia Commonwealth School of Medicine, Richmond, VA, USA
* Corresponding author. Division of Nephrology and Hypertension, Pediatric Specialists of Virginia, 3023 Hamaker Court, Suite 600, Fairfax, VA 22031.
E-mail address: Pseo-mayer@psvcare.org

Pediatr Clin N Am 66 (2019) 121–134
https://doi.org/10.1016/j.pcl.2018.08.010
0031-3955/19/© 2018 Elsevier Inc. All rights reserved.

homeostasis. Part skilled artisan, part workhorse, in the act of reabsorbing solutes, the kidneys expend a metabolic demand equal to that of the heart and twice that of the brain.[1]

The importance and complexity of ion reabsorption by the kidney is highlighted when this function is disrupted, as is the case in patients with congenital salt-losing tubulopathies. The most common variants are Bartter syndrome (BS) and Gitelman syndrome (GS), which affect the thick ascending limb (TAL) of Henle loop and the distal convoluted tubule (DCT), respectively. Other distinct salt-losing tubulopathies with unique features, such as transient neonatal BS and epilepsy, ataxia, sensorineural deafness, tubulopathy (EAST) syndrome, have also been identified. These are complex disorders with overlapping clinical and biochemical features due to defects in renal salt handling, and they remain therapeutically challenging despite major advances in knowledge about mechanism and genotypic correlations.[2]

Patients may present in the neonatal intensive care unit with prematurity and polyuria; in the emergency room with muscle weakness and rhabdomyolysis; or at a well-child examination with short stature, constipation, and nocturia. BS and GS and related salt-losing tubulopathies should be considered in a variety of settings in the pediatric patient with hypokalemic hypochloremic metabolic alkalosis.

HISTORY

In 1962, Dr Frederic Bartter described 2 African American patients with severe hypokalemic alkalosis, normotensive hyperaldosteronism, and hyperplasia and hypertrophy of the juxtaglomerular apparatus.[3] Several years later, Gitelman and colleagues[4] described a similar but distinct syndrome in 3 patients who had these findings and impaired renal conservation of magnesium. As more cases of suspected BS and GS were described, it was noted that the clinical symptoms correlated closely with those of chronic diuretic use. BS patients mimed the action of furosemide and GS patients mimed that of thiazide diuretics. Subsequently, renal ion transport channels were identified as having a role in disease mechanism, and clinical observations facilitated gene identification using gene candidate strategy.[5]

CLINICAL PRESENTATION

Although variants of BS and GS are genotypically distinct, there is considerable overlap in clinical presentation. Clinically, these tubulopathies are often categorized into several major groups: antenatal BS (ABS) or hyperprostaglandin E syndrome (HPES), classic BS (CBS), and GS. Other related syndromes (**Box 1**) have overlapping clinical features and so are included in this discussion. All share the characteristics of renal salt wasting, hypokalemic hypochloremic metabolic alkalosis, and low or normal blood pressure despite hyperreninemia and hyperaldosteronism. Neonates may present with polyhydramnios, prematurity, and poor growth. One ABS variant presents with transient hyperkalemia and acidosis.[6] Older children may present with symptoms of chronic hypokalemia, such as constipation, muscle cramps, and weakness, as well as poor growth, salt-craving, nocturia, and vomiting. Hypercalciuria, with or without medullary nephrocalcinosis, is present in some variants.

The differential diagnosis of hypokalemic hypochloremic metabolic alkalosis includes pyloric stenosis, diuretic use, congenital chloride diarrhea, laxative abuse, and cystic fibrosis. Other features (ie, age, medication history, and lack of gastrointestinal losses or pulmonary disease) can be helpful to distinguish between a salt-wasting tubulopathy and another cause. If diuretic use is not suspected, urinary chloride measurement, elevated in BS and GS, can decipher between renal and nonrenal causes of chloride loss.

Box 1
Types of Bartter syndrome, Gitelman syndrome, and related conditions

Disorder	OMIM, Gene	Gene Product	Inheritance	Features
BS Variants				
BS I (ABS, HPES)	601678, SLC12A1	NKCC2	AR	Polyhydramnios, prematurity, hypokalemic hypochloremic alkalosis, nephrocalcinosis, with or without concentrating defect
BS II (ABS with transient hyperkalemia and acidosis, HPES)	241200, KCNJ1	ROMK1	AR	Polyhydramnios, prematurity, transient hyperkalemia and acidosis, then hypokalemic hypochloremic alkalosis, nephrocalcinosis, with or without concentrating defect
BS III (CBS)	607364, CLCNKB	ClC-Kb	AR; many sporadic	Variable age at presentation with severity corresponding to type of gene mutation; hypokalemic hypochloremic alkalosis
BS IVa and BS IVb (ABS or HPES with sensorineural deafness)	602522, BSND CLCNKA, CLCNKB	Bartter ClC-Ka and ClC-Kb	AR	Polyhydramnios, prematurity, hypokalemic hypochloremic alkalosis, sensorineural deafness, with or without concentrating defect
BS V (transient ABS)	300971, MAGED2	MAGED2	XR	Severe polyhydramnios, hypokalemic hypochloremic alkalosis with symptoms resolving within the first few months of life
AD hypocalcemic hypercalciuria	601199, L125P	CaSR	AD	Hypocalcemic hypocalciuria, hypokalemic hypochloremic alkalosis, suppressed PTH
GS variants				
GS	263800, SLC12A3	NCC	AR	Present in later childhood or adulthood with weakness, lethargy, carpopedal spasm, hypokalemic alkalosis, hypomagnesemia, hypermagnesiuria and hypocalciuria
EAST syndrome (SeSAME)	612780, Kir4.1	KCNJ10	AR	Epilepsy, ataxia, sensorineural deafness, hypokalemic hypochloremic alkalosis
Other variants				
CLDN10 mutations	617579, CLDN10	Claudin-10	AR	Hypokalemic metabolic alkalosis with hypocalciuria but normal to elevated magnesium

Abbreviations: AD, autosomal dominant; AR, autosomal recessive; CaSR, calcium-sensing receptor; ClC-Ka, chloride channel-Ka; ClC-Kb, chloride channel-Kb; MAGED, melanoma-associated antigen-D2; NCC, thiazide-sensitive NaCl cotransporter; NKCC2, furosemide-sensitive Na-K-2Cl cotransporter; OMIM, online Mendelian inheritance in man; PTH, parathyroid hormone; ROMK, renal outer medullary K channel; SeSAME, seizures, sensorineural deafness, ataxia, mental retardation, and electrolyte imbalances; XR, X-linked recessive.

VARIANTS OF BARTTER AND GITELMAN SYNDROMES AND RELATED CONDITIONS

Classification schemes of BS, GS, and related syndromes are in evolution. Historically, patients were categorized by phenotypic characteristics (ABS vs CBS based on age and severity of presentation); however, emerging data about genetic variants and unique and distinct mechanisms of salt-wasting present a new gene-based framework for classification. Moreover, there is variation in clinical presentation even when the same gene is affected (eg, BS type III can present antenatally or later in life, with or without hypercalciuria). Mutation type also affects phenotype, offering an additional framework for categorization. As disease mechanisms and causes of phenotypic variation are further elucidated, classification schemes may use a combination of clinical and biochemical characteristics with gene mutation and affected transport mechanism. **Box 1** summarizes current acknowledged BS and GS types, as well as related variants, and lists gene mutations and products, as well as typical clinical characteristics. For the purposes of this article, the following discussion refers to typical manifestations of known types.

Antenatal Bartter Syndrome (Types I, II, IVa, and IVb)

BS type I is hallmarked by severe antenatal symptoms, with polyhydramnios noted during the second trimester.[6,7] Premature delivery between 29 to 36 weeks is common.[7] Characteristic BS facies include triangular face with prominent forehead, large eyes, protruding pinnae, and a drooping mouth with pouting expression, attributed to facial muscle weakness secondary to hypokalemia.[8] Infants have extreme polyuria with impaired renal concentrating capacity (sometimes leading to an erroneous diagnosis of nephrogenic diabetes insipidus [NDI]), and may experience life-threatening salt and water loss. In addition to hypokalemic hypochloremic alkalosis, patients may exhibit fever, vomiting, and failure to thrive secondary to increased prostaglandin E formation. Blood pressure is normal despite high levels of renin and aldosterone.[6] Hypercalciuria may cause development of nephrocalcinosis.[2,6,7,9,10]

BS type I is caused by inactivating mutations in the *SLC12A1* gene coding the furosemide-sensitive luminal Na-K-2Cl cotransporter (NKCC2) in the TAL of Henle loop (**Fig. 1**). In this segment, ion transport is driven by the electrochemical gradient generated by the basolateral Na-K-ATPase pump. This gradient facilitates transport of sodium, potassium, and chloride into the cell via NKCC2. Without transcellular transport of sodium chloride, there is no lumen-positive transepithelial voltage gradient to facilitate paracellular transport of sodium. This prevents generation of the corticomedullary osmotic gradient needed for urine concentration and causes hyposthenuria. Increased salt delivery to the distal nephron results in enhanced sodium reabsorption in the aldosterone sensitive segments, which is accompanied by excretion of potassium and hydrogen ions, causing hypokalemic metabolic alkalosis.

The NKCC2 transporter is also responsible for mediating chloride entry into the macula densa. A nonfunctioning transporter causes decreased chloride concentration in the fluid of the adjacent lumen, stimulating renin release. This compounds a hyperreninemic state already stimulated by salt wasting and volume contraction. Hyperaldosteronism further propagates hypokalemia, exaggerating metabolic alkalosis and impeding water reabsorption. Despite renin-angiotensin-aldosterone system (RAAS) activation, patients are typically normotensive. The reduced lumen-positive transmembrane potential is also responsible for a decrease of paracellular divalent cations, causing hypermagnesiuria and hypercalciuria, and often nephrocalcinosis.[11,12] Prostaglandin E2 is released in response to impaired sodium absorption in the TAL and may be measured at high levels in the urine and blood.

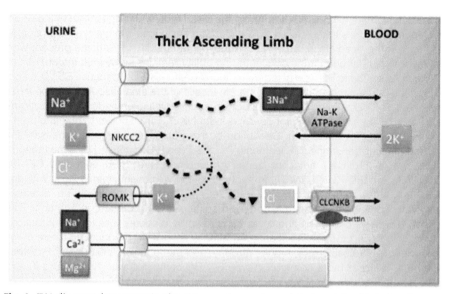

Fig. 1. TAL diagram demonstrating key transporters and associated proteins. Mutations in associated genes impact transporter activity and lead to clinical findings observed in Bartter syndrome. NKCC2 (affected in BS I), inhibited by loop diuretics, reabsorbs sodium, potassium and two chloride ions. ROMK (affected in BS II) recycles potassium to allow paracellular absorption of calcium and magnesium. CLCNKB (affected in BS III) and CLCNKA require Barttin (affected in BS IV) to reabsorb chloride. (*Adapted from* Kleta R, Bockenhauer D. Salt-Losing Tubulopathies in Children: What's New, What's Controversial? J Am Soc Nephrol 2018;29(3):727–39.)

Type II BS is unique because patients may demonstrate transient hyperkalemia. This variant is caused by mutations in the *KCNJ1* gene encoding renal outer medullary K channel (ROMK), also found in the TAL (see **Fig. 1**). ROMK is an inward rectifying potassium channel that ensures proper functioning of the NKCC2 by recycling potassium back into the luminal space. Loss of function results in decreased reabsorption of sodium chloride, and leads to the same sequelae seen in primary NKCC2 defects: polyhydramnios with massive salt wasting, hyponatremia, hypochloremia, volume contraction, metabolic alkalosis, hypercalciuria with nephrocalcinosis, hyperreninemia, hyperaldosteronism, and increased urinary prostaglandins. Hyperkalemia is likely due to the role of ROMK in potassium homeostasis in the cortical collecting duct.[6,7] This transient hyperkalemia, often associated with metabolic acidosis, mimics pseudohypoaldosteronism (PHA) type I,[2,7,11] although elevated potassium is transient in BS type II and sustained in patients with PHA I.[7]

Though typically considered CBS due to usual presentation later in life, BS type III is often not considered an antenatal variant. However, patients with BS type III have presented antenatally (see later discussion).[11,13]

Type IV BS, previously called ABS with sensorineural deafness, is comprised of 2 unique defects: type IVa (Barttin defect) and type IVB (mutations in basolateral chloride channel-Ka [ClC-Ka] and chloride channel-Kb [ClC-Kb]). Phenotypically, these conditions are indistinguishable. Neonates present with polyhydramnios, prematurity, polyuria, and severe salt wasting.[14] In contrast to types I and II, hypercalciuria may be transient, although when present it can still progress to medullary nephrocalcinosis.[5] Type IVA is caused by an inactivating mutation in the *BSND* gene, which encodes Barttin, an essential beta subunit of 2 chloride channels in the TAL, ClC-Ka and

ClC-Kb, which are expressed throughout the distal tubule. Barttin facilitates transport of chloride channels to the cell surface and mutations cause impaired release of chloride across the basolateral membrane in the TAL and DCT.[5,15] Patients present with polyhydramnios, though urine concentrating ability remains somewhat intact.[11,14]

A feature unique to BS type IV is sensorineural deafness[5,14,16] because *BSND* is also expressed in the cochlea, within the marginal cells of the stria vascularis. In the inner ear, the ClC-K- Barttin complex is responsible for recycling chloride ions, and mutations affect the ability of the chloride-dependent NKCC1 transporter to mediate transcellular passage of potassium. Disruption of this potassium gradient, necessary for hearing, causes sensorineural deafness.[16,17] BS Type IVB is caused by simultaneous mutations in 2 closely adjacent genes on chromosome 1p36 encoding ClC-Ka (*CLCNKA*) and ClC-Kb (*CLCNKB*). Phenotypically, these patients mimic those with defects in Barttin. Although mutations in *CLCNKB* manifest as CBS, no disease-associated defects have been reported in solitary ClC-Ka defects in humans. This defect, however, has been shown to cause a mild diabetes insipidus in knockout mice.[5,14,18] Renal biopsies in patients with type IV ABS show pronounced tissue damage, with glomerulosclerosis, tubular atrophy, and mononuclear infiltration.[5] Progressive renal failure is more common in type IV ABS compared with types I and II, and patients may require transplant.[16,19]

Classic Bartter Syndrome (Type III)

Historically, CBS was considered to have a milder phenotype than antenatal types; however, recent reports suggest this variant is more heterogeneous than previously described.[9,11,13] Type III BS is caused by a mutation in *CLCNKB*, the gene associated with ClC-Kb. Patients with CBS have a spectrum of phenotypic heterogeneity and may present with suspected ABS, CBS, or Gitelman-like syndrome, attributed to the distribution of the ClC-Kb channel throughout the nephron, particularly in the TAL, DCT, and early collecting duct.[5,9,11,13] Cases may present antenatally with polyhydramnios, or in early childhood with failure to thrive and lethargy, marked salt wasting, hypokalemia, polyuria, polydipsia, volume contraction, and muscle weakness.[9] Premature birth is less common but reported. Some cases may also present later in childhood or adulthood with incidental hypokalemia, hypomagnesemia, and/or hypocalciuria. Patients are usually normocalciuric and nephrocalcinosis is uncommon. Renal concentrating capacity is mostly preserved.[5,11,13] Despite often being considered the milder variant of BS, patients with type III typically have the most severe electrolyte abnormalities.

As with BS types I and II, defects in the ClC-Kb channel impair net sodium chloride reabsorption in the TAL and increase sodium chloride delivery to the distal nephron, causing salt wasting, volume contraction, and stimulation of the RAAS, with associated hypokalemic metabolic alkalosis.[9] Defective basolateral chloride efflux in the DCT decreases sodium chloride reabsorption via the sodium chloride cotransporter, causing a GS-like phenotype.[13] All CBS patients will have marked hypochloremia. The inconsistent genotypic-phenotypic correlation and multitude of mutation variants are current areas of investigation.[13,20]

Transient Neonatal Bartter Syndrome (Type V)

A curious type of transient ABS has been described in which infants have severe polyhydramnios, premature birth, extreme salt wasting, hypercalciuria, hyperreninemia, and hyperaldosteronism. However, in survivors, tubulopathy spontaneously improves within the first few months of life.[21–23] Laghmani and colleagues[23] performed whole exome sequencing in 16 such cases and discovered a nonsense mutation in the melanoma-associated antigen D2 (*MAGED2*), which affects expression and function of NKCC2 in the TAL. The transient nature of this variant raises questions about developmental differences in ion transport that could inform future targets of treatment.

Autosomal Dominant Hypocalcemic Hypercalciuria

Previously termed hypocalcemia with Bartter-like syndrome, the autosomal dominant hypocalcemic hypercalciuria variant is distinguished by an autosomal dominant inheritance pattern. Patients present with hypocalcemia and Bartter-like features: hypokalemia with metabolic alkalosis, hypercalciuria with nephrocalcinosis, hyperreninemia, and hyperaldosteronism. Hypocalcemia is associated with suppressed secretion of parathyroid hormone (PTH).[24] It may be difficult to differentiate between this disease and hypoparathyroidism on the basis of serum PTH levels and urinary calcium levels alone; however, it is important to distinguish because inadvertent treatment with vitamin D in these patients may lead to hypercalciuria, nephrocalcinosis, and renal impairment.[25] This variant is caused by a mutation in the extracellular basolateral calcium sensing receptor, which is expressed throughout most of the renal tubule but is predominantly in the TAL.[2] Gain-of-function mutations in this channel inhibit reabsorption of divalent cations into the renal tubule via paracellular transport, causing urinary loss of calcium and magnesium and PTH suppression. In addition, there is renal loss of sodium chloride with hypokalemia and secondary hyperaldosteronism, thought to be due to decreased sodium chloride transport in the TAL by direct inhibition of the NKCC2 or indirect inhibition of potassium via apical potassium channels.[26]

Gitelman Syndrome

GS, or familial hypokalemia-hypomagnesemia, is an autosomal recessive disorder characterized by hypokalemic metabolic alkalosis, hypomagnesemia, and hypocalciuria.[4] Symptoms usually occur after the age of 6 years[27] but may not present until adolescence or adulthood. Often, the diagnosis is fortuitous, with detection of incidental hypokalemia in a routine blood sample. Patients may complain of salt-craving, fatigue, weakness, dizziness, thirst, muscle weakness or cramps, palpitations, and nocturia. Chondrocalcinosis, pubertal delay, and tetany are other potential findings. Seizures, rhabdomyolysis, pseudogout, and pseudotumor cerebri have been reported.[27–29] Risk for prolonged QT and cardiac arrhythmias due to persistent hypokalemia and hypomagnesemia are concerns.[30–32] In 2016, a Kidney Disease: Improving Global Outcomes (KDIGO) consensus statement regarding GS was published, providing an initial framework to guide clinical quality and future investigations.[28]

GS is caused by biallelic inactivating mutations in the *SLC12A3* gene encoding the thiazide-sensitive sodium chloride cotransporter (NCC) in the DCT (**Fig. 2**). Greater than 350 mutations have been reported.[28] Decreased sodium chloride reabsorption by NCC-deficient cells leads to mild volume contraction and stimulation of RAAS cascade. Hyperaldosteronism will increase electrogenic sodium reabsorption in the cortical collecting duct (CCD) via the epithelial sodium channel and, in turn, increase secretion of potassium and hydrogen ions, causing hypokalemic metabolic alkalosis.[27] Passive calcium reabsorption in the proximal tubule and impaired sodium chloride reabsorption in the DCT indirectly downregulate the transient receptor potential cation channel subfamily M member 6 (TRPM6), leading to hypocalciuria and hypomagnesemia.[33] Chronic thiazide treatment has been described as akin to GS.[27]

Epilepsy, Ataxia, Sensorineural Deafness, Tubulopathy Syndrome

EAST syndrome manifests with the same electrolyte disturbances as GS but has additional distinct clinical features, including ataxia, seizures, and sensorineural deafness. It is caused by a loss-of-function mutation affecting *KCJN10*, which maintains the

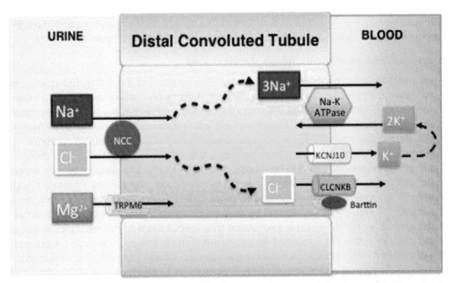

Fig. 2. DCT diagram. NCC, defective in Gitelman syndrome and the target of thiazide diuretics, reabsorbs sodium and chloride from the urine. Na-K-ATPase actively pumps sodium into the blood but requires KCNJ10 (affected in EAST syndrome) to maintain a basolateral potassium gradient. Chlroide enters the blood via CLCKNB (defective in BS III)..Magnesium is reabsorbed via action of TRPM6, the activity of which is indirectly impaired in GS. (*Adapted from* Kleta R, Bockenhauer D. Salt-Losing Tubulopathies in Children: What's New, What's Controversial? J Am Soc Nephrol 2018;29(3):727–39.)

intracellular potassium gradient in the DCT. *KCNJ10* is also expressed in glial cells in the brain, and alterations decrease the membrane potential, lowering the seizure threshold.[34] Seizures, sensorineural deafness, ataxia, mental retardation, and electrolyte imbalances (SeSAME) was the term previously used but has since been revised because difficulty communicating may not be related to intrinsic intellectual disability or mental retardation but rather to severe movement disorders affecting speech and written communication.[15]

Hypokalemic Alkalotic Salt-Losing Tubulopathies from CLDN10 Mutations

Recently, 2 patients with hypokalemic metabolic alkalosis were identified as having a novel cause of salt-wasting. The first presented in adulthood with chest pain, leading to diagnosis of hypokalemic metabolic alkalosis, due to presumed BS. She later developed hypocalciuria, suggestive of GS but had absence of hypomagnesemia and exaggerated response to thiazide, which are inconsistent with GS. Thus, whole exome sequencing was pursued and was notable for a novel mutation in *CLDN10*. The second patient presented in childhood with episodic hypokalemic metabolic alkalosis with illness; however, sequencing also revealed no sequence variants in *SLC12A3* or *CLCNKB*. Whole-exome sequencing identified a compound heterozygous mutation in *CLDN10*. This gene encodes the tight junction protein claudin-10, responsible for regulation of paracellular magnesium, calcium, and sodium permeability in the TAL.[35]

DIAGNOSIS

BS and GS comprise a spectrum with overlapping characteristics that can present with varying levels of severity, making diagnosis difficult. A careful history, physical examination, and laboratory evaluation should be undertaken (**Box 2**), with genetic

Box 2		
Preliminary workup in patient with suspected Bartter syndrome or Gitelman syndrome		
	Specimen or Test	**Expected Result**
Blood	Basic metabolic panel (Na, K, Cl, bicarbonate, BUN, creatinine, glucose)	Hyponatremia or normonatremia, hypokalemia, hypochloremia, metabolic alkalosis
	Renin	Elevated
	Aldosterone	Elevated
	Magnesium	Normal (BS), low (GS)
Urine	Potassium	Elevated (>2 mmol/mmol or >18 mEq/g)
	Spot potassium or creatinine ratio or transtubular potassium gradient[a]	Elevated (>2)
	Chloride	Elevated (>0.5%)
	Fractional excretion of chloride	Normal or low, consistent with isosthenuria or hyposthenuria
	Osmolality	
	Calcium	Elevated (BS), or low (GS)
	Calcium or creatinine ratio[b]	
Imaging	Renal ultrasound	May show nephrocalcinosis (BS I & II)

Abbreviations: BUN, blood urea nitrogen; Cl, chloride; K, potassium; Na, sodium.
[a] Only valid if urine osm > serum osm and urine Na greater than 25 mEq/L.
[b] Normal ranges vary; for reference ranges by age, see Blanchard et al., Kidney Int, 2018: 91, 24–33.

testing to be considered to confirm the fundamental defect and diagnosis. Age at diagnosis can help distinguish between an ABS variant and CBS or GS. In a premature neonate with polyuria and poor weight gain, it may be tempting to suspect NDI; however, these cases distinguish themselves from salt-wasting tubulopathies because NDI typically causes elevated serum sodium and lacks potassium and chloride urinary losses.[36] Furthermore, in NDI, urine osmolality is less than 100 mOsm/kg, whereas in BS it is typically not less than 160 mOsm/kg.[5] **Box 3** describes additional distinguishing characteristics that may refine diagnosis.

Biopsy is not typically pursued because clinical and genotypic diagnoses can be reached by other means. Findings feature juxtaglomerular hypertrophy and hyperplasia[3] but appearance rarely assists in distinguishing between the various genotypes. Renal biopsies in type IV BS patients have shown pronounced tissue damage with glomerular sclerosis, tubular atrophy, and mononuclear infiltration.[5]

MANAGEMENT

Acute management in dehydrated patients involves correcting water losses and repleting electrolytes. Chronically, patients require electrolyte supplementation and inhibition of prostaglandin production and/or the RAAS,[12] although comprehensive clinical studies examining efficacy and outcome are lacking. Patients with BS and GS are typically prescribed oral salt replacement therapy, although normalizing serum electrolytes with an ongoing tubular leak is challenging, optimal frequency of dosing is ill-defined, and serum levels greatly depend on the timing of last dose. In young children, oral sodium chloride replacement may be necessary early in life but increased dietary salt intake in older children is usually sufficient.[12] Potassium supplementation

Box 3
Features that distinguish Bartter and Gitelman syndrome variants

Variant	Age of Onset	Serum K	Serum Cl	Serum Mg	Serum Renin, Aldosterone	Urine Ca/Cr	Other Distinct Features
BS I	AN	Low	Low	Normal	High, high	High	—
BS II	AN	High, then low	Low	Normal	High, high	High	Transient hyperkalemia
BS III	N, C, A	Low	Very low	Normal	High, high	Low, normal, or high	—
BS IVa, IVb	AN	Low	Low	Normal	High, high	Normal or High	Sensorineural deafness
BS V	AN	Low	Low	Normal	High, high	—	Transient features
Hypocalcemic hypercalciuria	—	Low	Low	Normal	High, high	High	Family history, hypocalcemia, suppressed PTH
GS	C, A	Low	Low	Low	High, high	Low	—
EAST syndrome	—	Low	Low	Low	High, high	Low	Epilepsy, ataxia, sensorineural deafness

Abbreviations: A, adult; AN, antenatal; C, child; Ca/Cr, spot calcium to creatinine ratio; Mg, magnesium; N, neonate.

is often used, and GS patients also require high magnesium intake. Growth and pubertal delay has been shown to be reversible by adequate magnesium and potassium supplementation when combined with indomethacin,[37] although it is unclear what the specific target levels of potassium or magnesium should be.[15,28]

Antiprostaglandin mediators are paramount in management of ABS or HPES, in particular. Both indomethacin and selective cyclooxygenase (COX)-2 inhibitors (eg, rofecoxib and celecoxib) relieve symptoms of salt-losing tubulopathy, including hyperprostaglandinuria, secondary hyperaldosteronism, hypochloremic hypokalemic metabolic alkalosis, polyuria, and hypercalciuria.[38] Indomethacin is also associated with improved growth velocity in BS patients.[12,39] Monitoring of side effects is essential because indomethacin use has been associated with ulcers, necrotizing colitis, and gastrointestinal perforations in preterm infants.[40] Due to significant cardiovascular side effects, rofecoxib is no longer commercially available. It is also unclear whether and at what age COX-2 inhibitors should be discontinued.

The use of potassium-sparing diuretics in patients with BS and GS is controversial. Spironolactone, eplerenone, and amiloride may increase serum potassium levels, reverse metabolic alkalosis, and partially correct hypomagnesemia in patients. However, exacerbation of salt-wasting and risk of volume depletion are concerns. Thiazide diuretics are generally not recommended to treat hypercalciuria and nephrocalcinosis in patients with BS because they pose an increased risk of perpetuating volume depletion.[12]

Angiotensin converting enzyme inhibitor use has been reported in the treatment of BS. Enalapril has been shown to improve hypokalemia after 3 months of therapy, with partial correction of hypomagnesemia.[41,42] However, risk of hypotension remains a concern and should be part of the equation when evaluating risk versus benefit.[15,42]

Growth problems are a common presenting symptom in this population; therefore, when fluid, salt, and nutrition management has been optimized, growth hormone (GH) therapy should be considered. GH deficiency has been reported in concert with both BS and GS.[43,44] However, even in cases with normal insulin-like growth factor (IGF)-I and GH levels, patients often experience poor growth. Animal models suggest that chronic hypokalemia may inhibit pituitary GH secretion and may also cause tissue-specific alterations in IGF-I and GH metabolism.[45,46] Patients do respond to GH therapy,[44,47] although cost of GH treatment is a consideration.[48]

END-STAGE RENAL DISEASE TRANSPLANT

BS and GS rarely advance to end-stage renal disease (ESRD) and renal failure. In those who have progressed as a result of chronic nephropathy or medication side effects, renal transplant has proven successful.[49,50] Preemptive bilateral nephrectomy with subsequent transplantation has been performed in 2 patients with severe, debilitating ABS before the onset of ESRD in an effort to cure the underlying disease and improve quality of life,[51] though this is not standard practice.

SUMMARY

BS and GS patients demonstrate how dramatic the impact of impaired renal salt transport can be. Depending on the setting, certain red flags should prompt the clinician to consider these conditions, including polyhydramnios in the neonatal intensive care unit, chronic weakness exacerbated by gastrointestinal losses in the urgent setting, and poor growth identified at the well-child visit. Assessment of the basic metabolic panel and serum magnesium can be informative and can guide next steps. Neonatal and pediatric practitioners should consider these salt-losing tubulopathies in patients with unexplained hypokalemic hypochloremic metabolic alkalosis, especially when gastrointestinal losses and diuretic or laxative use are ruled out. Investigation of urinary potassium and urinary chloride measurement should be pursued and, if they are excessive, renal salt wasting should be implicated. Focused genetic testing may also be beneficial. Because they are uncommon, BS and GS remain therapeutically challenging and future advances in treatment will depend on collaborative efforts to systematically investigate options and better characterize genotypic-phenotypic correlations.

REFERENCES

1. Wang Z, Ying Z, Bosy-Westphal A, et al. Specific metabolic rates of major organs and tissues across adulthood: evaluation by mechanistic model of resting energy expenditure. Am J Clin Nutr 2010;92:1369–77.
2. Al Shibli A, Narchi H. Bartter and Gitelman syndromes: Spectrum of clinical manifestations caused by different mutations. World J Methodol 2015;5:55–61.
3. Bartter FC, Pronove P, Gill JR, et al. Hyperplasia of the juxtaglomerular complex with hyperaldosteronism and hypokalemic alkalosis. A new syndrome. 1962. J Am Soc Nephrol 1998;9:516–28.
4. Gitelman HJ, Graham JB, Welt LG. A new familial disorder characterized by hypokalemia and hypomagnesemia. Trans Assoc Am Physicians 1966;79:221–35.
5. Jeck N, Schlingmann KP, Reinalter SC, et al. Salt handling in the distal nephron: lessons learned from inherited human disorders. Am J Physiol Regul Integr Comp Physiol 2005;288:782.
6. Bhat YR, Vinayaka G, Sreelakshmi K. Antenatal Bartter syndrome: a review. Int J Pediatr 2012;2012:857136.
7. Finer G, Shalev H, Birk OS, et al. Transient neonatal hyperkalemia in the antenatal (ROMK defective) Bartter syndrome. J Pediatr 2003;142:318–23.
8. James T, Holland NH, Preston D. Bartter syndrome. Typical facies and normal plasma volume. Am J Dis Child 1975;129:1205–7.
9. Konrad M, Vollmer M, Lemmink HH, et al. Mutations in the chloride channel gene CLCNKB as a cause of classic Bartter syndrome. J Am Soc Nephrol 2000;11:1449–59.
10. Madrigal G, Saborio P, Mora F, et al. Bartter syndrome in Costa Rica: a description of 20 cases. Pediatr Nephrol 1997;11:296–301.
11. Peters M, Jeck N, Reinalter S, et al. Clinical presentation of genetically defined patients with hypokalemic salt-losing tubulopathies. Am J Med 2002;112:183–90.
12. Fremont OT, Chan JCM. Understanding Bartter syndrome and Gitelman syndrome. World J Pediatr 2012;8:25–30.
13. Seys E, Andrini O, Keck M, et al. Clinical and genetic spectrum of Bartter syndrome type 3. J Am Soc Nephrol 2017;28:2540–52.
14. Schlingmann KP, Konrad M, Jeck N, et al. Salt wasting and deafness resulting from mutations in two chloride channels. N Engl J Med 2004;350:1314–9.
15. Kleta R, Bockenhauer D. Salt-losing tubulopathies in children: what's new, what's controversial? J Am Soc Nephrol 2018;29(3):727–39.
16. Birkenhäger R, Otto E, Schürmann MJ, et al. Mutation of BSND causes Bartter syndrome with sensorineural deafness and kidney failure. Nat Genet 2001;29:310–4.
17. Estévez R, Boettger T, Stein V, et al. Barttin is a Cl- channel beta-subunit crucial for renal Cl- reabsorption and inner ear K+ secretion. Nature 2001;414:558–61.

18. Matsumura Y, Uchida S, Kondo Y, et al. Overt nephrogenic diabetes insipidus in mice lacking the CLC-K1 chloride channel. Nat Genet 1999;21:95–8.
19. Jeck N, Reinalter SC, Henne T, et al. Hypokalemic salt-losing tubulopathy with chronic renal failure and sensorineural deafness. Pediatrics 2001;108:E5.
20. García Castaño A, Pérez de Nanclares G, Madariaga L, et al. Poor phenotype-genotype association in a large series of patients with Type III Bartter syndrome. PLoS One 2017;12:e0173581.
21. Engels A, Gordjani N, Nolte S, et al. Angeborene passagere hyperprostaglandinurische tubulopathie bei zwei frühgeborenen geschwistern. Monatsschr Kinderheilkd 1991;139:185.
22. Reinalter S, Devlieger H, Proesmans W. Neonatal Bartter syndrome: spontaneous resolution of all signs and symptoms. Pediatr Nephrol 1998;12:186–8.
23. Laghmani K, Beck BB, Yang S, et al. Polyhydramnios, transient antenatal Bartter's syndrome, and MAGED2 mutations. N Engl J Med 2016;374:1853–63.
24. Watanabe S, Fukumoto S, Chang H, et al. Association between activating mutations of calcium-sensing receptor and Bartter's syndrome. Lancet 2002;360: 692–4.
25. Pearce SHS, Williamson C, Kifor O, et al. A familial syndrome of hypocalcemia with hypercalciuria due to mutations in the calcium-sensing receptor. N Engl J Med 1996;335:1115–22.
26. Vargas-Poussou R, Huang C, Hulin P, et al. Functional characterization of a calcium-sensing receptor mutation in severe autosomal dominant hypocalcemia with a Bartter-like syndrome. J Am Soc Nephrol 2002;13:2259–66.
27. Knoers, Nine VAM, Levtchenko EN. Gitelman syndrome. Orphanet J Rare Dis 2008;3:22.
28. Blanchard A, Bockenhauer D, Bolignano D, et al. Gitelman syndrome: consensus and guidance from a Kidney Disease: Improving Global Outcomes (KDIGO) controversies conference. Kidney Int 2017;91:24–33.
29. Smilde TJ, Haverman JF, Schipper P, et al. Familial hypokalemia/hypomagnesemia and chondrocalcinosis. J Rheumatol 1994;21:1515–9.
30. Scognamiglio R, Negut C, Calò LA. Aborted sudden cardiac death in two patients with Bartter's/Gitelman's syndromes. Clin Nephrol 2007;67:193–7.
31. Foglia PE, Bettinelli A, Tosetto C, et al. Cardiac work up in primary renal hypokalaemia-hypomagnesaemia (Gitelman syndrome). Nephrol Dial Transplant 2004;19:1398–402.
32. Bettinelli A, Borsa N, Bellantuono R, et al. Patients with biallelic mutations in the chloride channel gene CLCNKB: long-term management and outcome. Am J Kidney Dis 2007;49:91–8.
33. Nijenhuis T, Vallon V, van der Kemp AW, et al. Enhanced passive Ca2+ reabsorption and reduced Mg2+ channel abundance explains thiazide-induced hypocalciuria and hypomagnesemia. J Clin Invest 2005;115:1651–8.
34. Bockenhauer D, Feather S, Stanescu HC, et al. Epilepsy, ataxia, sensorineural deafness, tubulopathy, and KCNJ10 mutations. N Engl J Med 2009;360:1960–70.
35. Bongers EMHF, Shelton LM, Milatz S, et al. A novel hypokalemic-alkalotic salt-losing tubulopathy in patients with CLDN10 mutations. J Am Soc Nephrol 2017; 28(10):3118–28.
36. Bockenhauer D, Bichet DG. Pathophysiology, diagnosis and management of nephrogenic diabetes insipidus. Nat Rev Nephrol 2015;11:576–88.
37. Liaw LC, Banerjee K, Coulthard MG. Dose related growth response to indometacin in Gitelman syndrome. Arch Dis Child 1999;81:508–10.

38. Reinalter SC, Jeck N, Brochhausen C, et al. Role of cyclooxygenase-2 in hyper-prostaglandin E syndrome/antenatal Bartter syndrome. Kidney Int 2002;62: 253–60.
39. Vaisbich MH, Fujimura MD, Koch VH. Bartter syndrome: benefits and side effects of long-term treatment. Pediatr Nephrol 2004;19:858–63.
40. Marlow N, Chiswick ML. Neonatal Bartter's syndrome, indomethacin and necrotising enterocolitis. Acta Paediatr Scand 1982;71:1031–2.
41. Morales JM, Ruilope LM, Praga M, et al. Long-term enalapril therapy in Bartter's syndrome. Nephron 1988;48:327.
42. Hené RJ, Koomans HA, Dorhout Mees EJ, et al. Correction of hypokalemia in Bartter's syndrome by enalapril. Am J Kidney Dis 1987;9:200–5.
43. Boer LA, Zoppi G. Bartter's syndrome with impairment of growth hormone secretion. Lancet 1992;340:860.
44. Buyukcelik M, Keskin M, Kilic BD, et al. Bartter syndrome and growth hormone deficiency: three cases. Pediatr Nephrol 2012;27:2145–8.
45. Flyvbjerg A, Dørup I, Everts ME, et al. Evidence that potassium deficiency induces growth retardation through reduced circulating levels of growth hormone and insulin-like growth factor I. Metabolism 1991;40:769–75.
46. Gil-Peña H, Garcia-Lopez E, Alvarez-Garcia O, et al. Alterations of growth plate and abnormal insulin-like growth factor I metabolism in growth-retarded hypokalemic rats: effect of growth hormone treatment. Am J Physiol Renal Physiol 2009; 297:639.
47. Requeira O, Rao J, Baliga R. Response to growth hormone in a child with Bartter's syndrome. Pediatr Nephrol 1991;5:671–2.
48. Richmond E, Rogol AD. Current indications for growth hormone therapy for children and adolescents. Endocr Dev 2010;18:92–108.
49. Kim JY, Kim GA, Song JH, et al. A case of living-related kidney transplantation in Bartter's syndrome. Yonsei Med J 2000;41:662–5.
50. Calò LA, Marchini F, Davis PA, et al. Kidney transplant in Gitelman's syndrome. Report of the first case. J Nephrol 2003;16:144–7.
51. Chaudhuri A, Salvatierra O, Alexander SR, et al. Option of pre-emptive nephrectomy and renal transplantation for Bartter's syndrome. Pediatr Transplant 2006; 10:266–70.

Renal Tubular Acidosis

Robert Todd Alexander, MD, PhD[a], Martin Bitzan, MD[b,c],*

KEYWORDS

- Acid–base homeostasis • Bicarbonate • Renal Fanconi syndrome • Hyperkalemia
- Nephrocalcinosis • Ammonium • Urine anion gap

KEY POINTS

- Renal tubular acidosis should be suspected in poorly thriving young children with hyperchloremic and hypokalemic (in case of renal tubular acidosis types 1–3) normal anion gap metabolic acidosis, with or without syndromic features.
- Further workup is needed to determine the type of renal tubular acidosis and the presumed etiopathogenesis (eg, genetic forms, drug-induced, or secondary to autoimmune disorders), which will inform the treatment choices and prognosis.
- The risk of nephrolithiasis and calcinosis is linked to the presence (proximal renal tubular acidosis, negligible stone risk) or absence (distal renal tubular acidosis, high stone risk) of urine citrate excretion.

INTRODUCTION

The acid–base status is tightly controlled in the human body. Any deviation affects the physiologic milieu of cellular membranes, intracellular signaling, and metabolism, resulting in acute and long-term consequences on the cardiovascular system, bone health, and other tissue functions. A key player in the maintenance of acid–base homeostasis are the kidneys. The term renal tubular acidosis (RTA) describes a group of disorders caused by defects in the molecular machinery of the renal tubules that facilitates the reabsorption of bicarbonate (HCO_3^-), the secretion of protons (H^+), or both.[1]

Disclosure Statement: Dr. Alexander is is the Canada Research Chair in Renal Epithelial Transport Physiology and work in his laboratory is funded by grants from the Women and Children Health Research Institute (WCHRI), which is supported by the Stollery Children's Hospital Foundation, the Canadian Institutes of Health Research (CIHR, MOP 136891), the National Sciences and Engineering Research Council and the Kidney Foundation of Canada.

[a] Department of Pediatrics and Physiology, Stollery Children's Hospital, 11405-87 Avenue, Edmonton, Alberta T6G 1C9, Canada; [b] Division of Nephrology, Department of Pediatrics, The Montreal Children's Hospital, McGill University Health Centre, Room B RC.6651, Montreal, Quebec H4A 3J1, Canada; [c] Al Jalila Children's Hospital, Al Jadaf PO Box 7662, Dubai, UAE
* Corresponding author. Division of Nephrology, Department of Pediatrics, The Montreal Children's Hospital, McGill University Health Centre, Room B RC.6651, Montreal, Quebec H4A 3J1, Canada.
E-mail address: martin.bitzan@mcgill.ca

Pediatr Clin N Am 66 (2019) 135–157
https://doi.org/10.1016/j.pcl.2018.08.011
0031-3955/19/© 2018 Elsevier Inc. All rights reserved.

pediatric.theclinics.com

An adult consuming a normal western diet generates about 1 mmol of H^+ per kilogram of body weight that needs to be disposed of in a regulated fashion; the amount is 2 to 3 mmol per kilogram of body weight in growing children.[2–4] The kidney ensures whole body HCO_3^- homeostasis by producing HCO_3^- de novo from metabolizable organic anions, primarily in the proximal tubule, but also in other nephron segments. The generation of 2 NH_4^+ in the proximal tubule results in the release 2 NH_4^+.[5] Physiologically, NH_4^+ is partitioned so that about 50% end up in the circulation (renal vein) and the other 50% in the lumen, which undergoes recycling. Intraluminal ammonia binds and excretes hydrogen ions in the form of ammonium. Disturbances of these regulatory mechanisms by mutations of critical transporter molecules, nephro (tubulo) toxic agents or urinary tract obstruction can lead to distinct acid–base imbalances and their long-term clinical consequences, summarily known as RTA.

PHYSIOLOGY OF ACID–BASE REGULATION WITH EMPHASIS ON THE ROLE OF THE KIDNEY
Regulation of Acid–Base Homeostasis

A consequence of performing metabolic work is the generation of protons (H^+). Biological systems function optimally at a narrow pH range. It is, therefore, necessary for an organism to eliminate H^+ to maintain this homeostasis. Mammals, including humans, have adopted 3 general mechanisms to maintain the pH within this narrow physiologic range. The first is to produce and maintain an adequate supply of buffer, both within and outside of cells. The most important intracellular buffers are phosphate and proteins. The major extracellular buffer is bicarbonate. However, mineral bone is composed of hydroxyapatite ($Ca_{10}(PO_4)_6(OH)_2$), which can contribute buffer under acidotic conditions. The second mechanism regulating pH is respiration. Bicarbonate is in equilibrium with carbon dioxide and water ($HCO_3^- + H^+ \leftarrow \rightarrow H_2O + CO_2$); both of the substances on the right side of the equilibrium are expelled via the lungs. Consequently, alterations in respiration rapidly adjust plasma pH. Finally, the kidney eliminates protons directly in the urine, but also serves to generate new bicarbonate and to prevent it from being lost in the urine. These processes are outlined elsewhere in this article.

Proximal Renal Tubule and Bicarbonate Reabsorption

Bicarbonate is freely filtered at the glomerulus and must be reabsorbed to prevent its loss in the urine. The majority of bicarbonate is reabsorbed from the proximal tubule. This process depends on the secretion of acid into the proximal tubular lumen. The majority of protons are extruded in exchange for a sodium ion via the epithelial (apical) sodium proton (hydrogen) exchanger[6] isoform 3 (NHE3). A smaller quantity of protons is extruded into the lumen of this segment via a plasma membrane $H^+ATPase$.[7] Importantly in neonates and potentially older animals,[8] sodium proton exchange in the proximal tubule can also be mediated by NHE8, although this does not completely compensate for the loss of NHE3. The luminal conversion of H^+ and HCO_3^- into CO_2 and H_2O is facilitated by carbonic anhydrase 4 (CA4).[9,10]

$$H_+ + HCO_3 \rightleftarrows H_2CO_3 \overset{CA4}{\underset{CA2}{\rightleftarrows}} H_2O + CO_2$$

Water is then reabsorbed through aquaporin-1, which is expressed in the luminal and basolateral membrane of the proximal tubular cells.[8,11] Carbon dioxide does not require a protein transport mechanism to move across the cells; it is noteworthy, however, that aquaporin-1 has also been reported to facilitate transmembrane CO_2

movement.[12,13] Cytosolic carbonic anhydrase 2 (CA2) catalyzes intracellular H_2O and CO_2 back into a H^+ and HCO_3^-.[14,15] The proton is recycled across the apical membrane, whereas HCO_3^- is extruded together with Na^+ across the basolateral membrane via the electrogenic sodium bicarbonate cotransporter NBCe1 (solute linked carrier 4 A4; encoded by *SLC4A4*)[16–18] (**Fig. 1**). Bicarbonate escaping the proximal tubule[19] can be reclaimed by the thick ascending limb via a similar process involving NHE3.

Distal Nephron and Acid Secretion

Acid (proton) secretion occurs from type A (alpha) intercalated cells in the connecting tubule and collecting duct. Its secretion is mediated by the apically expressed plasma membrane H^+ATPase. H^+ is generated in the cytosol via conversion of H_2O and CO_2 into a proton and bicarbonate, a process catalyzed by carbonic anhydrase isoform 2, CA2.[15,20] This de novo–generated bicarbonate leaves the cell via the anion exchanger 1 (AE1, gene name *SLC4A1*) in the basolateral membrane.[21,22] Consequently, not only is acid extruded, but base is also generated via this process. H^+ is "trapped" in the

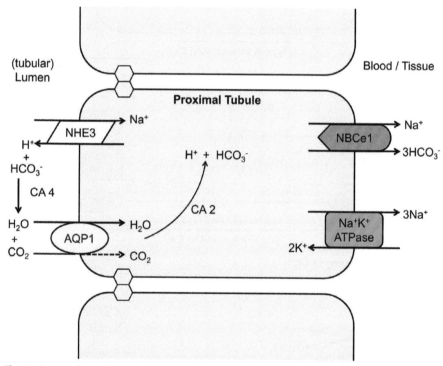

Fig. 1. Proximal tubule reabsorption of bicarbonate. The majority of filtered bicarbonate (HCO_3^-) is reabsorbed from the proximal tubule. It is first enzymatically converted to water and carbon dioxide (CO_2) by carbonic anhydrase 4 (CA4). The proton (H^+) is provided in exchange for sodium (Na^+) by the sodium protein exchanger isoform 3 (NHE3). Intracellular (cytosolic) CA2 converts water and CO_2 back into a proton, which is recycled via NHE3, and bicarbonate is extruded across the basolateral membrane of the cell, back into the circulation via the sodium bicarbonate cotransporter 1 (NBCe1). AQP1, aquaporin-1. (*Adapted from* Alexander RT, Bockenhauer D. Renal tubular acidosis. In: Geary DF, Schaefer F, editors. Pediatric kidney disease. Berlin: Springer; 2016. p. 973–91.)

lumen of the collecting duct through binding with ammonia (NH_3) to generate ammonium (NH_4^+)[19] (**Fig. 2**).

This buffering process is essential to maximize urinary acid excretion. Ammonia is concentrated in the lumen of the collecting duct via a recycling mechanism.[23] It is first generated from glutamine in the mitochondria of the proximal tubule and extruded into

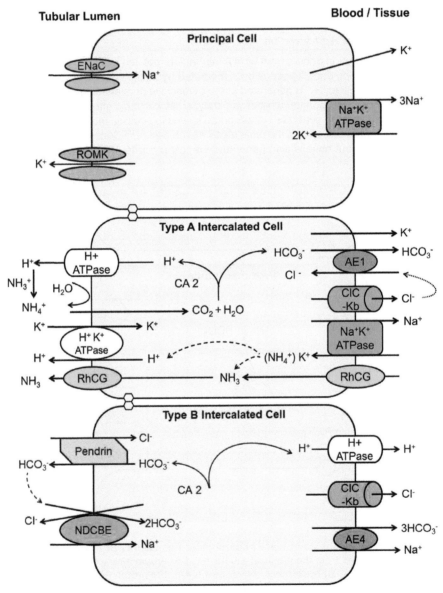

Fig. 2. Acid secretion in the collecting duct (CCD). Epithelial cells are depicted with their major physiologic roles in sodium, potassium, and acid–base regulation. AE1, anion exchanger 1 (SLC4A1); AE4, anion exchanger 4 (SLC4A9); ClC-Kb, chloride channel Kb; ENaC, epithelial sodium channel; NDCBE, sodium-driven chloride/bicarbonate exchanger; RhCG, Rhesus family C glycoprotein; ROMK, renal outer medullary potassium channel.

the tubular lumen via a sodium proton exchange mechanism.[24,25] This process also generates bicarbonate de novo. Luminal ammonium is absorbed across the epithelial cells in the loop of Henle and concentrated in the medullary interstitium.[26] Ammonia can then diffuse into the lumen of the collecting duct, down its concentration gradient, a process mediated by the Rhesus family C glycoprotein, a relative of the red blood cell antigen,[23] and combine with secreted protons to form ammonium (see **Fig. 2**).

CLINICAL MANIFESTATIONS AND BIOCHEMICAL FEATURES
Distal Renal Tubular Acidosis (Type 1 Renal Tubular Acidosis)

Type 1 (distal) RTA (dRTA) was the first form of RTA described.[1] It was reported as a clinical entity in 1935[27]; the designation as dRTA followed in 1951.[1,28] As the names imply, this tubular disorder is owing to the failure to secrete protons from type A intercalated cells in the connecting tubule and collecting duct.[1] It can be caused by several conditions including single gene defects, autoimmune diseases, such as Sjögren syndrome, drugs, or systemic disorders.[1,29–32] Drugs implicated in causing type 1 RTA include amphotericin B, vanadate, ifosfamide, lithium, and foscarnet. Distal RTA has also been seen in association with primary hyperparathyroidism and medullary sponge kidney (**Box 1**).[33] In (young) children presenting with type 1 RTA, single gene defects should be considered. Not surprisingly, given its requirement for the acidification of urine, mutations in 2 of the subunits of the plasma membrane H^+ATPase, $\alpha 4$ (gene name *ATPV0A4*) and $\beta 1$ (gene name *ATPV1B1*) or the anion exchanger isoform 1, AE1 (gene name *SLC4A1*) can cause isolated dRTA.[34–40] Mutation in carbonic anhydrase isoform 2 (gene name *CA2*) results in a mixed picture of both proximal renal tubular acidosis (pRTA) and dRTA.[14]

Children with genetic forms of dRTA present with failure to thrive and/or complications of the metabolic abnormalities caused by the disease. Blood tests typically demonstrate a normal anion gap metabolic acidosis (**Box 2**), often with hypokalemia.[41] These children have an inappropriately alkaline urine despite an acidic blood pH. dRTA is also commonly associated with hypercalciuria, nephrocalcinosis and/or nephrolithiasis (reviewed in[42]). Therefore, evaluation of pediatric kidney stone formers should include a blood gas analysis. Autosomal-recessive forms of dRTA are due to mutations in *ATP6V1B1* or *ATP6V0A4* that encode the $\beta 1$ and $\alpha 4$ subunits of the apical (vacuolar) H^+ ATPase.[40] These proteins are also expressed in the cochlea and endolymphatic sac of the ear.[37] Consequently, children with a mutation in either subunit suffer from sensorineural hearing loss.[37,40,43] Audiometry results may point to the molecular diagnosis and guide genetic testing. The described genetic defect can lead to distinct endolymphatic sac enlargement that can be recognized by an MRI of the inner ear.[44] Mutations of AE1 cause autosomal dominant or recessive dRTA.[35,45,46] A slightly longer isoform of AE1 is expressed in red blood cells. Owing to differential processing in red blood cells and type A intercalated cells, mutations in *AE1* typically cause only one disease or the other.[45] Patients with autosomal-dominant AE1 mutations tend to present later (ie, in adolescence or adulthood) and with less severe hypokalemia than those with autosomal recessive mutations; the latter are less common, cause more severe disease, and are more likely to be associated with hemolytic anemia.[47,48]

Autosomal-dominant mutations of AE1 can also underlie incomplete dRTA,[47] a term that describes individuals with normal acid–base status under physiologic conditions, but an inability to appropriately acidify their urine after an acid load. It

---

Box 1
Etiologies of distal (type 1) RTA

Primary/hereditary distal renal tubular acidosis (see Table 1)

Genetic abnormalities of the (apical) H^+ ATPase subunits

Variants of the gene encoding the (basolateral) anion exchanger 1 (AE1)

Variants of the gene encoding the cytosolic carbonic anhydrase 2

Autoimmune disorders

Sjögren syndrome

Lupus erythematosus

Autoimmune hepatitis

Rheumatoid arthritis

Polyarteritis nodosa

Nephrotoxic medications

Amphotericin B

Lithium, mercury

Trimethoprim

Ifosfamide

Vanadate

Foscarnet

Nonsteroidal analgesics

Hypercalciuria/nephrocalcinosis

Primary hyperparathyroidism

Hypothyroidism

Medullary sponge kidney

Tubular interstitial disorders

Obstructive uropathy

Pyelonephritis

Interstitial nephritis

Sickle cell disease

Others

Human immunodeficiency virus-associated nephropathy

Sarcoidosis

Amyloidosis

---

typically requires an ammonium chloride challenge or furosemide test to make this diagnosis.[31] Interestingly, patients with incomplete dRTA may also present with kidney stones, and dRTA should be considered in the differential diagnosis of hypercalciuria and nephrolithiasis.[36,45,49] Only recently have heterozygous mutations of the H^+ATPase β1 and α4 subunits been associated with incomplete dRTA[50,51] **(Table 1).**

> **Box 2**
> **Serum anion gap**
>
> The ionic balance is generally tightly regulated. For example, the loss of the anion bicarbonate leads to the displacement of chloride into the extracellular compartment.[127]
>
> The serum anion gap is calculated to estimate the concentrations of active ions using serum sodium, chloride and bicarbonate measurements that are readily available in clinical laboratories. Various components are not directly measured; hence the equation does not result in 0. The "gap" reflects unmeasured anions.
>
> $$\text{Serum anion gap} = Na^+ - (HCO_3^- + Cl^-)$$
>
> A normal serum anion gap is 12 to 16 mmol/L. The serum anion gap is increased in the presence of (unmeasured) ketones, lactate, salicylate, methanol, and so on.

Proximal Renal Tubular Acidosis (Type 2 Renal Tubular Acidosis)

Type 2 or pRTA is caused by a defect in proximal tubular bicarbonate reabsorption. Bicarbonate loss in the urine results in a normal anion gap metabolic acidosis. Hypokalemia is also present, similar to dRTA. However, distal acidification mechanisms remain in place allowing the patient to produce an acidic urine, that is, a urine pH of less than 5.5, when plasma bicarbonate concentrations are below the tubular reabsorption threshold. In contrast with distal tubular acidosis, patients with isolated pRTA do not develop nephrocalcinosis or kidney stones, likely because proximal citrate reabsorption is inhibited by alkaline luminal pH, which ensures sufficient urinary citrate excretion.[42,52–54]

Isolated pRTA is rare. The only known genetic abnormality underlying this disorder are mutations in the sodium bicarbonate cotransporter 1 (NBCe1, gene name *SLC4A4*). Children with this condition also have ocular abnormalities, such as band cataract, glaucoma, or band keratopathy[52,53,55,56] (see **Table 1**).

pRTA is more commonly seen as part of the renal Fanconi syndrome. The latter refers to a disorder of global proximal tubular dysfunction characterized by hypophosphatemia, glucosuria, low molecular weight proteinuria and amino aciduria in addition to (proximal) tubular acidosis. Examples of genetic diseases with prominent pRTA are nephropathic cystinosis, Lowe syndrome. and others, usually with a plethora of additional pathologies.[57,58] Acquired conditions include exposure to ifosfamide, cisplatin, and other tubulotoxic medications[59,60] (**Box 3**).

Combined (Mixed) Renal Tubular Acidosis (Type 3 Renal Tubular Acidosis)

Type 3 RTA combines clinical features of proximal and dRTA. It is a rare autosomal-recessive disorder that manifests with osteopetrosis, cerebral calcifications, nephrocalcinosis and nephrolithiasis, facial dysmorphism (hypertelorism, low set ears, and a depressed nasal bridge), conductive hearing loss and cognitive impairment.[61–64] The only known cause of this disease is a mutation in CA2.[14,65] The role of CA2 in proximal tubule bicarbonate absorption and in distal proton secretion accounts for the combined types of metabolic acidosis. CA2 is essential for osteoclast function, hence the overmineralization, that is, osteopetrosis.

Renal Tubular Acidosis with Hyperkalemia (Type 4 Renal Tubular Acidosis)

In contrast with RTA types 1 to 3, the defining feature of type 4 RTA is a high normal or increased plasma potassium level, not hypokalemia. Affected patients also have a normal anion gap metabolic acidosis. The primary abnormality is actual or effective hypoaldosteronism.[66] It results in sodium wasting from the collecting duct. Because

Table 1
Genetic causes of RTA

Protein Name	Gene Name	MIM #	Inheritance	Typical Clinical Features	Type of RTA
NBCe1	SLC4A4	603345, 604278	AR	Glaucoma, cataracts, band keratopathy	pRTA (type 2)
AE1	SLC4A1	109270, 179800, 611590	AD (less commonly AR)	Nephrocalcinosis, osteomalacia, rarely hemolytic anemia	dRTA (type 1)
β1 subunit of the H⁺ATPase	ATP6V1B1	267300	AR	Sensorineural hearing loss, nephrocalcinosis or nephrolithiasis	dRTA (type 1)
α4 subunit of the H⁺ATPase	ATP6V0A4	602722, 605239	AR	Late-onset sensorineural hearing loss, nephrocalcinosis or nephrolithiasis	dRTA (type 1)
CA2	CA2	611492, 259730	AR	Osteopetrosis	Combined distal/proximal RTA (type 3)

Abbreviations: AD, autosomal dominant; AR, autosomal recessive; *ATP6V0A4*, ATPase H + transporting V0 subunit A4; *ATP6V1B1*, ATPase H + transporting V1 subunit B1; CA2, *carbonic anhydrase 2*; dRTA, distal renal tubular acidosis; NBCe1, sodium bicarbonate cotransporter 1; RTA, renal tubular acidosis; SLC, solute-linked carrier.

Box 3
Etiologies of proximal (type 2) renal tubular acidosis

Isolated (primary) proximal renal tubular acidosis (see also Table 1)

Variants of the gene encoding the (basolateral) proximal
tubular sodium bicarbonate cotransporter sodium bicarbonate cotransporter 1[a]

Inherited disorders with (secondary) Fanconi syndrome

Cystinosis

Lowe syndrome

Wilson disease

Autoimmune disorders

Sjögren syndrome

Nephrotoxic medications

Ifosfamide

Cisplatin

Topiramate

Valproate

Acetazolamide

Aminoglycosides

Tetracyclines

Lead

Tubular interstitial disorders

Obstructive uropathy

Medullary cystic kidney disease

Others

Hypocalcemia

Amyloidosis

Multiple myeloma

Monoclonal gammopathy

Light chain deposition disease

[a] Associated with glaucoma, cataracts, or band keratopathy.

---

potassium and proton secretion in the collecting duct is coupled in this part of the nephron to sodium reabsorption (mainly via the principal cells), type 4 RTA results in hyperkalemic acidosis. Sodium reabsorption in the collecting duct occurs mainly through the aldosterone-regulated epithelial sodium channel ENaC. Normal ENaC function results in a lumen negative membrane potential that is, attenuated both by potassium secretion (through the renal outer medullary potassium channel) and by proton secretion by the plasma membrane $H^+ATPase$. Consequently, a failure to reabsorb sodium from the collecting duct also prevents H^+ secretion leading to metabolic acidosis (see **Fig. 2**).

A wide variety of conditions has been implicated in type 4 RTA in childhood.[31] The distally active diuretics spironolactone, amiloride, and triamterene cause RTA through their effects on collecting duct principal cells. Spironolactone and triamterene block (or compete with) the mineralocorticoid receptor leading to diminished ENaC expression, whereas amiloride blocks ENaC directly.[67] Type 4 RTA is also observed in patients with obstructive uropathy, pyelonephritis and, occasionally, lupus nephritis (**Box 4**). Genetic forms of hyperkalemic (type 4) RTA are known as pseudo-hypoaldosteronism because the plasma and urine electrolyte pattern resemble absence of aldosterone. Nevertheless, these patients typically present with increased serum aldosterone (and renin) concentrations.[68]

Box 4
Etiologies of hyperkalemic (type 4) renal tubular acidosis

Renal genetic causes

Variants of genes encoding proteins involved in the regulation of the epithelial sodium channel, including the mineralocorticoid receptor and intracellular signaling molecules

Bartter syndrome type 2

Adrenal insufficiency

Congenital adrenal hyperplasia (21-hydroxylase deficiency)

Adrenal suppression (hypoxia, sepsis)

Autoimmune adrenalitis

Addison disease

Autoimmune/related disorders

Lupus nephritis

Renal amyloidosis

Medication induced

Amiloride

Spironolactone

Triamterene

Eplerenone

Angiotensin-converting enzyme inhibitors

Angiotensin receptor blockers

Prostaglandin inhibitors

Calcineurin inhibitors (cyclosporine A, tacrolimus)

Nonsteroidal anti-inflammatory drugs

Heparin

Trimethoprim

Intrinsic renal disease

Chronic kidney disease

Obstructive uropathy

Pyelonephritis

Interstitial nephritis

Kidney transplant

This list is not comprehensive; association with various other diseases have been reported.

Type 1 pseudohypoaldosteronism is due to mineralocorticoid resistance. Patients display low blood pressure, hyponatremia, and hyperkalemia. There are 2 clinically distinct subtypes. The milder version is inherited as an autosomal-dominant condition and is due to loss of function mutations in the mineralocorticoid receptor gene NR3C2.[69,70] The more severe form is inherited as an autosomal-dominant disease. It is caused by mutations in 1 of the 3 ENaC subunits, either alpha, beta, or gamma,[71–74] and affects multiple tissues resulting in increased sodium concentration of sweat, saliva, and airway secretions. This has led at times to the erroneous diagnosis of cystic fibrosis.

Pseudohypoaldosteronism type II, also known as Gordon's syndrome, is a disorder characterized by hypertension and hyperkalemic RTA. Patients with this diagnosis have chloride-dependent sodium retention, and hypertension that is, very sensitive to thiazide therapy.[75] Thiazides inhibit sodium reabsorption through the sodium chloride cotransporter (NCC) in the distal convoluted tubule, upstream from the collecting duct. The pathogenesis of this disease involves increased sodium and chloride reabsorption from the distal convoluted tubule via NCC. Mutations in a number of genes including WNK1, WNK4, KLHL3, and CUL3 have been identified in patients with this condition.[76–79] The encoded proteins have all been implicated in the regulation of NCC activity or expression. The described mutations cause the stimulation NCC or prevention of its degradation, leading to increased sodium reabsorption from the distal convoluted tubule, volume expansion, and hypertension.[31] This process inhibits sodium reabsorption from the collecting duct and consequently potassium and proton excretion, that is, a hyperkalemic metabolic acidosis.

ACIDOSIS AND URINARY CALCIUM EXCRETION
Effect of Acidosis on Bone

Both acute and chronic metabolic acidosis (such as RTA) cause increased urinary calcium excretion. This is not likely due to increased intestinal calcium absorption, but a result of direct effects on bone.[80,81] There is an acute physiochemical effect and a more chronic cellular response. Bone is covered with negatively charged sites that bind both sodium and potassium. Protons can be exchanged acutely with these monovalent cations. Protons can rapidly dissolve hydroxyapatite and thereby buffer plasma pH and release calcium into blood and the urine.[82,83] Prolonged ($\geq$24 h) exposure to acid inhibits osteoblast and stimulates osteoclast activity,[84–86] which results in further calcium release from bone and calciuria.

Effect of Acidosis on the Renal Tubule

Metabolic acidosis causes calciuria via 2 mechanisms: the first is dissolution of bone and release of calcium into the circulation. This process results in increased glomerular filtration and decreased tubular reabsorption of calcium through feedback inhibition by elevated plasma calcium levels on the tubule (for a review, see[87]). The second mechanism is a direct effect of low cellular pH in the distal nephron. Although filtered calcium is reabsorbed predominantly from the proximal tubule and the thick ascending limb by a passive paracellular process, the ultimate amount of urinary calcium excretion is finely regulated in the distal convoluted and connecting tubule. This process occurs via an active transcellular process mediated by apical calcium influx through the calcium channel TRPV5.[88] Metabolic acidosis decreases calcium reabsorption from the distal nephron via decreasing TRPV5 expression.[89–92] Studies in TRPV5 knockout mice suggest that acidosis (ie, increased distal tubular cytosolic pH) directly impairs distal transcellular calcium reabsorption.[92]

Renal Tubular Acidosis and Urinary Calcium Excretion

Given the previous discussion, patients with type 2 RTA would be expected to develop hypercalciuria, nephrolithiasis, and nephrocalcinosis as is observed in patients with type 1 RTA.[93] This is not, however, the case. This seeming discrepancy has been explained in part by the differences in urinary citrate excretion.[42] Citrate binds calcium and prevents it from precipitating as a calcium oxalate or calcium phosphate salt. A luminal alkaline pH found in RTA type 2 patients inhibits proximal tubular citrate reabsorption, which enhances the urinary excretion of citrate.[94] Patients with pRTA thus have increased urinary citrate, which might prevent the precipitation of calcium along the tubule. Moreover, increased luminal pH in the distal nephron might also enhance TRPV5 activity resulting in increased calcium reabsorption and decreased urinary calcium excretion.[95]

DIAGNOSIS AND DIFFERENTIAL DIAGNOSES OF RENAL TUBULAR ACIDOSIS

The presence of hypokalemic hyperchloremic metabolic acidosis and a normal plasma anion gap in a patient with a normal glomerular filtration rate are suggestive of RTA. A similar electrolyte constellation can be seen in patients with gastrointestinal bicarbonate losses, for example, owing to profuse watery diarrhea, pancreatic fistula, nasojejunal suctioning, or chronic laxative use. Children with RTA may present with poor growth, volume depletion, fatigue, or lethargy. Alternatively, RTA may be diagnosed incidentally owing to an abnormal blood gas analysis.[96]

Distal Renal Tubular Acidosis

Type 1 RTA is defined by the inability of the distal tubular segments to adequately acidify the urine, which leads to inappropriately alkalized urine in the presence of metabolic acidosis. Patients typically present with hyperchloremic normal serum anion gap metabolic acidosis and hypokalemia, hypercalciuria, and normal glomerular filtration rate. Patients may also demonstrate nephrocalcinosis. The key feature of dRTA is the inability of the kidney to excrete protons as ammonium (NH_4^+). Some authors suggest that the ammonium excretion be used for the classification of RTAs.[97] Hypokalemia of dRTA is partly due to increased secretion through the apical renal outer medullary potassium channel to support ENaC mediated Na^+ reabsorption (see **Fig. 2**) and augmented by aldosterone secretion owing to volume depletion. Hypokalemia can be severe and occasionally present as muscle paralysis.[98]

Of note, pRTA may also present with inappropriately high urine pH at plasma bicarbonate concentrations above the bicarbonate threshold. The definite diagnosis of dRTA requires demonstration of the acidification defect, which is commonly done indirectly, by calculating the urine anion gap as a surrogate for ammonium measurements in the urine[99–101] (**Box 5**). A negligible or positive urine anion gap in the context of metabolic acidosis is suggestive of dRTA reflecting the absence of ammonium excretion[102] (**Fig. 3**).

The diagnosis of dRTA is relatively straightforward when the child presents with classical clinical and biochemical findings. Incomplete forms of dRTA can pose a diagnostic challenge, because the urine acidification defect is only apparent after a physiologic challenge. Two diagnostic studies have been used to confirm the diagnosis, either loading with ammonium chloride[90,100,102] or the administration of a loop diuretic, for example, furosemide.[102–104] In the first scenario, patients with (incomplete) dRTA will develop metabolic acidosis owing to a lack of proton secretion in the collecting duct (**Fig. 4**). In the second scenario, the loop diuretic will lead to increased distal

---

Box 5
Urine anion gap (UAG)

Calculation of the urine anion gap is an indirect method to estimate urinary ammonium (NH_4^+) excretion. UAG is only useful (and valid) for the differential diagnosis of patients with normal anion gap hyperchloremic metabolic acidosis (NAGMA).[1,99–102]
It is determined by subtracting the sum of easily measurable anions from the sum of cations in the urine. The formula resembles the determination of the plasma anion gap.
$UAG = Na^+ + K^+ - Cl^-$
Note: In relatively acidic urine (pH < 6.5), the urine bicarbonate concentration (U [HCO_3^-]) is essentially zero and its effect on the UAG is, therefore, negligible.
Unmeasured, and generally negligible are the urine anions sulfate and phosphate and the cations calcium and magnesium. NH_4^+ constitutes the major urine cation, and its excretion is accompanied by chloride as $NH_4^+Cl^-$.
Systemic metabolic acidosis leads physiologically to large urinary ammonium excretion, which serves to trap secreted protons. It is identified by a negative UAG owing to the increased Cl^- excretion that accompanies the unmeasured cation NH_4^+. This scenario is commonly seen in children with severe diarrhea and NAGMA or after acid or NH_4Cl loading.
A small or positive UAG in a patient with NAGMA indicates failure to acidify the urine (see example).
The UAG helps to diagnose patients with proximal renal tubular acidosis when the plasma bicarbonate level is below the bicarbonate threshold. The UAG is negative, because the distal acidification mechanism (proton secretion by type A intercalated cells) is intact.
NH_4^+ excretion and UAG calculation in a study with human volunteers and patients[a]

Group	Net Acid (μmol/min)	U pH	U NH_4^+ (mmol/L)	U Na^+	U K^+	U Cl^-	UAG
Healthy controls	26	6.0	14	NA	NA	NA	41
Controls, acid loaded[b]	73	4.9	35	119	86	233	−27
Diarrhea	59	5.6	42	31	25	76	−20
Type 1 renal tubular acidosis	7.2	6.5	7	70	35	79	23
Type 4 renal tubular acidosis	31	6.1	9	64	23	57	30

Urine bicarbonate and protons are in equilibrium with water and CO_2. Urine pH and [HCO_3^-] must be measured in a fresh sample, ideally saved under oil to prevent diffusion of CO_2, which leads to a shift of the equation to the right and an increase in pH.
 [a] Extracted from Batlle et al.[100]
 [b] Controls received ammonium chloride for 3 days.

Na^+ uptake via ENaC, which creates a favorable gradient for proton secretion by the neighboring type A intercalated cells in the collecting duct (see **Fig. 2**). The procedure has been standardized by the additional administration of a mineralocorticoid, for example, fludrocortisone.[102–104] With both studies, patients with dRTA fail to acidify their urine (see **Fig. 4**).

The differential diagnoses of primary dRTA include acquired disorders, such as autoimmune diseases, idiopathic hypercalciuria, nephrocalcinosis, or nephrotoxic medications (see **Box 1**). Patients with suspected or proven dRTA should undergo audiometry (see **Table 1**).

Proximal (Type 2) Renal Tubular Acidosis

Tubular losses of bicarbonate typically lead to alkaline urine owing to defective (restricted) proximal tubular reabsorption. Distal delivery of nonreabsorbed anion (HCO_3^-) obligates the excretion of Na^+ and K^+, which leads to volume depletion, compensatory aldosterone secretion, and (additional) potassium loss in the urine. However, when the plasma bicarbonate concentration falls below the threshold of tubular

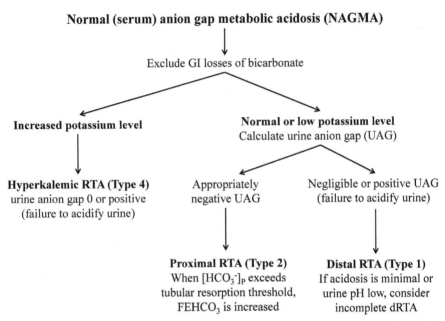

Fig. 3. Algorithm to aid in the differentiation between normal anion gap metabolic acidosis (NAGMA) owing to renal (renal tubular acidosis [RTA]) or extrarenal causes. dRTA, distal renal tubular acidosis; FEHCO₃, fractional excretion of bicarbonate; GI, gastrointestinal.

bicarbonate reabsorption, the urine pH decreases to or less than 5.5, because the distal nephron (collecting duct) maintains the ability to acidify the urine. This differentiates pRTA from dRTA. To diagnose pRTA definitively, tubular bicarbonate reabsorption (or fractional excretion of bicarbonate) is assessed at high and low plasma bicarbonate

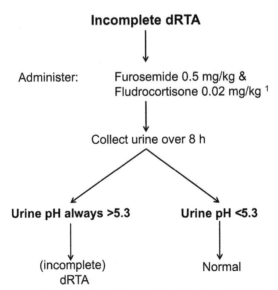

Fig. 4. Diagnostic approach to (suspected) incomplete distal renal tubular acidosis (dRTA). For practical details, see text. (*Adapted from* Alexander RT, Bockenhauer D. Renal tubular acidosis. In: Geary DF, Schaefer F, editors. Pediatric kidney disease. Berlin: Springer; 2016. p. 973–91.)

concentrations. A fractional excretion greater than 15% (or some authors even suggest >5%)[31,105] in the presence of a metabolic acidosis is diagnostic (**Box 6**).

Tubular bicarbonate excretion can be measured while infusing NaHCO$_3$. Sodium bicarbonate is administered intravenously to increase blood bicarbonate concentrations by 2 mmol/L until urine pH exceeds 5.8. Urine bicarbonate excretion increases at a specific serum bicarbonate concentration, which indicates the bicarbonate threshold[31,106] (see **Box 6**). The physiologic bicarbonate threshold is approximately 22 mmol/L in infants and 25 mmol/L in older children.[106,107] A threshold of less than 20 mmol/L is consistent with pRTA. To rationalize this concept, if the bicarbonate threshold is 16 mmol/L, the patient will stop losing bicarbonate and be able to acidify the urine to less than 5.5 at a plasma HCO$_3^-$ concentration of less than or equal to 16 mmol/L. Detailed protocols for functional testing can be found elsewhere.[102]

MANAGEMENT AND PROGNOSIS OF CHILDREN WITH RENAL TUBULAR ACIDOSIS
Treatment of Children with Distal Renal Tubular Acidosis

Treatment goals are adequate growth and prevention of bony abnormalities, kidney stones, and nephrocalcinosis.[41,59] Hypercalciuria is associated with hypocitruria in patients with dRTA.[108] Alkali therapy is preferably prescribed in the form of potassium or Na/K citrate. Rarely is alkali therapy in excess of 5 mmol/kg/d needed to correct the metabolic acidosis.[41] The ENaC blocker amiloride may be offered to patients with persistent hypokalemia. A comprehensive, interdisciplinary approach is recommended for children with dRTA complicated by hearing loss, hemolytic anemia, or kidney stones.

Treatment of Children with Proximal Renal Tubular Acidosis

The first-line treatment for patients with isolated (genetic) pRTA is supplementation of alkali losses.[109,110] Efforts to increase plasma bicarbonate concentrations are especially relevant in growing children. Depending on the individual bicarbonate threshold, patients may need large quantities of alkali to normalize the blood pH, generally 5 to 15 mmol/kg/d.[59] The amount of bicarbonate required can be decreased by adding a thiazide diuretic.[111] Thiazide-induced inhibition of the apical NaCl cotransporter

---

Box 6
Fractional excretion of bicarbonate

Calculating the fractional excretion of bicarbonate (FEHCO$_3$) is useful in the differential diagnosis of suspected renal tubular acidosis.

$$FEHCO_3\ (\%) = \frac{[HCO_3]_U \times [Cr]_S}{[HCO_3]_S \times [Cr]_U} \times 100$$

Tubular bicarbonate reabsorption (or conversely, fractional excretion of bicarbonate) is assessed at high and low serum HCO$_3^-$ concentrations.

A FEHCO$_3$ of greater than 15% (or by some authors even >5%) in the presence of metabolic acidosis is diagnostic for proximal renal tubular acidosis.[31,105]

To confirm the diagnosis, serum HCO$_3^-$ is increased to 18 or 20 mmol/L with an intravenous infusion of NaHCO$_3$ at 0.5 to 1 mmol/kg/h. The urine pH (initially expected to be low) will increase to greater than or equal to 7.5 when the threshold for HCO$_3$ reabsorption is reached. In patients with proximal renal tubular acidosis, the FEHCO$_3$ will exceed 15% or 20% as determined by this formula. Online calculators are available.

NCC in the distal convoluted tubule results in mild volume depletion, which is thought to increase bicarbonate reabsorption in the loop of Henle and the proximal tubule. Unfortunately, this therapy can worsen preexisting hypokalemia, because it will increase sodium flow to the collecting duct and enhance sodium absorption there, consequently increasing K excretion. K^+ (and alkali) supplementation is preferably given in the form of potassium citrate.[31]

Treatment of Children with Type 4 Renal Tubular Acidosis

Therapeutic management depends on the etiology of the disorder. Underlying kidney diseases should be treated, for example, effective intermittent catherization in children with a dysfunctional bladder. In addition, offending medications should be discontinued. The plasma pH can be corrected with alkali therapy using sodium salts, which may be supplemented with additional NaCl in the presence of sodium wasting. Thiazide diuretics are effective in patients with pseudohypoaldosteronism type 2 (Gordon syndrome).[75,112,113]

Prognosis of Proximal and Distal Renal Tubular Acidosis

Data on the long-term outcome of children with isolated pRTA are limited, owing to the rarity of this disease. Chronic kidney disease and end-stage renal disease have not been reported (in contrast with dRTA). Whereas high-dose alkali therapy and other measures improve plasma pH and growth, normal plasma bicarbonate concentrations are difficult to maintain in pRTA.[114] The prognosis of renal Fanconi syndrome is varied and depends on its etiology. Details can be found elsewhere.[60,115–118]

The prognosis of dRTA, if diagnosed and treated early, is favorable with preserved glomerular filtration rate and improved growth.[119,120] However, delayed diagnosis and persistent acidosis may result in growth impairment, severe bone deformities and, rarely chronic kidney disease.[119,121–124] Alkali therapy does not improve or prevent hearing loss.[125] The outcome of acquired forms of both proximal and dRTA depends on the treatment of the etiology, including the protection from repeated exposure.[126]

SUMMARY

RTA should be suspected in poorly thriving young children with hyperchloremic and hypokalemic (in case of RTA types 1–3) normal anion gap metabolic acidosis, with or without syndromic features. Further workup is needed to determine the type of RTA and the presumed etiopathogenesis (eg, genetic forms, drug-induced, or secondary to autoimmune disorders), which will inform the treatment choices and prognosis. The risk of nephrolithiasis and calcinosis is linked to the presence (pRTA, negligible stone risk) or absence (dRTA, high stone risk) of urine citrate excretion. New formulations of slow-release alkali and potassium combination supplements are currently being tested that are expected to simplify treatment and lead to sustained acidosis correction compared with traditional supplements.

ACKNOWLEDGMENTS

The authors thank Mr. Giuseppe Pascale for help with the artwork.

REFERENCES

1. Rodriguez Soriano J. Renal tubular acidosis: the clinical entity. J Am Soc Nephrol 2002;13(8):2160–70.
2. Halperin ML, Jungas RL. Metabolic production and renal disposal of hydrogen ions. Kidney Int 1983;24(6):709–13.

3. Kildeberg P, Engel K, Winters RW. Balance of net acid in growing infants. Endogenous and transintestinal aspects. Acta Paediatr Scand 1969;58(4): 321–9.

4. Chan JC. The influence of dietary intake on endogenous acid production. Theoretical and experimental background. Nutr Metab 1974;16(1):1–9.

5. Kurtz I. Molecular mechanisms and regulation of urinary acidification. Compr Physiol 2014;4(4):1737–74.

6. Schultheis PJ, Clarke LL, Meneton P, et al. Renal and intestinal absorptive defects in mice lacking the NHE3 Na^+/H^+ exchanger. Nat Genet 1998;19(3): 282–5.

7. Zimolo Z, Montrose MH, Murer H. H+ extrusion by an apical vacuolar-type H(+)-ATPase in rat renal proximal tubules. J Membr Biol 1992;126(1):19–26.

8. Schnermann J, Chou CL, Ma T, et al. Defective proximal tubular fluid reabsorption in transgenic aquaporin-1 null mice. Proc Natl Acad Sci U S A 1998;95(16): 9660–4.

9. Rector FC Jr, Carter NW, Seldin DW. The mechanism of bicarbonate reabsorption in the proximal and distal tubules of the kidney. J Clin Invest 1965;44: 278–90.

10. Brown D, Zhu XL, Sly WS. Localization of membrane-associated carbonic anhydrase type IV in kidney epithelial cells. Proc Natl Acad Sci U S A 1990;87(19): 7457–61.

11. Vallon V, Verkman AS, Schnermann J. Luminal hypotonicity in proximal tubules of aquaporin-1-knockout mice. Am J Physiol Renal Physiol 2000;278(6): F1030–3.

12. Cooper GJ, Boron WF. Effect of PCMBS on CO_2 permeability of Xenopus oocytes expressing aquaporin 1 or its C189S mutant. Am J Physiol 1998;275(6 Pt 1):C1481–6.

13. Endeward V, Musa-Aziz R, Cooper GJ, et al. Evidence that aquaporin 1 is a major pathway for CO_2 transport across the human erythrocyte membrane. FASEB J 2006;20(12):1974–81.

14. Sly WS, Hewett-Emmett D, Whyte MP, et al. Carbonic anhydrase II deficiency identified as the primary defect in the autosomal recessive syndrome of osteopetrosis with renal tubular acidosis and cerebral calcification. Proc Natl Acad Sci U S A 1983;80(9):2752–6.

15. Spicer SS, Sens MA, Tashian RE. Immunocytochemical demonstration of carbonic anhydrase in human epithelial cells. J Histochem Cytochem 1982;30(9): 864–73.

16. Damkier HH, Nielsen S, Praetorius J. Molecular expression of SLC4-derived Na+-dependent anion transporters in selected human tissues. Am J Physiol Regul Integr Comp Physiol 2007;293(5):R2136–46.

17. Krapf R, Alpern RJ, Rector FC Jr, et al. Basolateral membrane Na/base cotransport is dependent on CO_2/HCO_3 in the proximal convoluted tubule. J Gen Physiol 1987;90(6):833–53.

18. Petrovic S, Dubose TD Jr. Missense mutations and proximal RTA. Have we reached a new threshold? Focus on "missense mutation T485S alters NBCe1-A electrogenicity causing proximal renal tubular acidosis". Am J Physiol Cell Physiol 2013;305(4):C373–4.

19. Hamm LL, Simon EE. Roles and mechanisms of urinary buffer excretion. Am J Physiol 1987;253(4 Pt 2):F595–605.

20. Brown D, Roth J, Kumpulainen T, et al. Ultrastructural immunocytochemical localization of carbonic anhydrase. Presence in intercalated cells of the rat collecting tubule. Histochemistry 1982;75(2):209–13.

21. Han JS, Kim GH, Kim J, et al. Secretory-defect distal renal tubular acidosis is associated with transporter defect in H(+)-ATPase and anion exchanger-1. J Am Soc Nephrol 2002;13(6):1425–32.

22. Stehberger PA, Shmukler BE, Stuart-Tilley AK, et al. Distal renal tubular acidosis in mice lacking the AE1 (band3) Cl-/HCO3- exchanger (slc4a1). J Am Soc Nephrol 2007;18(5):1408–18.

23. Wagner CA, Devuyst O, Belge H, et al. The rhesus protein RhCG: a new perspective in ammonium transport and distal urinary acidification. Kidney Int 2011;79(2):154–61.

24. Good DW, Burg MB. Ammonia production by individual segments of the rat nephron. J Clin Invest 1984;73(3):602–10.

25. Kinsella JL, Aronson PS. Interaction of NH4+ and Li+ with the renal microvillus membrane Na+-H+ exchanger. Am J Physiol 1981;241(5):C220–6.

26. Weiner ID, Verlander JW. Recent advances in understanding renal ammonia metabolism and transport. Curr Opin Nephrol Hypertens 2016;25(5):436–43.

27. Lightwood R. Calcium infarction of the kidneys in infants. Arch Dis Child 1935; 10:205–6.

28. Pines KL, Mudge GH. Renal tubular acidosis with osteomalacia; report of 3 cases. Am J Med 1951;11(3):302–11.

29. Breedveld FC, Haanen HC, Chang PC. Distal renal tubular acidosis in polyarteritis nodosa. Arch Intern Med 1986;146(5):1009–10.

30. Both T, Zietse R, Hoorn EJ, et al. Everything you need to know about distal renal tubular acidosis in autoimmune disease. Rheumatol Int 2014;34(8):1037–45.

31. Alexander RT, Bockenhauer D. Renal tubular acidosis. In: Geary DF, Schaefer F, editors. Pediatric kidney disease. Berlin: Springer Berlin Heidelberg; 2016. p. 973–91.

32. Both T, Dalm VA, van Hagen PM, et al. Reviewing primary Sjogren's syndrome: beyond the dryness - From pathophysiology to diagnosis and treatment. Int J Med Sci 2017;14(3):191–200.

33. Fabris A, Lupo A, Ferraro PM, et al. Familial clustering of medullary sponge kidney is autosomal dominant with reduced penetrance and variable expressivity. Kidney Int 2013;83(2):272–7.

34. Bruce LJ, Cope DL, Jones GK, et al. Familial distal renal tubular acidosis is associated with mutations in the red cell anion exchanger (Band 3, AE1) gene. J Clin Invest 1997;100(7):1693–707.

35. Karet FE, Gainza FJ, Gyory AZ, et al. Mutations in the chloride-bicarbonate exchanger gene AE1 cause autosomal dominant but not autosomal recessive distal renal tubular acidosis. Proc Natl Acad Sci U S A 1998;95(11):6337–42.

36. Jarolim P, Shayakul C, Prabakaran D, et al. Autosomal dominant distal renal tubular acidosis is associated in three families with heterozygosity for the R589H mutation in the AE1 (band 3) Cl-/HCO3- exchanger. J Biol Chem 1998; 273(11):6380–8.

37. Karet FE, Finberg KE, Nelson RD, et al. Mutations in the gene encoding B1 subunit of H+-ATPase cause renal tubular acidosis with sensorineural deafness. Nat Genet 1999;21(1):84–90.

38. Hahn H, Kang HG, Ha IS, et al. ATP6B1 gene mutations associated with distal renal tubular acidosis and deafness in a child. Am J Kidney Dis 2003;41(1): 238–43.

39. Ruf R, Rensing C, Topaloglu R, et al. Confirmation of the ATP6B1 gene as responsible for distal renal tubular acidosis. Pediatr Nephrol 2003;18(2):105–9.
40. Stover EH, Borthwick KJ, Bavalia C, et al. Novel ATP6V1B1 and ATP6V0A4 mutations in autosomal recessive distal renal tubular acidosis with new evidence for hearing loss. J Med Genet 2002;39(11):796–803.
41. Batlle D, Haque SK. Genetic causes and mechanisms of distal renal tubular acidosis. Nephrol Dial Transplant 2012;27(10):3691–704.
42. Alexander RT, Cordat E, Chambrey R, et al. Acidosis and urinary calcium excretion: insights from genetic disorders. J Am Soc Nephrol 2016;27(12):3511–20.
43. Karet FE, Finberg KE, Nayir A, et al. Localization of a gene for autosomal recessive distal renal tubular acidosis with normal hearing (rdRTA2) to 7q33-34. Am J Hum Genet 1999;65(6):1656–65.
44. Rink N, Bitzan M, O'Gorman G, et al. Endolymphatic sac enlargement in a girl with a novel mutation for distal renal tubular acidosis and severe deafness. Case Rep Pediatr 2012;2012:605053.
45. Tanphaichitr VS, Sumboonnanonda A, Ideguchi H, et al. Novel AE1 mutations in recessive distal renal tubular acidosis. Loss-of-function is rescued by glycophorin A. J Clin Invest 1998;102(12):2173–9.
46. Sritippayawan S, Sumboonnanonda A, Vasuvattakul S, et al. Novel compound heterozygous SLC4A1 mutations in Thai patients with autosomal recessive distal renal tubular acidosis. Am J Kidney Dis 2004;44(1):64–70.
47. Rysava R, Tesar V, Jirsa M Jr, et al. Incomplete distal renal tubular acidosis co-inherited with a mutation in the band 3 (AE1) gene. Nephrol Dial Transplant 1997;12(9):1869–73.
48. Ribeiro ML, Alloisio N, Almeida H, et al. Severe hereditary spherocytosis and distal renal tubular acidosis associated with the total absence of band 3. Blood 2000;96(4):1602–4.
49. Cheidde L, Vieira TC, Lima PR, et al. A novel mutation in the anion exchanger 1 gene is associated with familial distal renal tubular acidosis and nephrocalcinosis. Pediatrics 2003;112(6 Pt 1):1361–7.
50. Imai E, Kaneko S, Mori T, et al. A novel heterozygous mutation in the ATP6V0A4 gene encoding the V-ATPase a4 subunit in an adult patient with incomplete distal renal tubular acidosis. Clin Kidney J 2016;9(3):424–8.
51. Zhang J, Fuster DG, Cameron MA, et al. Incomplete distal renal tubular acidosis from a heterozygous mutation of the V-ATPase B1 subunit. Am J Physiol Renal Physiol 2014;307(9):F1063–71.
52. Igarashi T, Inatomi J, Sekine T, et al. Mutations in SLC4A4 cause permanent isolated proximal renal tubular acidosis with ocular abnormalities. Nat Genet 1999;23(3):264–6.
53. Igarashi T, Inatomi J, Sekine T, et al. Novel nonsense mutation in the Na^+/HCO_3^- cotransporter gene (SLC4A4) in a patient with permanent isolated proximal renal tubular acidosis and bilateral glaucoma. J Am Soc Nephrol 2001;12(4):713–8.
54. Lemann J Jr, Adams ND, Wilz DR, et al. Acid and mineral balances and bone in familial proximal renal tubular acidosis. Kidney Int 2000;58(3):1267–77.
55. Horita S, Yamada H, Inatomi J, et al. Functional analysis of NBC1 mutants associated with proximal renal tubular acidosis and ocular abnormalities. J Am Soc Nephrol 2005;16(8):2270–8.
56. Dinour D, Chang MH, Satoh J, et al. A novel missense mutation in the sodium bicarbonate cotransporter (NBCe1/SLC4A4) causes proximal tubular acidosis

and glaucoma through ion transport defects. J Biol Chem 2004;279(50): 52238–46.

57. Bokenkamp A, Ludwig M. The oculocerebrorenal syndrome of Lowe: an update. Pediatr Nephrol 2016;31(12):2201–12.

58. Cherqui S, Courtoy PJ. The renal Fanconi syndrome in cystinosis: pathogenic insights and therapeutic perspectives. Nat Rev Nephrol 2017;13(2):115–31.

59. Haque SK, Ariceta G, Batlle D. Proximal renal tubular acidosis: a not so rare disorder of multiple etiologies. Nephrol Dial Transplant 2012;27(12):4273–87.

60. Kitterer D, Schwab M, Alscher MD, et al. Drug-induced acid-base disorders. Pediatr Nephrol 2015;30(9):1407–23.

61. Shah GN, Bonapace G, Hu PY, et al. Carbonic anhydrase II deficiency syndrome (osteopetrosis with renal tubular acidosis and brain calcification): novel mutations in CA2 identified by direct sequencing expand the opportunity for genotype-phenotype correlation. Hum Mutat 2004;24(3):272.

62. Ismail EA, Abul Saad S, Sabry MA. Nephrocalcinosis and urolithiasis in carbonic anhydrase II deficiency syndrome. Eur J Pediatr 1997;156(12):957–62.

63. Muzalef A, Alshehri M, Al-Abidi A, et al. Marble brain disease in two Saudi Arabian siblings. Ann Trop Paediatr 2005;25(3):213–8.

64. Fathallah DM, Bejaoui M, Lepaslier D, et al. Carbonic anhydrase II (CA II) deficiency in Maghrebian patients: evidence for founder effect and genomic recombination at the CA II locus. Hum Genet 1997;99(5):634–7.

65. Bolt RJ, Wennink JM, Verbeke JI, et al. Carbonic anhydrase type II deficiency. Am J Kidney Dis 2005;46(5):A50, e71-53.

66. Karet FE. Mechanisms in hyperkalemic renal tubular acidosis. J Am Soc Nephrol 2009;20(2):251–4.

67. Frindt G, Yang L, Uchida S, et al. Responses of distal nephron Na(+) transporters to acute volume depletion and hyperkalemia. Am J Physiol Renal Physiol 2017;313(1):F62–73.

68. Riepe FG. Pseudohypoaldosteronism. Endocr Dev 2013;24:86–95.

69. Geller DS, Rodriguez-Soriano J, Vallo Boado A, et al. Mutations in the mineralocorticoid receptor gene cause autosomal dominant pseudohypoaldosteronism type I. Nat Genet 1998;19(3):279–81.

70. Sartorato P, Lapeyraque AL, Armanini D, et al. Different inactivating mutations of the mineralocorticoid receptor in fourteen families affected by type I pseudohypoaldosteronism. J Clin Endocrinol Metab 2003;88(6):2508–17.

71. Chang SS, Grunder S, Hanukoglu A, et al. Mutations in subunits of the epithelial sodium channel cause salt wasting with hyperkalaemic acidosis, pseudohypoaldosteronism type 1. Nat Genet 1996;12(3):248–53.

72. Kerem E, Bistritzer T, Hanukoglu A, et al. Pulmonary epithelial sodium-channel dysfunction and excess airway liquid in pseudohypoaldosteronism. N Engl J Med 1999;341(3):156–62.

73. Saxena A, Hanukoglu I, Saxena D, et al. Novel mutations responsible for autosomal recessive multisystem pseudohypoaldosteronism and sequence variants in epithelial sodium channel alpha-, beta-, and gamma-subunit genes. J Clin Endocrinol Metab 2002;87(7):3344–50.

74. Strautnieks SS, Thompson RJ, Gardiner RM, et al. A novel splice-site mutation in the gamma subunit of the epithelial sodium channel gene in three pseudohypoaldosteronism type 1 families. Nat Genet 1996;13(2):248–50.

75. Schambelan M, Sebastian A, Rector FC Jr. Mineralocorticoid-resistant renal hyperkalemia without salt wasting (type II pseudohypoaldosteronism): role of increased renal chloride reabsorption. Kidney Int 1981;19(5):716–27.

76. Wilson FH, Disse-Nicodeme S, Choate KA, et al. Human hypertension caused by mutations in WNK kinases. Science 2001;293(5532):1107–12.

77. Boyden LM, Choi M, Choate KA, et al. Mutations in kelch-like 3 and cullin 3 cause hypertension and electrolyte abnormalities. Nature 2012;482(7383): 98–102.

78. Louis-Dit-Picard H, Barc J, Trujillano D, et al. KLHL3 mutations cause familial hyperkalemic hypertension by impairing ion transport in the distal nephron. Nat Genet 2012;44(4):456–60. S451–3.

79. Santos F, Gil-Pena H, Alvarez-Alvarez S. Renal tubular acidosis. Curr Opin Pediatr 2017;29(2):206–10.

80. Lemann J Jr, Litzow JR, Lennon EJ. The effects of chronic acid loads in normal man: further evidence for the participation of bone mineral in the defense against chronic metabolic acidosis. J Clin Invest 1966;45(10):1608–14.

81. Martin HE, Jones R. The effect of ammonium chloride and sodium bicarbonate on the urinary excretion of magnesium, calcium, and phosphate. Am Heart J 1961;62:206–10.

82. Bushinsky DA, Levi-Setti R, Coe FL. Ion microprobe determination of bone surface elements: effects of reduced medium pH. Am J Physiol 1986;250(6 Pt 2): F1090–7.

83. Bushinsky DA, Wolbach W, Sessler NE, et al. Physicochemical effects of acidosis on bone calcium flux and surface ion composition. J Bone Miner Res 1993;8(1):93–102.

84. Bushinsky DA. Net calcium efflux from live bone during chronic metabolic, but not respiratory, acidosis. Am J Physiol 1989;256(5 Pt 2):F836–42.

85. Krieger NS, Sessler NE, Bushinsky DA. Acidosis inhibits osteoblastic and stimulates osteoclastic activity in vitro. Am J Physiol 1992;262(3 Pt 2):F442–8.

86. Bushinsky DA. Stimulated osteoclastic and suppressed osteoblastic activity in metabolic but not respiratory acidosis. Am J Physiol 1995;268(1 Pt 1):C80–8.

87. Alexander RT, Rievaj J, Dimke H. Paracellular calcium transport across renal and intestinal epithelia. Biochem Cell Biol 2014;92(6):467–80.

88. Hoenderop JG, van Leeuwen JP, van der Eerden BC, et al. Renal Ca^{2+} wasting, hyperabsorption, and reduced bone thickness in mice lacking TRPV5. J Clin Invest 2003;112(12):1906–14.

89. Sutton RA, Wong NL, Dirks JH. Effects of metabolic acidosis and alkalosis on sodium and calcium transport in the dog kidney. Kidney Int 1979;15(5):520–33.

90. Wong NL, Quamme GA, Dirks JH. Actions of parathyroid hormone are not impaired during chronic metabolic acidosis. J Lab Clin Med 1985;105(4):472–8.

91. Dubb J, Goldberg M, Agus ZS. Tubular effects of acute metabolic acidosis in the rat. J Lab Clin Med 1977;90(2):318–23.

92. Nijenhuis T, Renkema KY, Hoenderop JG, et al. Acid-base status determines the renal expression of Ca^{2+} and Mg^{2+} transport proteins. J Am Soc Nephrol 2006; 17(3):617–26.

93. Norman ME, Feldman NI, Cohn RM, et al. Urinary citrate excretion in the diagnosis of distal renal tubular acidosis. J Pediatr 1978;92(3):394–400.

94. Brennan S, Hering-Smith K, Hamm LL. Effect of pH on citrate reabsorption in the proximal convoluted tubule. Am J Physiol 1988;255(2 Pt 2):F301–6.

95. Lambers TT, Oancea E, de Groot T, et al. Extracellular pH dynamically controls cell surface delivery of functional TRPV5 channels. Mol Cell Biol 2007;27(4): 1486–94.

96. Yaxley J, Pirrone C. Review of the diagnostic evaluation of renal tubular acidosis. Ochsner J 2016;16(4):525–30.

97. Kamel KS, Briceno LF, Sanchez MI, et al. A new classification for renal defects in net acid excretion. Am J Kidney Dis 1997;29(1):136–46.

98. Jha R, Muthukrishnan J, Shiradhonkar S, et al. Clinical profile of distal renal tubular acidosis. Saudi J Kidney Dis Transpl 2011;22(2):261–7.

99. Goldstein MB, Bear R, Richardson RM, et al. The urine anion gap: a clinically useful index of ammonium excretion. Am J Med Sci 1986;292(4):198–202.

100. Batlle DC, Hizon M, Cohen E, et al. The use of the urinary anion gap in the diagnosis of hyperchloremic metabolic acidosis. N Engl J Med 1988;318(10):594–9.

101. Batlle D, Ba Aqeel SH, Marquez A. The urine anion gap in context. Clin J Am Soc Nephrol 2018;13(2):195–7.

102. Santos F, Ordonez FA, Claramunt-Taberner D, et al. Clinical and laboratory approaches in the diagnosis of renal tubular acidosis. Pediatr Nephrol 2015; 30(12):2099–107.

103. Smulders YM, Frissen PH, Slaats EH, et al. Renal tubular acidosis. Pathophysiology and diagnosis. Arch Intern Med 1996;156(15):1629–36.

104. Walsh SB, Shirley DG, Wrong OM, et al. Urinary acidification assessed by simultaneous furosemide and fludrocortisone treatment: an alternative to ammonium chloride. Kidney Int 2007;71(12):1310–6.

105. Brown D, Hirsch S, Gluck S. Localization of a proton-pumping ATPase in rat kidney. J Clin Invest 1988;82(6):2114–26.

106. Edelmann CM, Soriano JR, Boichis H, et al. Renal bicarbonate reabsorption and hydrogen ion excretion in normal infants. J Clin Invest 1967;46(8):1309–17.

107. Soriano JR, Boichis H, Edelmann CM Jr. Bicarbonate reabsorption and hydrogen ion excretion in children with renal tubular acidosis. J Pediatr 1967; 71(6):802–13.

108. Caruana RJ, Buckalew VM Jr. The syndrome of distal (type 1) renal tubular acidosis. Clinical and laboratory findings in 58 cases. Medicine (Baltimore) 1988;67(2):84–99.

109. Nash MA, Torrado AD, Greifer I, et al. Renal tubular acidosis in infants and children. Clinical course, response to treatment, and prognosis. J Pediatr 1972; 80(5):738–48.

110. McSherry E, Morris RC Jr. Attainment and maintenance of normal stature with alkali therapy in infants and children with classic renal tubular acidosis. J Clin Invest 1978;61(2):509–27.

111. Rampini S, Fanconi A, Illig R, et al. Effect of hydrochlorothiazide on proximal renal tubular acidosis in a patient with idiopathic "de Toni-Debre-Fanconi syndrome. Helv Paediatr Acta 1968;23(1):13–21.

112. Gordon RD, Geddes RA, Pawsey CG, et al. Hypertension and severe hyperkalaemia associated with suppression of renin and aldosterone and completely reversed by dietary sodium restriction. Australas Ann Med 1970;19(4):287–94.

113. Achard JM, Disse-Nicodeme S, Fiquet-Kempf B, et al. Phenotypic and genetic heterogeneity of familial hyperkalaemic hypertension (Gordon syndrome). Clin Exp Pharmacol Physiol 2001;28(12):1048–52.

114. Kari JA, El Desoky SM, Singh AK, et al. The case | renal tubular acidosis and eye findings. Kidney Int 2014;86(1):217–8.

115. Kiran BV, Barman H, Iyengar A. Clinical profile and outcome of renal tubular disorders in children: a single center experience. Indian J Nephrol 2014;24(6): 362–6.

116. Nesterova G, Williams C, Bernardini I, et al. Cystinosis: renal glomerular and renal tubular function in relation to compliance with cystine-depleting therapy. Pediatr Nephrol 2015;30(6):945–51.

117. Bockenhauer D, Kleta R. Renal Fanconi syndromes and other proximal tubular disorders. In: Geary DF, Schaefer F, editors. Pediatric kidney disease. Berlin: Springer; 2016. p. 883–904.
118. Quigley R, Wold MTF. Renal tubular acidosis in children. In: Avner ED, Harmon WE, Niaudet P, et al, editors. Pediatric nephrology, vol. 2. Heidelberg (Germany): Springer; 2016. p. 1273–306.
119. Santos F, Chan JC. Renal tubular acidosis in children. Diagnosis, treatment and prognosis. Am J Nephrol 1986;6(4):289–95.
120. Besouw MTP, Bienias M, Walsh P, et al. Clinical and molecular aspects of distal renal tubular acidosis in children. Pediatr Nephrol 2017;32(6):987–96.
121. Donckerwolcke R, Yang WN, Chan JC. Growth failure in children with renal tubular acidosis. Semin Nephrol 1989;9(1):72–4.
122. Bagga A, Bajpai A, Gulati S, et al. Distal renal tubular acidosis with severe bony deformities and multiple fractures. Indian Pediatr 2001;38(11):1301–5.
123. Bajpai A, Bagga A, Hari P, et al. Long-term outcome in children with primary distal renal tubular acidosis. Indian Pediatr 2005;42(4):321–8.
124. Vivante A, Lotan D, Pode-Shakked N, et al. Familial autosomal recessive renal tubular acidosis: importance of early diagnosis. Nephron Physiol 2011;119(3): p31–9.
125. Bajaj G, Quan A. Renal tubular acidosis and deafness: report of a large family. Am J Kidney Dis 1996;27(6):880–2.
126. Hall AM, Bass P, Unwin RJ. Drug-induced renal Fanconi syndrome. QJM 2014; 107(4):261–9.
127. Sharma S, Aggarwal S. Hyperchloremic acidosis. Treasure Island (FL): Stat-Pearls; 2018.

Fanconi Syndrome

John W. Foreman, MD

KEYWORDS

• Fanconi syndrome • Proximal tubule • Cystinosis • Dent disease • Lowe syndrome

KEY POINTS

- Fanconi syndrome is a global disorder of the proximal tubule.
- In children, this principally caused by inborn errors of metabolism and in adults it is usually caused by drugs and toxins.
- Treatment consists of treating the underlying disorder or removal of the toxin and replacing the lost electrolytes and volume.

INTRODUCTION

In the 1930s, de Toni, Debré, and coworkers and Fanconi independently described several children with the combination of renal rickets, glycosuria, and hypophosphatemia. Fanconi syndrome, also called the DeToni, Debré, Fanconi syndrome, now refers to a global dysfunction of the proximal tubule leading to excessive urinary excretion of amino acids, glucose, phosphate, bicarbonate, uric acid, and other solutes reabsorbed by this nephron segment (**Table 1**). When severe, these losses lead to acidosis, dehydration, electrolyte imbalances, rickets, osteomalacia, and growth failure. Numerous inherited or acquired disorders are associated with Fanconi syndrome (**Table 2**).

ETIOLOGY AND PATHOGENESIS

The sequence of events leading to Fanconi syndrome is incompletely defined and probably varies with each cause. Possible mechanisms include widespread abnormality of most or all of the proximal tubule carriers, "leaky" brush border or basolateral cell membrane, inhibited or abnormal Na^+, K^+-ATPase pump, impaired mitochondrial energy generation, or other cell organelle dysfunction. The most common cause of Fanconi syndrome in children is an inborn error of metabolism, whereas in adults the most common cause of Fanconi syndrome is an endogenous or exogenous toxin.

CLINICAL MANIFESTATIONS
Aminoaciduria

Aminoaciduria is a cardinal feature of Fanconi syndrome. Virtually every amino acid is found in excess in the urine, thus the term generalized aminoaciduria. There are no

Department of Pediatrics, Duke University School of Medicine, Erwin Road, Durham, NC 27710, USA
E-mail address: john.foreman@duke.edu

Pediatr Clin N Am 66 (2019) 159–167
https://doi.org/10.1016/j.pcl.2018.09.002
0031-3955/19/© 2018 Elsevier Inc. All rights reserved.

Table 1
Signs and symptoms of Fanconi syndrome

Metabolic Abnormalities	Clinical Features
Glycosuria	Rickets, osteomalacia
Generalized Aminoaciduria	Growth retardation
Hypophosphatemia	Polyuria
Hyperchloremic metabolic acidosis	Dehydration
Hypokalemia	Low-molecular-weight proteinuria
Hypouricemia	Muscle weakness
Hypocarnitinemia	

clinical consequences, however, because the losses are trivial, 0.5 to 1.0 g/d, in relation to the dietary intake.

Glycosuria

Glycosuria is another of the cardinal features of Fanconi syndrome and results from impaired tubular reabsorption of glucose. It is often one of the first diagnostic clues. As with aminoaciduria, glycosuria rarely causes symptoms, such as weight loss or hypoglycemia.

Hypophosphaturia

Hypophosphatemia, secondary to impairment in phosphate reabsorption, is a common finding in Fanconi syndrome. Elevated parathyroid hormone and low vitamin D levels also may play a role in the phosphaturia of Fanconi syndrome, although these hormonal abnormalities are not always present. A few patients have impaired conversion of 25-hydroxyvitamin D to 1,25-hydroxyvitamin D; metabolic acidosis, another feature of Fanconi syndrome, may also impair this conversion. Another mechanism for the hypophosphatemia is impairment of the megalin-dependent reabsorption and degradation of filtered parathyroid hormone. Hypophosphatemia often leads to significant bone disease, presenting with pain, fractures, rickets, or growth failure.

Urinary Bicarbonate Wasting/Hyperchloremic Metabolic Acidosis

Hyperchloremic metabolic acidosis, another feature of Fanconi syndrome, is a result of impaired bicarbonate reabsorption by the proximal tubule (proximal or type 2 renal

Table 2
Causes of Fanconi syndrome

Inherited Causes	Acquired Causes
Cystinosis	Drugs: cisplatin, ifosfamide, tenofovir, cidofovir, adefovir, didanosine, gentamicin, azathioprine, valproic acid, suramin, streptozocin, ranitidine
Galactosemia	
Hereditary fructose intolerance	
Tyrosinemia	Heavy metals: lead, cadmium
Wilson disease	Dysproteinemias: multiple myeloma, Sjögren syndrome, light chain proteinuria, amyloidosis
Lowe syndrome	
Dent disease	Chinese herbal medicine: aristolochic acid
Glycogenosis	Toluene: Glue sniffing
Mitochondrial cytopathies	Nephrotic syndrome
	Renal transplantation
Idiopathic	Acute tubular necrosis

tubular acidosis). This impaired reabsorption can lead to the loss of more than 30% of the normal filtered load of bicarbonate, but serum $[HCO_3^-]$ usually remains between 12 and 18 mmol/L.

Natriuresis and Kaliuresis

Natriuresis and kaliuresis are common in Fanconi syndrome and can give rise to significant, even life-threatening, problems. These electrolyte losses are in part related to impaired bicarbonate reabsorption, with the subsequent urinary excretion of sodium and potassium ions with the bicarbonate. In some cases, sodium and potassium losses are so great that metabolic alkalosis and hyperaldosteronism result, simulating Bartter syndrome despite the underlying impaired bicarbonate reabsorption.

Polyuria and Polydipsia

Polyuria, polydipsia, and frequent bouts of severe dehydration are common symptoms in young patients with Fanconi syndrome.

Growth Retardation

Growth retardation in children with Fanconi syndrome is multifactorial. Hypophosphatemia, rickets, and acidosis contribute to growth failure, as do chronic hypokalemia and extracellular volume contraction.

Proteinuria

Proteinuria is usually minimal, except when Fanconi syndrome develops in association with the nephrotic syndrome. Typically, only low-molecular-weight proteins (<30,000 Da) are excreted, such as vitamin D and A–binding proteins, enzymes, immunoglobulin light chains, and hormones.

INHERITED CAUSES OF FANCONI SYNDROME
Cystinosis

Cystinosis, or cystine storage disease, is characterized biochemically by excessive intracellular storage, particularly in lysosomes, of the amino acid cystine.[1] Three different types of cystinosis can be distinguished based on clinical course and age at onset and the intracellular cystine content. Benign or adult cystinosis is associated with cystine crystals in the cornea and bone marrow only, as well as a mild elevation in intracellular cystine levels; no renal disease is evident in benign, adult cystinosis. In contrast, infantile or nephropathic cystinosis, the most common form of cystinosis, is associated with the highest intracellular levels of cystine and the earliest onset of renal disease. In the intermediate or adolescent form, intracellular cystine levels are between those of the infantile and adult forms, with a later onset of renal disease.

Etiology and pathogenesis
Cystinosis is an autosomal-recessive disease caused by a mutation in the *CTNS* gene, which codes for the lysosomal membrane protein, cystinosin, that mediates the transport of cystine out of the lysosome.[2] Recently, cystinosin has been shown to play a role in other cellular processes besides lysosomal cystine transport and may explain the persistence of the Fanconi syndrome despite cystine depletion.[3]

Clinical manifestations
The first clinical symptoms and signs in nephropathic cystinosis are those of Fanconi syndrome and usually appear in the second one-half of the first year of life. Rickets is common after the first year of life, along with growth failure. The growth failure occurs

before the glomerular filtration rate (GFR) decreases and despite correction of electrolyte and mineral deficiencies. The GFR invariably declines and, in untreated children, end-stage renal disease occurs by late childhood.

Photophobia is another common symptom that occurs by 3 years of age and is progressive. Older patients with cystinosis may develop visual impairment and blindness.

Common late complications of cystinosis include hypothyroidism, splenomegaly, hepatomegaly, decreased visual acuity, swallowing difficulties, pulmonary insufficiency, and corneal ulcerations.[4] Less frequently, older patients have developed insulin-dependent diabetes mellitus, myopathy, and progressive neurologic disorders. Decreased brain cortex has also been noted on imaging in some patients. Older patients may develop vascular calcification, especially of the coronary arteries, which can lead to myocardial ischemia.

Diagnosis
The diagnosis is based on the demonstration of elevated intracellular levels of cystine, usually in white blood cells or skin fibroblasts. Patients with nephropathic and intermediate cystinosis have intracellular cystine levels that exceed 2 nmol half-cystine/mg protein (normal <0.2 nmol half-cystine/mg protein). A slit-lamp demonstration of corneal crystals strongly suggests the diagnosis[2] (**Fig. 1**). A prenatal diagnosis can be made with amniocytes or chorionic villi.

Treatment
Nonspecific therapy for infantile cystinosis consists of vitamin D therapy and replacement of the urinary electrolyte losses, followed, in due course, by the management of the progressive renal failure. Cysteamine therapy lowers tissue cystine levels and slows the decrease in the GFR, especially if started before 2 years of age.[5] Cysteamine therapy also improves linear growth, but not the Fanconi syndrome. The most common problems associated with cysteamine therapy are nausea, vomiting, and the medication's foul odor and taste. Treatment should begin with a low dose of cysteamine soon after the diagnosis is made, increased during 4 to 6 weeks to 60 to 90 mg/kg/d in 4 divided doses as close to every 6 hours as possible, with the goal of achieving and maintaining a cystine level of less than 2.0 and preferably less than 1.0 mmol half-cystine/mg protein. A long-acting formulation of cysteamine is now available that allows twice-daily dosing. A 50-mmol/L solution of cysteamine applied

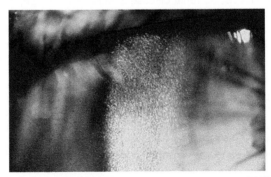

Fig. 1. Corneal opacities in cystinosis. Tinsel-like refractile opacities in the cornea of a patient with cystinosis under slit-lamp examination. (*From* Foreman JW. Cystinosis and the Fanconi syndrome. In: Avner ED, Harmon WE, Niaudet P, editors. Pediatric nephrology. 5th edition. Philadelphia: Lippincott Williams & Wilkins; 2004. p. 789; with permission.)

topically onto the eye has proved useful in depleting the cornea of cystine crystals, but it requires administration 6 to 12 times a day to be effective.

Successful renal transplantation reverses the renal failure and Fanconi syndrome but does not seem to improve the extrarenal manifestations of cystinosis. Cysteamine therapy should be continued after transplantation.

Galactosemia

Galactosemia is an autosomal recessively inherited disorder of galactose metabolism caused by decreased activity of the enzyme galactose 1-phosphate uridyltransferase. Affected infants ingesting milk containing lactose, the most common source of galactose in the diet, rapidly develop vomiting, diarrhea, failure to thrive, cataracts, jaundice, and, ultimately, hepatic cirrhosis. Galactose intake leads within days to hyperaminoaciduria, albuminuria, and glycosuria, which is principally galactosuria and not glycosuria. Galactosemia is treated by elimination of galactose from the diet with resolution of Fanconi syndrome in a few days.

Hereditary Fructose Intolerance

Hereditary fructose intolerance is another autosomal-recessive disorder of carbohydrate metabolism associated with Fanconi syndrome caused by a deficiency of the B isoform of the enzyme fructose 1-phosphate aldolase. Symptoms of hereditary fructose intolerance appear at weaning when fruit, vegetables, and sweetened cereals that contain fructose or sucrose are introduced. Children with this disorder experience nausea, vomiting, and symptoms of hypoglycemia or even convulsion, shock, and acute kidney injury shortly after the ingestion of fructose. The Fanconi syndrome is only present after exposure to fructose. Treatment of hereditary fructose intolerance involves strict avoidance of foods containing fructose and sucrose.

Glycogenosis

Most patients with glycogen storage disease and Fanconi syndrome have an autosomal-recessive disorder characterized by heavy glycosuria and increased glycogen storage in the liver and kidney, known as the Fanconi-Bickel syndrome or glycogen storage disease type XI, or glucose-losing syndrome, because the glucose losses can be massive.[6] The defect is deficient activity of the sugar transporter GLUT2, which facilitates sugar exit from the basolateral side of the proximal tubule and intestinal cell and sugar entry and exit from the hepatocyte and pancreatic β cell. A few patients with type I glycogen storage disease have mild Fanconi syndrome but not Fanconi-Bickel syndrome. The therapy for this disorder is directed at the renal solute losses, treatment of rickets (which can be severe), and frequent feeding to prevent ketosis. Uncooked cornstarch has been shown to lessen the hypoglycemia and to improve growth.

Tyrosinemia

Hereditary tyrosinemia type I, also known as hepatorenal tyrosinemia, is an autosomal-recessive defect of tyrosine metabolism caused by deficient activity of fumaryl acetoacetate hydrolase affecting the kidneys and peripheral nerves but especially the liver. Decreased or absent fumaryl acetoacetate hydrolase activity leads ultimately to the formation of succinyl acetone, which may be the cause of the Fanconi syndrome in tyrosinemia. A diet low in phenylalanine and tyrosine dramatically improves the renal tubular dysfunction and nitisinone is useful in preventing further renal and hepatic dysfunction.[7]

Wilson Disease

Wilson disease is an autosomal-recessive disorder of copper metabolism caused by a defect in the P-type copper–transporting adenosine triphosphatase ATP7B that affects the liver, kidney, and central nervous system, leading excessive copper storage in numerous tissues.[8] The Fanconi syndrome usually appears before the onset of hepatic failure. Hypercalciuria with development of renal stones and nephrocalcinosis also have been reported. Besides proximal tubular dysfunction, abnormalities in distal tubular function, decreased concentrating ability, and distal renal tubular acidosis (type 1 renal tubular acidosis) have also been observed. Treatment with penicillamine, 1.0 to 1.5 g/d, reverses the renal dysfunction and may reverse the hepatic and neurologic disease, depending on the degree of damage before the onset of therapy.

Lowe Syndrome

Lowe syndrome (oculocerebrorenal syndrome) is an X-linked disorder caused by deficient activity of phosphatidyl inositol 4,5-bisphosphate 5-phosphatase, OCRL1, involved with cell trafficking and signaling. Lowe syndrome is characterized by congenital cataracts and glaucoma, severe mental retardation, neonatal hypotonia, and renal abnormalities.[9] The Fanconi syndrome is followed by progressive renal impairment, but end-stage renal disease usually does not occur until the third to fourth decade of life. Only symptomatic treatment is available.

Dent Disease

Dent disease is an X-linked recessive disorder characterized by low-molecular-weight proteinuria, hypercalciuria, nephrolithiasis, nephrocalcinosis, and rickets.[10,11] Affected males often have aminoaciduria, phosphaturia, and glycosuria. Renal failure is common and may occur by late childhood. Hemizygous females usually have only proteinuria and mild hypercalciuria. Most patients have a defect in the renal ClC-5 chloride channel. Dent disease type 2 is clinically similar, except there is a mutation in the same gene that causes Lowe syndrome, although patients with Dent type 2 disease do not have the brain or eye involvement seen in Lowe syndrome. Lack of the C1C-5 channel activity interferes with protein reabsorption from the tubule through the megalin-cubilin receptor system and cell surface receptor recycling and may explain the phosphaturia, glycosuria, and aminoaciduria.

Mitochondrial Cytopathies

Mitochondrial cytopathies are a diverse group of diseases with abnormalities in mitochondrial DNA that lead to mitochondrial dysfunction in various tissues and widespread clinical abnormalities, including neurologic disorders, retinitis pigmentosa, diabetes mellitus, pancreatic insufficiency, anemia, hepatic disease, and cardiomyopathy.[12]

   The most common renal manifestation associated with mitochondrial cytopathies is Fanconi syndrome, although a number of patients have been described with focal segmental glomerulosclerosis and corticosteroid-resistant nephrotic syndrome. There is little to offer these patients in terms of definitive therapy, although supplementation with menadione, ubidecarenone, riboflavin, and ascorbic acid has been found to benefit some patients.

Idiopathic Fanconi Syndrome

A number of patients develop Fanconi syndrome in the absence of any known cause. Not all the features of Fanconi syndrome may be present when the patient is first seen, but appear over time. Idiopathic Fanconi syndrome can be inherited in an autosomal-dominant, autosomal-recessive, or even X-linked pattern. However, most cases occur sporadically, with no evidence of genetic transmission. The prognosis is variable, and some patients develop chronic renal failure 10 to 30 years after onset of symptoms. A few patients that have undergone renal transplantation have had recurrence of the Fanconi syndrome, suggesting an extrarenal cause.

ACQUIRED CAUSES OF FANCONI SYNDROME

Numerous substances can injure the proximal renal tubule. Injury can range from an incomplete Fanconi syndrome to acute tubular necrosis or end-stage renal disease. The extent of the tubular damage varies depending on the type of toxin, amount ingested, and host susceptibility. A careful history of possible toxin exposure and recent medications is important in patients with tubular dysfunction. **Table 2** lists the more common causes of acquired Fanconi syndrome.

Heavy Metal Intoxication

A major cause of proximal tubular dysfunction is acute heavy metal intoxication, principally lead and cadmium. In lead poisoning, the renal tubular dysfunction, mainly aminoaciduria and mild glycosuria and phosphaturia, is usually overshadowed by the development of chronic kidney disease and involvement of other organs, especially the central nervous system.[13] Fanconi syndrome associated with cadmium poisoning is associated with severe bone pain, giving rise to the name *itai-itai* (ouch-ouch) disease for its occurrence in Japanese patients affected by industrial contamination of the soil.[14]

Cancer Chemotherapy Agents

A number of cancer chemotherapy agents have been associated with Fanconi syndrome and renal tubular dysfunction, especially cisplatin and ifosfamide. The nephrotoxicity of both cisplatin and ifosfamide is dose dependent and often irreversible. Besides the usual manifestations of Fanconi syndrome, cisplatin toxicity is characterized by hypermagnesuria that leads to hypomagnesemia, which can be extremely severe, persistent, and difficult to treat.[15,16]

Other Drugs and Toxins

Exposure to a wide range of toxins may give rise to Fanconi syndrome, often in association with a reduced GFR, including 6-mercaptopurine, toluene (glue sniffing), and Chinese herbal medicines containing *Aristolochia* species.[17] There have also been anecdotal reports associating Fanconi syndrome with valproic acid (valproate), suramin, gentamicin, and ranitidine. Antiviral medications, especially antiretroviral agents such as tenofovir, are an increasingly common cause of Fanconi syndrome.[18]

Dysproteinemias

Dysproteinemia from multiple myeloma, light chain proteinuria, Sjögren syndrome, and amyloidosis is sometimes associated with Fanconi syndrome, which seems to be correlated with urinary free light chains that can cause proximal tubule dysfunction through intracellular crystallization or lysosomal dysfunction.[19]

Glomerular Disease

The nephrotic syndrome has rarely been associated with the Fanconi syndrome. Most of these patients have focal segmental glomerulosclerosis, and the occurrence of Fanconi syndrome heralds a poor prognosis.

Table 3	
General treatment of Fanconi syndrome	
Supplement	**Dose Range**
Bicarbonate	2–10 mEq/kg/d
Potassium	1–5 mEq/kg/d
Phosphate	500–3000 mg/d
Carnitine	50–100 mg/kg/d
Calcitriol	0.1–0.25 µg/d

Titrate doses to normalize serum levels, except for calcitriol.

After Acute Kidney Injury

Tubular dysfunction can occur during recovery from acute kidney injury from any cause, whether or not a known tubular toxin was originally implicated and is usually transient.

After Renal Transplantation

Fanconi syndrome has occurred rarely after renal transplantation. The pathogenesis probably is multifactorial, including sequelae of acute tubular necrosis, rejection, nephrotoxic drugs, ischemia from renal artery stenosis, and residual hyperparathyroidism.

TREATMENT OF FANCONI SYNDROME

Therapy, whenever possible, should be directed at the underlying causes of Fanconi syndrome. In addition, therapy is directed at the renal solute losses and at the bone disease often present in these patients (**Table 3**). The proximal renal tubular acidosis (type 2 renal tubular acidosis) usually requires large doses of alkali for correction. Potassium supplementation usually is also needed, especially if there is a significant renal tubular acidosis. A few patients will require sodium supplementation along with potassium. Magnesium supplementation may be required. Adequate fluid intake is essential. Correction of hypokalemia and its effect on the concentrating ability of the distal tubule may lessen the polyuria.

Hypophosphatemia should be treated with 1 to 3 g/d of oral phosphate with the goal of normalizing serum phosphate concentrations. Many patients with Fanconi syndrome will require supplemental vitamin D for the adequate treatment of the rickets and osteomalacia. Supplemental calcium is indicated in those with hypocalcemia after supplemental vitamin D is started. Hyperaminoaciduria, glycosuria, proteinuria, and hyperuricosuria usually do not lead to clinical difficulties and do not require specific treatment. Carnitine supplementation, to compensate for the urinary losses, may improve muscle function and lipid profiles, but the evidence is inconsistent.

REFERENCES

1. Emma F, Nesterova G, Langman C, et al. Nephropathic cystinosis: an international consensus document. Nephrol Dial Transplant 2014;(Suppl 4):87–94.
2. Town M, Jean G, Cherqui S, et al. A novel gene encoding an integral membrane protein is mutated in nephropathic cystinosis. Nat Genet 1998;18:319–24.
3. Andrzejewska Z, Nevo N, Thomas L, et al. Cystinosin is a component of the vacuolar H+-ATPase-Ragulator-Rag complex signaling controlling mammalian target of rapamycin complex 1. J Am Soc Nephrol 2016;27:1678–88.

4. Gahl WA, Balog JZ, Kleta R. Nephropathic cystinosis in adults: natural history and effects of oral cysteamine therapy. Ann Intern Med 2007;147:241–50.
5. Kleta R, Gahl WA. Pharmacological treatment of nephropathic cystinosis with cysteamine. Expert Opin Pharmacother 2004;5:2255–62.
6. Santer S, Steinmenn B, Schaub J. Fanconi-Bickel syndrome: a congenital defect of facilitative glucose transport. Curr Mol Med 2002;2:213–27.
7. de Laet C, Dionisi-Vici C, Leonard JV, et al. Recommendations for the management of tyrosinaemia type I. Orphanet J Rare Dis 2013;8:8.
8. Weiss KH, Stemmel W. Evolving perspectives in Wilson disease: diagnosis, treatment and monitoring. Curr Gastroenterol Rep 2012;14:1–7.
9. Shurman SJ, Scheinman SJ. Inherited cerebrorenal syndromes. Nat Rev Nephrol 2009;5:529–38.
10. Edvardsson VO, Goldfarb DS, Lieske JC, et al. Hereditary causes of kidney stones and chronic kidney disease. Pediatr Nephrol 2013;28:1923–42.
11. Schaeffer C, Creatore A, Rampoldi L. Protein trafficking defects in inherited kidney diseases. Nephrol Dial Transplant 2014;29:iv33–44.
12. Emma F, Montini G, Parikh SM, et al. Mitochondrial dysfunction in inherited renal disease and acute kidney injury. Nat Rev Nephrol 2016;12:267–80.
13. Barbier O, Jacquillet G, Tauc M, et al. Effect of heavy metals on and the handling by, the kidney. Nephron Physiol 2005;99:105–10.
14. Prozialeck WC, Edwards JR. Mechanisms of cadmium-induced proximal tubule injury: new insights with implications for biomonitoring and therapeutic interventions. J Pharmacol Exp Ther 2012;343:2–12.
15. Skinner R. Nephrotoxicity–what do we know and what don't we know? J Pediatr Hematol Oncol 2011;33:128–34.
16. Karasawa T, Steyger PS. An integrated view of cisplatin-induced nephrotoxicity and ototoxicity. Toxicol Lett 2015;237:219–27.
17. Vanherweghem JL, Nortier JL. Aristolochic acid nephropathy: a worldwide problem. Kidney Int 2008;74:158–69.
18. Milburn J, Jones R, Levy JB. Renal effects of novel antiretroviral drugs. Nephrol Dial Transplant 2016;32:434–9.
19. Luciani A, Sirac C, Terryn S, et al. Impaired lysosomal function underlies monoclonal light chain-associated renal Fanconi syndrome. J Am Soc Nephrol 2016;27:2049–61.

Update on Dent Disease

Abdulla M. Ehlayel, MD[a], Lawrence Copelovitch, MD[b],*

KEYWORDS

- Dent disease • *CLCN5* • *OCRL1* • Nephrolithiasis • Chronic kidney disease

KEY POINTS

- Dent disease is an X-linked renal proximal tubular disorder characterized by low molecular weight proteinuria, hypercalciuria, and nephrocalcinosis.
- Mutations in both the *CLCN5* and *OCRL1* genes have been associated with the Dent phenotype and are now classified as Dent-1 and Dent-2, respectively.
- Nephrolithiasis, chronic kidney disease/proteinuria, and variable features of Fanconi syndrome are common.
- 30% to 80% of affected men develop end-stage kidney disease in the third to fifth decade of life, but our understanding of the precise pathophysiology and effective treatment regimens remains elusive.

CLINICAL EVALUATION
Historical Perspective

Dent disease is a renal proximal tubular disorder characterized by low molecular weight (LMW) proteinuria, hypercalciuria, and nephrocalcinosis. Nephrolithiasis, chronic kidney disease (CKD), and variable manifestations of other proximal tubule dysfunctions are frequently observed. In 1964, Dent and Friedman[1] described 2 unrelated male individuals with "hypercalciuric rickets"; the first presented with rickets, acidosis, and hypercalciuria, and the second with failure to thrive, rickets, and an intellectual disability. In the 1990s, the genetic underpinnings of the condition began to be appreciated. Wrong and colleagues[2] described a familial form of renal Fanconi syndrome in 25 patients from 5 different families. They termed the condition "Dent disease" and suggested that it was inherited in an X-linked fashion. Shortly thereafter, the first gene associated with the condition, *CLCN5*, was identified and fully characterized.[3,4] It was subsequently recognized that a subset of several previously described syndromes were associated with mutations in the same voltage-gated chloride channel. These included X-linked recessive nephrolithiasis in North America,[5] X-linked recessive hypophosphatemic rickets in Europe,[6] and the idiopathic LMW

[a] Division of Nephrology, The Children's Hospital of Philadelphia, 3401 Civic Center Boulevard, Philadelphia, PA 19104, USA; [b] Division of Nephrology, The Children's Hospital of Philadelphia, Perelman School of Medicine at the University of Pennsylvania, 3400 Civic Center Boulevard, Philadelphia, PA 19104, USA
* Corresponding author.
E-mail address: copelovitch@email.chop.edu

Pediatr Clin N Am 66 (2019) 169–178
https://doi.org/10.1016/j.pcl.2018.09.003
0031-3955/19/© 2018 Elsevier Inc. All rights reserved.
pediatric.theclinics.com

proteinuria of Japanese children.[7,8] Ongoing investigations of patients with Dent disease without *CLCN5* mutations revealed that many had mutations in the *OCRL1* gene also located on the X-chromosome.[9] Perhaps somewhat fittingly, it was ultimately recognized that the first patient described by Dent and Friedman[1] had a mutation in the *CLCN5* gene and the second had mutation in *OCRL1*.[10] To properly classify the Dent phenotype associated with *OCRL1* mutations, the term Dent-2 was coined. Those with the originally described *CLCN5* were classified as having Dent-1. Importantly, mutations in the *OCRL1* gene are also seen in patients with Oculocerebrorenal Syndrome, otherwise known as Lowe Syndrome (LS). LS is a rare genetic disorder with an estimated prevalence of 1 in 500,000.[11] It is classically associated with a renal tubulopathy/Fanconi syndrome, congenital cataracts, hypotonia, and intellectual disability.

Presentation

Historically, patients with Dent disease present in childhood with symptoms related to or with nephrolithiasis, osteomalacia, or rickets associated with asymptomatic (LMW) proteinuria. Patients may have short stature, which is typically mild and subclinical in Dent-1 and more pronounced in Dent-2.[12] In addition, polyuria, polydipsia, and salt craving have been described.[13] Patients with Dent-2 may have mild intellectual impairment, developmental delay, and subclinical cataracts. These findings are typically less severe as compared with those with classic LS. In the genomic era there are an increasing number of patients present with asymptomatic proteinuria (ranging from low grade to nephrotic range) discovered incidentally on testing performed for screening or other purposes. A poorly characterized family history of renal disease in male individuals on the maternal side may subsequently become apparent. Occasionally, patients present with either CKD or end-stage kidney disease (ESKD) and are diagnosed retrospectively.

Patients also may present with signs and symptoms related to hypercalciuria or nephrolithiasis.[14] Clinical manifestations include hematuria (microscopic or gross), dysuria, and flank or abdominal pain. Hypercalciuria also may be asymptomatic and is present in 75% to 90% of patients with genetically confirmed Dent disease.[12,15] A higher excretion rate of calcium is observed in children compared with adults,[16] and hypercalciuria tends to decrease as the glomerular filtration rate (GFR) declines.[17] Nephrocalcinosis is seen in approximately 75% of male patients with Dent-1 disease and 40% with Dent-2.[12] The presence and severity of nephrocalcinosis has not been shown to correlate with the likelihood of developing CKD.[16,17] Approximately 30% to 50% of male patients ultimately develop kidney stones,[16,17] with considerable interfamilial and intrafamilial variability.[14] The calculi are typically composed of calcium oxalate and/or calcium phosphate. An estimated 50% of female carriers have hypercalciuria, and nephrolithiasis has infrequently been reported.[18]

Symptomatic disease occurs almost exclusively in male patients. Female carriers of the disease may have LMW proteinuria and hypercalciuria, but rarely if ever develop CKD. To date, only one female patient has been described with ESKD in a kindred with Dent disease, based on historical information; however, a comprehensive evaluation (LMW protein, urine calcium) was not available.[2] To our knowledge, only 3 additional heterozygous women with CKD have been described.[19]

Patients with Dent disease have varying degrees of proximal tubular dysfunction. Virtually all patients have LMW proteinuria. Only 2 patients with a known pathogenic mutation in the *CLCN5* gene have been described without LMW proteinuria. The first was and adult male patient with isolated hypercalciuria despite a pathogenic mutation,[20] and the second was diagnosed at the age of 1.3 years based on family history.[19] Whether he will eventually develop LMW proteinuria is not known.[1] The most commonly tested LMW proteins include β_2-microglobulin, α_1-microglobulin and retinol-binding protein (RBP). Generally, the loss of these proteins is not known to be associated with any clinical manifestations; however, there are several reports indicating that urinary loss of RBP in Dent disease may contribute to the development of episodic night blindness.[13,21]

Additional manifestations of proximal tubular dysfunction may be present with variable frequencies (**Table 1**). These include kaliuresis/hypokalemia, phosphaturia/hypophosphatemia, aminoaciduria, glycosuria, and uricosuria/hypouricemia. Hypomagnesemia and acidosis/impaired urinary acidification may be present, but are relatively less common findings. Although patients with Dent disease and LS share some common renal manifestations, several phenotypic discrepancies have been observed. Renal tubular acidosis is more severe and clinically significant in LS, whereas hypercalciuria, nephrocalcinosis, and nephrolithiasis are relatively less common.[13]

Differential diagnosis

In children presenting with rickets or osteomalacia and features of proximal tubule dysfunction, both inherited and acquired causes of Fanconi syndrome should be investigated. Cystinosis, galactosemia, hereditary fructose intolerance, glycogen storage diseases, and mitochondrial myopathies generally must be excluded. Acquired causes related to either medications, such as tenofovir, or toxins, including lead, should be considered. The presence of proximal tubular dysfunction in the absence of acidosis should prompt the evaluation for Dent disease. Dent disease should be considered in patients presenting with proteinuria and/or focal glomerulosclerosis, particularly in male patients without edema or hypoalbuminemia, and in patients with a family history of renal disease in male patients on the maternal side.[10,22] The differential diagnosis for hypercalciuria, nephrocalcinosis, and recurrent nephrolithiasis in the context of normal serum calcium is extensive and includes idiopathic hypercalciuria, medullary sponge kidney, prematurity, furosemide or topiramate exposure, ketogenic diet, distal renal tubular acidosis, familial hypomagnesemia with hypercalciuria and nephrocalcinosis, Bartter syndrome, and hereditary hypophosphatemic rickets with hypercalciuria.[23] Dent disease has rarely been reported in patients with a Bartter-like phenotype presenting with hypokalemic metabolic alkalosis, normal blood pressures, and nephrocalcinosis.[24]

Disease Course

Most male patients with Dent disease develop CKD, with an estimated decline in GFR of 1.0 to 1.6 mL/min per 1.73 m^2 per year.[17] Approximately 30% to 80% of affected male

Table 1		
Frequency of proximal tubular abnormalities in Dent disease		
Serum and Urinary Findings	**Dent-1,[19] %**	**Dent-2[9,17,26,46–49]**
Hypouricemia	34	25% (1/4)
Aminoaciduria	48	38% (15/40)
Glycosuria	26	16% (7/44)
Hypokalemia	37	12% (3/26)
Hypophosphatemia	36	7% (3/42)
Hypomagnesemia	13	0% (0/5)
Acidosis	9	10% (5/50)

The numbers in parenthesis indicate numbers of patients with abnormality / number of patients with Dent-2.
Data from Refs.[9,17,19,26,46–49]

patients develop ESKD between ages 30 and 50 years[18]; however, male patients progressing to ESKD have been described as late as the sixth to seventh decades of life.[2] Importantly, there may be tremendous variability in the onset and progression of CKD within affected members of the same family. Approximately 50% of patients will develop nephrotic-range proteinuria without evidence of nephrotic syndrome.[17,25] Patients with declining renal function and ESKD eventually require renal replacement therapy. Patients with LS typically progress to ESKD at a faster rate than those with Dent disease. Analysis of known OCRL1 mutations suggests that all Dent-2 mutations fall into 1 of 2 classes that do not overlap with mutations associated with LS. All Dent-2–associated missense mutations lie within the phosphatidylinositol phosphate 5-phosphatase domain (exons 9–15), whereas all of the other mutations (nonsense and frameshift) are found within the first 7 exons of the gene. In contrast, all LS mutations fall primarily in exons 9 to 22 and are generally predicted to result in a more significant reduction in OCRL1 function. It has been speculated that the premature termination mutations observed in Dent-2 might still allow a somewhat functional protein if transcription resumed at exon 8, which potentially could occur variably in different tissues, resulting in the preserved function in the eye and brain seen in Dent-2 but not LS.[26] In addition, it is also conceivable that modifier genes may compensate for the OCRL deficiency[12] in Dent-2, thereby producing a milder phenotype than LS.

LABORATORY EVALUATION
Laboratory Parameters

Children with suspected Dent disease should be evaluated for proximal tubular dysfunction, hypercalciuria, nephrocalcinosis, renal calculi, and CKD. Laboratory studies should include serum and urine investigations that assess for GFR, hypokalemia, hypophosphatemia, acidosis, hypouricemia, glycosuria, aminoaciduria, LMW proteinuria, hypercalciuria, and overt proteinuria.

Tubular proteinuria is defined as increased excretion of both LMW proteins and albumin in the context of proximal renal tubular dysfunction.[20] LMW proteins refers to proteins that have a molecular weight (MW) less than albumin and include β_2-microglobulin (MW 12 kDa), α_1-microglobulin (MW 30 kDa), RBP (MW 21 kDa), and urine protein 1 (Clara Cell Protein, MW 20 kDa). Proteins with an MW <20 kDa are filtered across the glomerular basement membrane and largely reabsorbed in the proximal tubule. RBP is considered the optimum protein for detection of LMW proteinuria and is typically increased $\sim 10^5$-fold above the normal range in affected male patients.[20] β_2-microglobulin is typically increased $\sim 10^4$-fold above the normal range, but may be unstable in acidic urine (pH <5.5).[27]

Hypercalciuria appears to be the most important risk factor for development of nephrocalcinosis and kidney stones.[16] Testing for hypercalciuria is challenging in the pediatric age group. Ideally, a 24-hour urine sample should be analyzed, but this may not be feasible before the child is toilet trained. Spot measurement of the urine calcium-to-creatinine ratio is a practical alternative to assess for hypercalciuria using age-appropriate norms. Urinary excretion of both oxalate and citrate are typically within normal limits.[15] Although hypercalciuria is a major feature of Dent disease, the progression to CKD has been observed in the absence of nephrocalcinosis[17,28] and likely occurs through other mechanisms.

Histology

The histologic findings in Dent disease are generally nonspecific and may involve both the glomeruli and tubulointerstitium. In the largest study to date of 30 renal biopsies, focal global glomerular sclerosis and tubulointerstitial fibrosis were the most common findings and were observed in 83% and 60% of specimens, respectively.[29] Tubulointerstitial inflammation, tubular atrophy, and nephrocalcinosis also may be observed. Histologic evidence of nephrocalcinosis was seen observed in 20%, and focal segmental glomerulosclerosis was found in 6% to 7% of biopsies. Importantly, there are several reports of patients presenting with isolated proteinuria and a normal GFR in whom biopsy findings of either focal global sclerosis or focal segmental glomerulosclerosis have been observed.[10,22] Immune complex deposits are generally absent on immunofluorescence studies and foot process effacement may be observed on electron microscopy. Renal biopsy findings associated with lower GFR at biopsy include higher percentages of globally sclerotic glomeruli, foot process effacement, and interstitial inflammation, whereas steeper annual GFR decline is associated with foot process effacement.[29]

GENETICS

Dent disease is caused by mutations in either the *CLCN5* or *OCRL1* genes, both located on the X-chromosome. Dent-1 refers to patients with mutations in the *CLCN5* gene, and is found in 60% of patients with the clinical phenotype. An additional 15% to 20% are due to mutations in *OCRL1* and are known as Dent-2.[9,30] Genetic heterogeneity caused by yet to be identified genetic mutations are assumed to be responsible for the remaining cases.[31]

Dent-1

Dent-1 is caused by inactivating mutations in the *CLCN5* gene located on the short arm of the X-chromosome (Xp11.22). *CLCN5* encodes CLC-5, a chloride proton exchanger mainly found in the renal and intestinal epithelia. In the kidney, CLC-5 is mostly expressed in the proximal tubule and α-intercalated cells of the collecting duct.[32] More than 130 different *CLCN5* mutations have been identified, with most being either missense or nonsense mutations.[33] The type of mutation (missense, nonsense, or frameshift) does not seem to reliably predict disease outcome or prognosis.[17]

Dent-2

The *OCRL1* gene is located on the long arm of the X-chromosome (Xq25) and encodes a lipid phosphatase that hydrolyzes phosphatidyl-inositol 4,5-bisphosphate (PIP_2).[14] Mutations in the *OCRL1* gene are also seen in LS, suggesting that Dent-2 disease may be a milder variant of LS.[34]

PATHOPHYSIOLOGY
Chloride Exchanger

The CLC family is a group of chloride-specific ion channels and transporters that were initially described in the early 1990s. Three CLC subfamilies are found in animals, with 13 individual CLC proteins having been described to date. CLC proteins generally function as either Cl^- channels or Cl^-/H^+ exchangers,[32] and have been associated with neuromuscular (myotonia congenita, *CLCN1*), bone (osteopetrosis, *CLCN7*), and renal diseases (Bartter disease, *CLCNKB*, and Dent disease-1, *CLCN5*) in which anion transport is critical.

Endocytic Pathway

CLC-5 is expressed in the proximal tubule, the thick ascending limb of the loop of Henle, and the intercalated cells of the collecting ducts.[35] Reabsorption of filtered

LMW proteins is mediated by the megalin and cubilin receptors in the proximal tubule cells. They form a multireceptor complex on the apical brush border and bind different ligands, including LMW proteins.[36] Under normal circumstances, ligands bind to these receptors leading to endocytosis. The endosome is progressively acidified by an H^+-ATPase, leading to dissociation of the receptor ligand complex and subsequent degradation of the ligand in the lysosome.[14] The chloride exchanger CLC-5 is believed to either dissipate the positive charge gradient in the endosome or drive proton entry directly into the proximal tubular cells where the tubular luminal chloride content is high, resulting in proton entry into the endosome and thereby playing an essential role in the endocytotic pathway.

Studies of CLC-5 knockout mice demonstrate abnormal endosomal function.[37,38] In addition to, the potential role of maintaining endosomal acidification described previously it has also been hypothesized that CLC-5 plays a role in recycling megalin and cubilin to the brush border, which is critical for normal endosomal function.[35,39] Recent studies in zebrafish suggest that *OCRL1* is also involved in the renal tubular endocytotic pathway.[40] The accumulation of PIP_2 due to decreased *OCRL1* activity is thought to alter cell signaling involved in endocytosis. This may also affect intracellular trafficking of proteins and actin polymerization, leading to disruption of certain cell-cell contacts in the proximal tubule,[41] thereby providing a potential explanation for the similar phenotype observed.

Mouse models suggest that impaired endocytosis may lead to decreased proximal tubular reabsorption of parathyroid hormone (PTH). The accumulation of PTH in the urine of the late proximal tubule may result in internalization of the sodium-phosphate–dependent transporter IIa receptors, thereby promoting phosphaturia.[14] The mechanisms contributing to hypercalciuria have not been fully elucidated. A possible explanation is that the high urinary PTH causes increased activity of the 1α-hydroxylase enzyme in the proximal tubule. The resulting increased conversion of 25(OH)-vitamin D3 to 1,25 (OH)-vitamin D3 would thereby enhance intestinal calcium reabsorption and ultimately promote hypercalciuria.[39]

MANAGEMENT
Current Therapies

Current interventions are aimed at slowing the progression of CKD and decreasing hypercalciuria and its complications. Treatment of the hypercalciuria is mainly achieved through low sodium diet and thiazide diuretics. The use of thiazide diuretics has not been evaluated in randomized controlled trials but has been showed to reduce hypercalciuria by more than 40% in the short term[42]; however, use may be limited by the development of hypotension or hypokalemia. Dietary calcium restriction is not recommended, as decreased intake may compromise bone health and increase risk of nephrolithiasis. Hypokalemia, acidosis, and/or hypophosphatemia should be treated with supplementation. Treatment with vitamin D should be used carefully to avoid exacerbation of hypercalciuria. High-citrate diet has been shown to delay progression of CKD in a mouse model,[43] but has not been evaluated in humans. Although citrate therapy is used in patients with LS to treat the acidosis, the benefit in Dent disease has yet to be proven, as urinary citrate excretion is generally normal.

Angiotensin-converting enzyme inhibitors (ACEIs) and angiotensin receptor blockers (ARBs) have been used in patients with proteinuria.[10,17,22,25] Given that Dent disease is a primarily a nonglomerular disease, the rationale to using ACEI/ARB therapy is unclear. The long-term effects of ACEI and ARB therapy in Dent disease have not been studied. In a retrospective review of 8 patients treated with

ACEI/ARB therapy, 2 had significant reductions in proteinuria, 4 had no change in proteinuria, 1 had to be discontinued because of rapidly rising creatinine, and 1 had no follow-up data. Two of the 3 patients followed for at least 3 years had a substantial decline in GFR.[25]

Future Therapies/Diagnostics

Although our understanding of the genetics and pathophysiology of Dent disease have evolved considerably since Dent and Friedman's[1] original description, our ability to effectively treat the condition has remained elusive. Furthermore, Dent disease likely remains underdiagnosed in individuals with both CKD and renal calculi due to a general lack of awareness and the absence of a readily available screening tool. The development of urinary proteome analysis may prove to be a useful tool in diagnosing patients with a variety of renal conditions in a noninvasive fashion. Recently, Santucci and colleagues[44] studied a large family with Dent disease. Analysis of more than 1000 samples revealed a specific cluster of proteins in the urine of affected patients as compared with carrier female individuals and healthy subjects. The identification of this specific profile has implications for increasing our diagnostic capacity as well as the ability to noninvasively monitor both progression and efficacy of medical intervention.

As with many genetic conditions, the potential of gene editing, exon skipping, gene replacement, medications that suppress stop codons, medications with the ability to rescue nonfunctional proteins, and bone marrow transplantation to deliver functional proteins and rescue damaged organs are exciting potential therapies. Recently, a CIC-5 knockout mouse model transplanted with wild-type bone marrow showed improvement in proximal tubular dysfunction and rescue of megalin receptor expression on the apical membrane. Nanotubular extensions were observed between the engrafted bone marrow–derived cells and proximal tubule cells, providing a potential explanation for the rescue mechanism.[45] Whether this could ultimately have clinical application to human patients remains to be evaluated.

REFERENCES

1. Dent CE, Friedman M. Hypercalcuric rickets associated with renal tubular damage. Arch Dis Child 1964;39(205):240–9.

2. Wrong OM, Norden AGW, Feest TG. Dent's disease; a familial proximal renal tubular syndrome with low-molecular-weight proteinuria, hypercalciuria, nephrocalcinosis, metabolic bone disease, progressive renal failure and a marked male predominance. QJM 1994;87(8):473–93.

3. Fisher SE, Black GC, Lloyd SE, et al. Isolation and partial characterization of a chloride channel gene which is expressed in kidney and is a candidate for Dent's disease (an X-linked hereditary nephrolithiasis). Hum Mol Genet 1994;3(11): 2053–9. Available at: http://pubman.mpdl.mpg.de/pubman/item/escidoc: 529621:6.

4. Fisher SE, Van Bakel I, Lloyd SE, et al. Cloning and characterization of CLCN5, the human kidney chloride channel gene implicated in dent disease (an X-linked hereditary nephrolithiasis). Genomics 1995;29(3):598–606.

5. Frymoyer PA, Scheinman SJ, Dunham PB, et al. X-linked recessive nephrolithiasis with renal failure. N Engl J Med 1991;325(10):681–6.

6. Bolino A, Devoto M, Enia G, et al. Genetic mapping in the Xp11.2 region of a new form of X-linked hypophosphatemic rickets. Eur J Hum Genet 1993;1(4):269–79.

7. Igarashi T, Hayakawa H, Shiraga H, et al. Hypercalciuria and nephrocalcinosis in patients with idiopathic low-molecular-weight proteinuria in Japan: is the disease identical to Dent's disease in United Kingdom? Nephron 1995;69(3):242–7. Available at: http://www.ncbi.nlm.nih.gov/pubmed/7753256.

8. Akuta N, Lloyd SE, Igarashi T, et al. Mutations of CLCN5 in Japanese children with idiopathic low molecular weight proteinuria, hypercalciuria and nephrocalcinosis. Kidney Int 1997;52(4):911–6.

9. Hoopes RR, Shrimpton AE, Knohl SJ, et al. Dent disease with mutations in OCRL1. Am J Hum Genet 2005;76(2):260–7.

10. Frishberg Y, Dinour D, Belostotsky R, et al. Dent's disease manifesting as focal glomerulosclerosis: is it the tip of the iceberg? Pediatr Nephrol 2009;24(12):2369–73.

11. Loi M. Lowe syndrome. Orphanet J Rare Dis 2006;1(1):1–5.

12. Bökenkamp A, Böckenhauer D, Cheong H II, et al. Dent-2 disease: a mild variant of Lowe syndrome. J Pediatr 2009;155(1):94–9.

13. Bhardwaj S, Thergaonkar R, Sinha A, et al. Phenotype of Dent disease in a cohort of Indian children. Indian Pediatr 2016;53(11):977–82.

14. Claverie-Martín F, Ramos-Trujillo E, García-Nieto V. Dent's disease: clinical features and molecular basis. Pediatr Nephrol 2011;26(5):693–704.

15. Ludwig M, Utsch B, Balluch B, et al. Hypercalciuria in patients with CLCN5 mutations. Pediatr Nephrol 2006;21(9):1241–50.

16. Scheinman SJ. X-linked hypercalciuric nephrolithiasis: clinical syndromes and chloride channel mutations. Kidney Int 1998;53(1):3–17.

17. Blanchard A, Curis E, Guyon-Roger T, et al. Observations of a large Dent disease cohort. Kidney Int 2016;90(2):430–9.

18. Devuyst O, Thakker RV. Dent's disease. Orphanet J Rare Dis 2010;5(1):28.

19. Mansour-Hendili L, Blanchard A, Le Pottier N, et al. Mutation update of the CLCN5 gene responsible for Dent disease 1. Hum Mutat 2015;36(8):743–52.

20. Norden AGW, Scheinman SJ, Deschodt-Lanckman MM, et al. Tubular proteinuria defined by a study of Dent's (CLCN5 mutation) and other tubular diseases. Kidney Int 2000;57(1):240–9.

21. Sethi SK, Ludwig M, Kabra M, et al. Vitamin A responsive night blindness in Dent's disease. Pediatr Nephrol 2009;24(9):1765–70.

22. Copelovitch L, Nash MA, Kaplan BS. Hypothesis: Dent disease is an underrecognized cause of focal glomerulosclerosis. Clin J Am Soc Nephrol 2007;2(5):914–8.

23. Copelovitch L. Urolithiasis in children: medical approach. Pediatr Clin North Am 2012;59(4):881–96.

24. Bogdanović R, Draaken M, Toromanović A, et al. A novel CLCN5 mutation in a boy with Bartter-like syndrome and partial growth hormone deficiency. Pediatr Nephrol 2010;25(11):2363–8.

25. van Berkel Y, Ludwig M, van Wijk JAE, et al. Proteinuria in Dent disease: a review of the literature. Pediatr Nephrol 2017;32(10):1851–9.

26. Shrimpton AE, Hoopes RR, Knohl SJ, et al. OCRL1 mutations in Dent 2 patients suggest a mechanism for phenotypic variability. Nephron - Physiol 2009;112(2):27–36.

27. Bernard AM, Moreau D, Lauwerys R. Comparison of retinol-binding protein and beta 2-microglobulin determination in urine for the early detection of tubular proteinuria. Clin Chim Acta 1982;126(1):1–7.

28. Hoopes J, Hueber PA, Reid J, et al. CLCN5 chloride-channel mutations in six new North American families with X-linked nephrolithiasis. Kidney Int 1998;54(3):698–705.

29. Wang X, Anglani F, Beara-Lasic L, et al. Glomerular pathology in Dent disease and its association with kidney function. Clin J Am Soc Nephrol 2016;11(12): 2168–76.

30. Böckenhauer D, Bökenkamp A, Nuutinen M, et al. Novel OCRL mutations in patients with Dent-2 disease. J Pediatr Genet 2012;1(1):15–23.

31. Hoopes RR, Raja KM, Koich A, et al. Evidence for genetic heterogeneity in Dent's disease. Kidney Int 2004;65(5):1615–20.

32. Poroca DR, Pelis RM, Chappe VM. ClC channels and transporters: structure, physiological functions, and implications in human chloride channelopathies. Front Pharmacol 2017;8(MAR):1–25.

33. Pusch M, Zifarelli G. ClC-5: Physiological role and biophysical mechanisms. Cell Calcium 2015;58(1):57–66.

34. Levin-Iaina N, Dinour D. Renal disease with OCRL1 mutations: Dent-2 or Lowe syndrome? J Pediatr Genet 2012;1(1):3–5.

35. Devuyst O, Jouret F, Auzanneau C, et al. Chloride channels and endocytosis: new insights from Dent's disease and ClC-5 knockout mice. Nephron Physiol 2005; 99(3):p69–73.

36. Nielsen R, Christensen EI, Birn H. Megalin and cubilin in proximal tubule protein reabsorption: from experimental models to human disease. Kidney Int 2016; 89(1):58–67.

37. Piwon N, Gunther W, Schwake M, et al. ClC-5 Cl–channel disruption impairs endocytosis in a mouse model for Dent's disease. Nature 2000;408(6810): 369–73.

38. Wang SS, Devuyst O, Courtoy PJ, et al. Mice lacking renal chloride channel, CLC-5, are a model for Dent's disease, a nephrolithiasis disorder associated with defective receptor-mediated endocytosis. Hum Mol Genet 2000;9(20): 2937–45.

39. Günther W, Piwon N, Jentsch TJ. The ClC-5 chloride channel knock-out mouse—an animal model for Dent's disease. Pflügers Arch - Eur J Physiol 2003;445(4): 456–62.

40. Oltrabella F, Pietka G, Ramirez IB-R, et al. The Lowe syndrome protein OCRL1 is required for endocytosis in the zebrafish pronephric tubule. PLOS Genet 2015; 11(4):e1005058.

41. Suchy SF, Nussbaum RL. The deficiency of PIP2 5-phosphatase in Lowe syndrome affects actin polymerization. Am J Hum Genet 2002;71(6):1420–7.

42. Raja KA, Schurman S, D'Mello RG, et al. Responsiveness of hypercalciuria to thiazide in Dent's disease. J Am Soc Nephrol 2002;13(12):2938–44.

43. Cebotaru V, Kaul S, Devuyst O, et al. High citrate diet delays progression of renal insufficiency in the ClC-5 knockout mouse model of Dent's disease. Kidney Int 2005;68(2):642–52.

44. Santucci L, Candiano G, Anglani F, et al. Urine proteome analysis in Dent's disease shows high selective changes potentially involved in chronic renal damage. J Proteomics 2016;130:26–32.

45. Gabriel SS, Belge H, Gassama A, et al. Bone marrow transplantation improves proximal tubule dysfunction in a mouse model of Dent disease. Kidney Int 2017;91(4):842–55.

46. Utsch B, Bökenkamp A, Benz MR, et al. Novel OCRL1 mutations in patients with the phenotype of Dent disease. Am J Kidney Dis 2006;48(6):942–54.

47. Tasic V, Lozanovski VJ, Korneti P, et al. Clinical and laboratory features of Macedonian children with OCRL mutations. Pediatr Nephrol 2011;26(4):557–62.

48. Zaniew M, Bökenkamp A, Kołbuc M, et al. Long-term renal outcome in children with OCRL mutations: retrospective analysis of a large international cohort NDT Advance Access. Nephrol Dial Transpl 2016;1–11. https://doi.org/10.1093/ndt/gfw350.
49. Li F, Yue Z, Xu T, et al. Dent disease in Chinese children and findings from hetero-zygous mothers: phenotypic heterogeneity, fetal growth, and 10 novel mutations. J Pediatr 2016;174(20110171110047):204–10.e1.

Hypophosphatemic Rickets

Martin Bitzan, MD[a],*, Paul R. Goodyer, MD[b]

KEYWORDS

- FGF23 • Hypophosphatemia • Klotho • Osteomalacia • PHEX • Phosphate
- Vitamin D • X-linked hypophosphatemia

KEY POINTS

- Hypophosphatemia disorders can be divided conceptionally into those with increased fibroblast growth factor 23 (FGF23) levels (caused by mutations of extrarenal factors or by tumors) and those with normal or suppressed FGF23 (due to mutations tubular phosphate transporters). Rickets are the consequence of dysregulated phosphate transport and/or FGF23 excess.
- X-linked hypophosphatemia is due to a hemizygous dominant mutation of the *phosphate-regulating endopeptidase homolog, X-linked* gene leading to unregulated FGF23 production.
- Disease manifestations (rickets, leg bowing, growth delay; osteomalacia, enthesopathies, tooth decay; tertiary hyperparathyroidism), differential diagnoses (inherited forms, tumor-induced osteomalacia), and therapeutic goals change with age.
- Conventional treatment with phosphate supplements and pharmacologic doses of active vitamin D may require the addition of growth hormone and calcimimetics. New biological therapeutics, including FGF23 targeting monoclonal antibodies or recombinant receptor blockers, are being developed and becoming available.
- Lastly, identification of genetic mutations associated with hypophosphatemia syndromes has contributed to our understanding of the pathogenesis and potential treatment of hypercalciuria, nephrocalcinosis, and renal stones disease.

INTRODUCTION

The endocrinologist Fuller Albright has been credited with the first description of hypophosphatemic rickets (HR) that failed to respond to high doses of vitamin D. The diagnostic label vitamin D–resistant rickets was later changed into X-linked HR (XLHR). The currently preferred term is X-linked hypophosphatemia (XLH).[1,2] In up to 85% of familial and sporadic cases of HR, specific disease-causing genetic variants can be identified.[2,3] The molecular defect underlying XLHR, a mutation in *phosphate*

Disclosure Statement: No disclosures.
[a] Department of Pediatrics, The Montreal Children's Hospital, McGill University Health Centre, 1001 Boulevard Décarie, Room B RC.6164, Montreal, Quebec H4A 3J1, Canada; [b] The Research Institute of the McGill University Health Centre, 1001 Boulevard Décarie, Room EM1.2232, Montreal, Quebec H4A3J1, Canada
* Corresponding author.
E-mail address: martin.bitzan@mcgill.ca

Pediatr Clin N Am 66 (2019) 179–207
https://doi.org/10.1016/j.pcl.2018.09.004
0031-3955/19/© 2018 Elsevier Inc. All rights reserved.

pediatric.theclinics.com

(PO$_4$)-regulating endopeptidase homolog, X-linked (PHEX), was reported in 1995.[4] How the product of the mutated PHEX gene leads to hypophosphatemia is not yet entirely solved. An autosomal dominant form of HR was subsequently traced to an activating mutation in the gene encoding fibroblast growth factor 23 (FGF23).[5,6]

XLHR is the most common of genetically defined hypophosphatemic disorders and serves as the prototype of hereditary PO$_4$-wasting conditions. This review focuses on the physiologic aspects of PO$_4$ regulation and the genetic and clinical therapeutic aspects of XLHR. Other hypophosphatemia syndromes are briefly presented.

PHOSPHATE HOMEOSTASIS

Phosphorus, the most abundant anion in the body,[7] is an essential element for numerous cellular molecules, including nucleic acids, proteins, and lipids. It is critical for bone formation, and it is involved in acid-base regulation and cellular physiology. Rickets is a disease of the growth plate due to insufficient availability of PO$_4$ (inorganic phosphorus [Pi]). It only affects growing children.[2] PO$_4$ deficiency may be due to poor absorption from the gut or renal wasting.

The average adult body contains about 700 g of phosphorus: 85% is found in skeletal bones and teeth, 14% in soft tissues, and only 1% is present in the extracellular fluid, which is in equilibrium with the major phosphorus stores.[2] Plasma PO$_4$ is bound to proteins and lipids (16%), whereas the remainder is present as orthophosphate or free Pi, which exists as monovalent H$_2$PO$_4^-$ and divalent HPO$_4^{2-}$ in a 1:4 M ratio at physiologic pH and is filtered into the Bowman space of the glomerulus.[8]

The primary organ involved in the maintenance of the serum PO$_4$ concentration is the kidney.[9] The overall phosphorus balance is accomplished by intestinal absorption and renal excretion, which is regulated by the serum PO$_4$ level, vitamin D, parathyroid hormone (PTH), and phosphatonins (Fig. 1). The ability of a cell to sense changes in extracellular PO$_4$ levels is critical for Pi homeostasis and skeletal mineralization. Recent work has provided evidence for the molecular basis of the long-postulated Pi sensing mechanism and for intracellular signaling by extracellular PO$_4$.[8]

Phosphorus Absorption

Intestinal absorption of phosphorus is nutrition dependent. Only 30% of PO$_4$ absorption is controlled by active 1,25-dihydroxycholecalciferol (1,25(OH)$_2$D or calcitriol), which contrasts with the tight regulation of PO$_4$ reabsorption in the kidney.[10] Requirements of Pi are highest during the third trimester of gestation and in infants to support adequate skeletal bone mineralization.[11] Nutritional uptake of phosphorus in the gut is approximately 16 mg per kilogram of body weight in children[2] or 800 to 1500 mg per day in adults. Pi transport across the epithelial brush border membrane is mediated almost entirely by the sodium-dependent PO$_4$ cotransporter II (NaPi-IIb) transporter (encoded by SLC34A2; solute carrier family 34 (sodium phosphate), member 2). Because PO$_4$ is bound to polyvalent cations in the gut, including Ca^{2+} and Mg^{2+}, only about two-thirds of the ingested PO$_4$ is absorbed.[11] The daily turnover of PO$_4$ in skeletal bone, due to physiologic remodeling, amounts to 3 mg/kg (200 mg in adults).[2]

Phosphorus Excretion

The major site of Pi excretion is the kidney (900 mg daily in adults consuming an average diet).[12] P$_i$ passes freely through the glomerular filtration barrier. Its concentration in the Bowman space (the glomerular filtrate) equates the concentration of total free PO$_4$ in plasma.[13] Between 80% and 97% of the filtered PO$_4$ load is reabsorbed from the tubular lumen (fractional tubular reabsorption of PO$_4$ [TRP]), mainly in the proximal convoluted

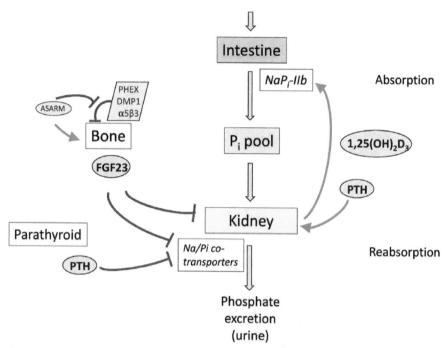

Fig. 1. PO$_4$ homeostasis. For details, see text and cited references. $\alpha5\beta3$, $\alpha5\beta3$-integrin, *ASARM*, acidic serine- and aspartate-rich motif peptides; *DMP1*, dentin matrix protein-1.

segments; the remainder (3%–20%) is excreted in the final urine (fractional excretion of PO$_4$ [FEPO$_4$]). Both can be calculated from simultaneously measured creatinine and PO$_4$ concentrations in plasma and in urine (see later discussion). There is no reabsorption in the loop of Henle. The extent and mechanisms of reabsorption in the distal tubule, if any, is controversial and may be limited to conditions of PO$_4$ deprivation.[13] Tubular PO$_4$ reabsorption is a saturable process. When the PO$_4$ concentration in the glomerular filtrate exceeds the physiologic threshold, PO$_4$ excretion increases linearly with an increase in glomerular filtration rate (GFR) (and the filtered load).[13,14]

PO$_4$ reabsorption is regulated by PTH and phosphatonins, mainly endocrine FGF23.[11] PO$_4$ leaves the proximal tubular epithelial cells via a postulated electrogenic PO$_4$-anion exchanger (**Fig. 2**).[13,15]

Phosphate Transporters

Reabsorption of PO$_4$ from the tubular lumen is a unidirectional, transcellular process.[16] Apical entry into the proximal tubular epithelial cells against the intracellular/tubular concentration gradient is facilitated by sodium/ PO$_4$ cotransporters. The tubular capacity of PO$_4$ reabsorption depends on the abundance of Na/Pi cotransporters in the proximal tubular epithelial cell apical brush border membrane. Physiologically important Pi transporters in the kidney belong to 2 isoforms of the SLC34 family of solute carriers, the type II cotransporters NaPi-IIa (*SLC34A1*; solute carrier family 34 (sodium phosphate), member 1) and NaPi-IIc (*SLC34A3*; solute carrier family 34 (sodium phosphate), member 3) and the type III sodium-dependent PO$_4$ symporter PiT-2 (*SLC20A2*; solute carrier family 20 member 2)[6,7,11,17–19] (**Table 1**).

Physiologically, expression of NaPi-IIa and NaPi-IIc is highest in early convoluted proximal tubules (S1 segment) and in juxtamedullary nephrons but spreads to the

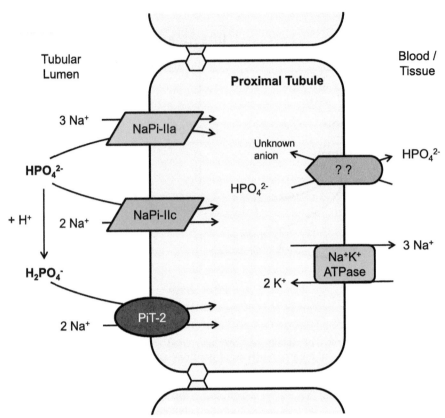

Fig. 2. Schematic drawing of proximal tubular phosphate transport. Three apical (luminal) cotransporters mediate phosphate reabsorption. They differ with respect to valence of PO_4, stoichiometry of Na^+ and PO_4, electrogenicity, and pH gating. The affinities of NaPi-IIa, NaPi-IIc and PiT-2 are approximately 300 to 2000-fold higher for PO_4 than for Na^+. PO_4 leaves the proximal tubular epithelial cell via a postulated electrogenic PO_4 anion exchanger. Acidosis leads to the addition of a hydrogen ion to divalent PO_4 and inhibition (direct pH gating) of Na^+coupled PO_4 transport by type II cotransporters (Na-IIa and Na-IIc). (*Adapted from* Curthoys NP, Moe OW. Proximal tubule function and response to acidosis. Clin J Am Soc Nephrol 2014;9(9):1627–38.)

late proximal tubule (S2/S3 segments) and to superficial nephrons during PO_4 depletion.[6,20] The 3 Pi transporters have differential sensitivities to pH and regulation by dietary Pi intake and phosphaturic hormones. Type II transporters are selective for divalent PO_4 (HPO_4^{2-}), while type III transporters favour monovalent PO_4 ($H_2PO_4^-$)[19] (see **Fig. 2**). A third member of the SLC34 family, NaPi-IIb, is expressed in the luminal brush border of the small intestine but also in the lungs and testis.[13] The type III PO_4 transporter PiT-1 (*SLC20A1*) is expressed ubiquitously.[21–23] PiT-1 and PiT-2 facilitate Pi sensing and intracellular signaling.[8] Studies in PiT-2 knockout mice suggest that PiT-2 is involved in normal bone development and growth and that it plays a role in cortical and trabecular bone metabolism, likely by regulating PO_4 transport and mineralization processes in the bone.[23] In humans, mutations in *SLC20A2* have been linked to familial idiopathic basal ganglia calcification and fetal growth restriction, among others (see **Table 1**).[24]

Table 1
Renal phosphate transporters

Transporter/Channel[a]	Gene Chromosomal Location MIM	Protein Expression	Function, Mechanism	Comments, Disease Associations
Type II				
NaPi-IIa (NPT2a) Na$^+$ coupled PO$_4$ transporter (Na/Pi cotransporter)	*SLC34A1* 5q35.3 *612286	(Apical) brush border of proximal tubular epithelial cell (predominantly S1 segment)	Accounts for 70%-80% of renal tubular PO$_4$ reabsorption (in mice) Risk gene for kidney stones[19] Transport stoichiometry 3:1 Na$^+$: divalent HPO$_4{}^{2-}$ per transport cycle (electrogenic)	Overlapping syndrome of hypophosphatemia, hypercalcemia, and nephrocalcinosis NPHLOP1# 182309 FRTS2# 613388 HCINF2# 616963
NaPi-IIc (NPT2c)	*SLC34A3* 9q34.3 *609826	Physiologically exclusively along proximal tubular epithelium of deep nephrons (also expressed in bone, with unclear function)	Accounts for 10% of PO$_4$ reabsorption Transport stoichiometry 2:1 Na$^+$: divalent HPO$_4{}^{2-}$ per transport cycle (electroneutral)	Hereditary hypophosphatemic rickets with hypercalciuria (HHRH # 24530) Isolated hypercalciuria and nephrolithiasis[131,133]
NaPi-IIb (NPT2b)	*SLC34A2* 4p15.2 *604217	Broad expression: Intestine Lung (alveolar type II epithelial cells)	Intestinal Pi absorption Alveolar surfactant production Transport stoichiometry 3:1 Na$^+$: divalent HPO$_4{}^{2-}$ per transport cycle (electrogenic)	Pulmonary alveolar microlithiasis (autosomal recessive)
Type III				
PiT-1 (Na-dependent Pi transporter [symporter]-1) Glvr-1	*SLC20A1* 2q14.1 *137570	Ubiquitous	Small contribution to tubular PO$_4$ transport Pi sensing	Major P$_i$ transporter in brain[22]
PiT-2	*SLC20A2* 8p11.21 *158378	Colocalize to brush border of proximal tubule (with NaPi-IIa and NaPi-IIc)	Transports mainly monovalent PO$_4^-$ (H$_2$PO$_4^-$) Pi-dependent secretion of FGF23 Pi sensing	Basal ganglial calcification[134] No known defect of renal PO$_4$ handling[19]

Abbreviation: Glvr-1, Gibbon ape leukemia virus receptor-1.

[a] Mutations in 2 other genes may directly affect renal PO$_4$ transport, *NHERF1* (Na/H exchanger factor-1 or SLC9A3R1 [MIM * 604990]; see also **Fig. 5**), associated with nephrolithiasis, osteoporosis, and hypophosphatemia (NPHLOP2),[135,136] and *XPR1* (xenotropic and polytrophic retrovirus receptor [MIM *605237]), associated with basal ganglia calcifications.[134]

Regulation of Phosphate Transport and Serum Concentration

Multiple mechanisms regulate Pi transport. PTH, calcitonin, glucocorticoids, and other drugs, such as calcineurin inhibitors, as well as acidosis inhibit tubular reabsorption. In contrast, growth hormone, IGF-1 and insulin, thyroid hormone, and hypocalcemia and PO_4 depletion lead to increased Pi reabsorption.

Important regulators of the serum PO_4 level are PTH and phosphatonins.[13] The latter are humoral factors with phosphaturic activity. They inhibit PO_4 reabsorption and decrease the level of $1,25(OH)_2D$. PTH and phosphatonins (foremost FGF23) diminish PO_4 reabsorption by decreasing the abundance of apically expression Na/Pi cotransporters, which augments phosphaturia.[25–27] The drivers of PTH and phosphatonin secretion are serum calcium, PO_4, and $1,25(OH)_2D$ concentrations (**Fig. 3**).

Fibroblast growth factor 23

FGF23 is a glycoprotein of 32 kD, produced and secreted by osteoblasts and osteocytes.[28,29] The description of its hormonal, phosphaturic function in 2000[30] established the importance of bones as an endocrine tissue.[31] Synthesis and secretion of FGF23 is stimulated by elevated serum Pi concentrations and $1,25(OH)_2D$[29,32–36] (see **Fig. 3**). The full-length protein, encoded by 3 exons, includes an N-terminal hydrophobic, FGF homology domain, and a C-terminal domain that interacts with αKlotho to form the FGF/Klotho-FGFR receptor complex (see later discussion). Intact FGF23 is cleaved at the amino acid residues Arg (176)-X-X-Arg (179)/Ser (180) recognition sequence, which generates 2 inactive (N- and C-terminal) fragments[28] (**Fig. 4**).

The precise mechanism underlying FGF23 dysregulation, for example, in XLH and tumor-induced osteomalacia is still being worked out.[37] Recent studies suggest that iron deficiency stimulates *FGF23* gene transcription, with the involvement of hypoxia-inducible factor 1 (HIF1α).[37–39] FGF23 signaling diminishes sodium-dependent Pi reabsorption; it also inhibits 1α-hydroxylase (CYP27B1) and increases 24-hydroxylase activity, both of which reduce the availability of $1,25(OH)_2D$ (see **Fig. 3**). Reduced availability of active D_3 limits calcium absorption in the gut and calcium reabsorption in renal tubules.

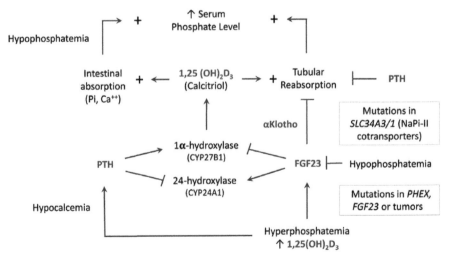

Fig. 3. Regulation of FGF23, αKlotho, PTH, calcitriol, phosphate and calcium. Stimulatory and inhibitory effects are indicated.

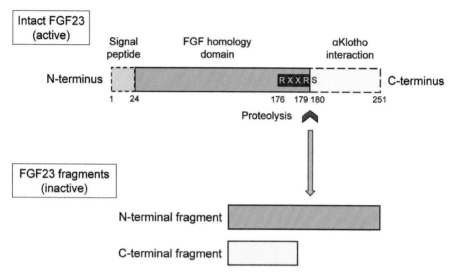

Fig. 4. The FGF23 molecule with the cleavage $R_{176}XXR_{179}$ recognition motif. The N-terminal signal peptide is removed before secretion from osteocytes/osteoblasts. Proteolytic cleavage of FGF23 between Arg179 and Ser180 generates 2 inactive (N- and C-terminal) fragments. (*Adapted from* Kinoshita Y, Fukumoto S. X-linked hypophosphatemia and FGF23-related hypophosphatemic diseases: prospect for new treatment. Endocr Rev 2018;39(3):274–91; and Gonciulea AR, De Beur JSM. Fibroblast growth factor 23-mediated bone disease. Endocrinol Metab Clin North Am 2017;46(1):19–39.)

Klotho

αKlotho has been originally described in 1997 as the product of a gene named *KL* or *KLOTHO*; its mutation resulted in premature aging of transgenic mice who also presented growth retardation, vascular calcification, and osteomalacia, among others.[40,41] The name is derived from the goddess of fate in Greek mythology who spins the thread of life.[40]

In humans, αKlotho exists as a full-length, single-pass (trans)membrane form and a pleiotropic, soluble (shed) extracellular form (sKlotho).[41,42] αKlotho is highly expressed in kidneys, parathyroid gland, choroid plexus, and sinoatrial node and minimally in bone and cartilage.[43] Both the transmembrane form and soluble Klotho interact with the FGF receptor in proximal tubular cells converting it to a high-affinity receptor for FGF23[41,42,44,45] (**Fig. 5**). Signaling of the FGF23-FGFR-Klotho complex leads to the internalization and degradation of NaP_i-IIa and NaP_i-IIc in the proximal tubule, inhibition of $1,25(OH)_2D$ synthesis, and increased 24-hydroxylase activity.[44,46,47] sKlotho influences Na^+-K^+-ATPase activity in the basolateral membrane, which leads to an increased Na^+ ion gradient and enhanced transepithelial calcium transport in the kidney and the choroid plexus in the brain.[48] sKlotho also plays a direct role in calcium homeostasis by regulating the transient receptor potential vanilloid type 5 (TRPV5) calcium channel at the apical membrane of the distal convoluted and connecting tubular cells responsible for calcium reabsorption in the distal nephron.[18,49–51]

Phosphate regulating endopeptidase homolog, X-linked

PHEX comprises 18 exons and codes for an 86.5 kD, type II membrane protein with an N-terminal cytoplasmic tail, a transmembrane domain, and a long extracellular C-terminus.[52] The PHEX protein is a member of the neutral endopeptidase family of zinc metalloproteinases that mediate the activation or degradation of peptide

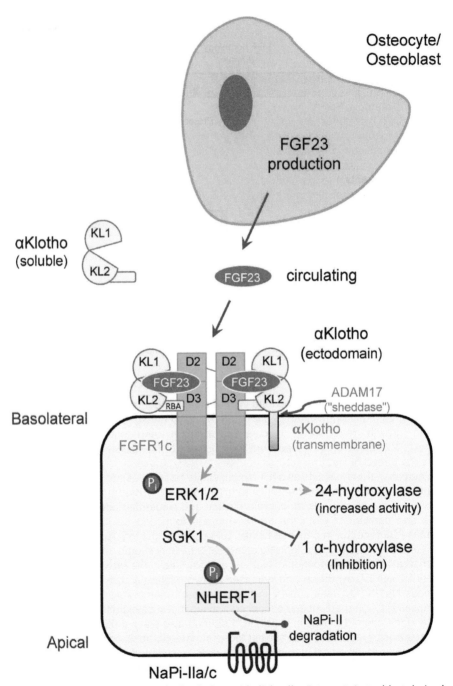

Fig. 5. FGF23 signaling in proximal tubular epithelial cells. Osteocyte/osteoblast-derived, endocrine FGF23 binds to the FGF receptor, FGFR1c and its coreceptor, αKlotho. The FGF23-FGFR-Klotho complex is stabilized by the receptor-binding arm (RBA) of Klotho. This ternary complex dimerizes via heparan sulfate (*stick lines*) to form a quaternary complex, which enables intracellular signal transduction. The kidney is the main source of

hormones.[4] It is expressed in osteoblasts and osteoclasts of skeletal bones and in teeth (odontoblasts) and parathyroid glands as well as lung, brain, ovary, testicle, and muscle but not in kidneys.[53,54] It binds to matrix extracellular phosphoglyco-protein (MEPE) and relieves the inhibitory effect of these proteins on bone mineral-ization.[55] The interaction between PHEX, dentin matrix protein-1 (DMP1), and $\alpha_5\beta_3$-integrin, which form a trimeric complex on the osteocyte plasma membrane, regu-lates and restricts FGF23 expression, whereas acidic serine- and aspartate-rich motif (ASARM) peptides, derived from MEPE and other bone and dental matrix pro-teins, competitively inhibit the trimeric complex and increase FGF23 expres-sion.[37,56] Inactivating mutations in PHEX lead to an accumulation of ASARM peptide, a substrate for PHEX and a strong inhibitor of mineralization, and increased circulating levels of FGF23 that result in phosphaturia, hypophosphate-mia, and suppression of 25-hydroxyvitamin D to 1,25 dihydroxy-vitamin D conver-sion $(1,25(OH)_2D)$.[55,57–59]

Parathyroid hormone

PTH is an important hormonal effector of PO_4 and calcium homeostasis. It regulates renal PO_4 handling and bone turnover and amplifies the effects of vitamin D.[13] Low serum Ca^{++} concentrations trigger rapid release of PTH from secretory granules in para-thyroid gland chief cells via the calcium-sensing receptor.[60,61] PTH mobilizes PO_4 from skeletal bones into the blood stream, possibly by enhancing osteoclastic bone resorp-tion.[62] It induces the expression of 1α-hydroxylase in the proximal tubule of the kidney and the generation of $1,25(OH)_2D$ in a variety of tissues, including osteoblasts.[63]

PTH binding to its receptors on proximal tubular epithelial cells leads to dimin-ished abundance of apical proximal tubular NaPi-II cotransporters and diminished reabsorption of filtered Pi along the proximal tubule.[64] It also interferes with PO_4 reabsorption through the inhibition of basolateral Na^+-K^+-ATPase, which removes intracellular sodium in exchange for potassium. The basolateral exclusion of Na^+ is required to allow active transport of PO_4 across the apical membrane, which gen-erates the necessary Na^+ gradient (see **Fig. 2**). PTH causes phosphaturia within mi-nutes by impeding the apical Pi transport.[65]

HYPOPHOSPHATEMIA, RICKETS, AND OSTEOMALACIA
Clinical Findings

The clinical presentation of hypophosphatemia syndromes depends on the duration of hypophosphatemia and the age of patients (infancy and childhood vs adulthood).

---

circulating (soluble) Klotho, which is derived from the large extracellular (ecto) domain of transmembrane αKlotho via membrane-anchored proteases, such a ADAM17. Circulating FGF23 binds to FGFR1 and Klotho in tightly fitting grooves between D2/D3 and KL1/KL2 do-mains, respectively.[42] FGF23 signaling is mediated by transmembrane or sKLotho complexed with FGFR. FGF23 binding FGFR-Klotho complex stabilization via the RBA activates extracel-lular signal-regulated kinases 1 and 2 (ERK1/2) and serum/glucocorticoid-regulated kinase-1 (SGK1). αKlotho (transmembrane) or αKlotho (soluble or ectodomain) both signal ERK phos-phorylation. The resultant Na^+/H^+ exchange regulatory cofactor-1 (NHERF1 or SLC9A3 regu-lator 1) phosphorylation triggers degradation of membrane-bound sodium phosphate cotransporters NaPi-IIa and NaPi-IIc. FGF23 binding and receptor signaling also leads to in-hibition of 1a-hydroxylase CYP27B1 expression and activation of 24-hydroxylase in proximal tubular epithelial cells, resulting in decreased calcitriol levels. PTH signals through activation of protein kinase A (PKA) and C (PKC), which results in the phosphorylation of NHERF1, but stimulates 1α-hydroxylase and inhibits 24-hydroxylase. (Data from Refs.[41,42,46])

Different forms of hypophosphatemia cause similar, albeit not identical, clinical features and radiographical changes. Bone pain and deformities, fractures, disproportionate short stature, and dental abscesses are predominantly seen in chronically hypophosphatemic children. Adults may present with osteomalacia, bone pain, stiffness, and enthesopathy.[59,66,67]

Bone

Osteoblasts regulate the synthesis of bone matrix and bone mineralization, including the deposition of hydroxyapatite ($Ca_3(PO_4)_2Ca(OH)_2$). Multinucleated osteoclasts are responsible for bone resorption.[68] Healthy bone and bone development depend on the coordinated activities of osteoblasts and osteoclasts who receive input from PTH, calcitriol and FGF23, among others, and the transport of calcium and PO_4 in and out of zones of bone remodeling.[68,69] The epiphyseal growth plate influences longitudinal bone growth.[62] Growth velocity is the result of chondrocyte proliferation, matrix production, and chondrocyte function.[62,70]

HYP is the murine homolog of human *PHEX*. The HYP mouse, a model for (human) XLH, demonstrates substantial abnormalities in the growth plate.[4] The primary defect in these mice is impaired osteoblast-dependent mineralization.[62,71] Circulating FGF23-like fibroblast growth factors directly inhibit the proliferation and differentiation of chondrocytes at the growth plate. suggesting that growth plate maturation and bone formation are regulated by PO_4 and FGF23.[62,72]

HYPOPHOSPHATEMIA SYNDROMES

From a mechanistic and conceptual viewpoint, hypophosphatemia syndromes can be divided into those with increased FGF23 levels and those with normal or suppressed FGF23. Hypophosphatemia with increased FGF23 levels is caused by extrarenal factors, whereas hypophosphatemia with normal or suppressed FGF23 is due to mutations in genes encoding tubular PO_4 transporters. Rickets are the consequence of dysregulated PO_4 transport. Inherited disorders of renal PO_4 handling contrast with acquired hypophosphatemia syndromes due to insufficient dietary intake or absorption or due to tubulotoxic drugs or hormonally active tumors.[73]

The most common inherited form of hypophosphatemia and rickets is X-linked dominant hypophosphatemic rickets (XLH or XLHR; OMIM 307800) with a prevalence of 1 per 20,000 general population.[74] It accounts for approximately 80% of familial cases of hypophosphatemia[7] and serves as the prototype of defective tubular PO_4 transport due to extrarenal defects resulting in unregulated FGF23 activity.

Hypophosphatemia Disorders with Increased Fibroblast Growth Factor 23 Activity (Extrarenal Inherited Defects That Impact on Renal Phosphate Reabsorption)

X-linked hypophosphatemia

XLH is caused by loss-of-function mutations in *PHEX* (Xp22.1). Loss of PHEX is thought to cause phosphaturia by suppressing expression of NaPi transporters in the proximal tubule. Sustained tubular loss of PO_4 leads to profound hypophosphatemia, low mineral density.[75,76] Leg deformity and short stature (disproportional dwarfism with predominant shortening of lower limbs) are the consequences of decreased incorporation of PO_4 into growing bone and subtle dysregulation of renal $1,25(OH)_2D$ synthesis.[2,62]

Presentation X-linked hypophosphatemia is a dominant genetic disease. Hemizygous females who inherit a dysfunctional (mutated) *PHEX* allele have renal PO_4 wasting and severe bone deformities indistinguishable from affected (heterozygous) males.[77] The incidence is 4 to 5 per 100,000 live births.[78] During fetal life, bone is protected by maternal blood PO_4 levels (presuming the mother is unaffected) and the newborn skeleton is radiologically normal.[79] FGF23-driven phosphaturia is evident within the first few weeks of life, confirmed by TRP,[80] and serum PO_4 decreases to less than the normal range within the first month (Goodyer P, unpublished data, 2018). Serum PO_4 reaches a nadir less than 1 mM by about 6 months of age and the secondary increase in alkaline PO_4 increases to about 3 to 6 times the upper limit of normal. Interestingly, the TRP improves as serum PO_4 (and the filtered load of PO_4) declines and the calculation of the tubular maximum reabsorption of PO_4 (TmP)/GFR is needed to identify the mutant renal phenotype. The TmP/GFR ratio corresponds to the theoretic lower limit of serum PO_4 less than which all filtered PO_4 would be reabsorbed, assuming that the PO_4 concentration in serum is equal to its concentration in the glomerular filtrate. It can be calculated as $TmP/GFR = SPO_4 - (UPO_4 \times SCr/UCr)$ where UPO_4 denotes urine PO_4, and SCr and UCr serum and urine creatinine concentrations, respectively.[47,81] Although serum calcium and 1,25 $(OH)_2D$ levels are normal, nearly half of affected newborns with XLH have slightly elevated PTH levels, reflecting subtle dysregulation of $1,25(OH)_2D$. Skeletal deformities emerge in the second half of the first year of life because of the weight load on the undermineralized bone. Long bone metaphyses show fuzziness of the growth zone with cupping. Long bones exhibit decreased mineralization amid coarse, sclerotic trabeculae. Radiographs show frontal bossing of the skull, widening of the wrist, and bowing of the legs, which compromise body length. The angle between the femur and hip becomes progressively more oblique, and leg bowing may produce either valgus or varus deformities. The cancellous compartment of long bones (trabecular bone), particularly the tibia, is undermineralized (**Fig. 6**).[2,82] Without therapy, linear growth decelerates until 4 to 5 years of age.[79]

Early oral phosphate/calcitriol therapy Early intervention with balanced oral PO_4/calcitriol supplementation ameliorates hypophosphatemia, gradually reduces serum alkaline phosphatase, accelerates linear growth,[79] and minimizes the severity of skeletal deformity. However, excessive oral PO_4 load without additional calcitriol decreases serum ionized calcium and causes secondary hyperparathyroidism that adds to the FGF23-induced phosphaturia. One approach to balanced oral PO_4/calcitriol therapy is to introduce therapy as soon as the diagnosis is confirmed and monitor the following parameters every 1 to 3 months:

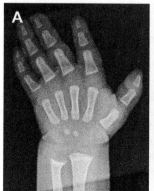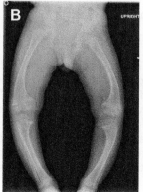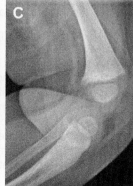

Fig. 6. Child with radiographic changes due to XLH demonstrating (*A*) Cupping of metaphyses of the wrist, (*B*) typical bowing of legs (varus deformity) and undermineralization of the trabecular (cancellous) bones, and (*C*) ragged (frayed) metaphysis of the femur.

- Oral PO_4 supplements should be introduced gradually over 1 to 2 months to allow for upregulation of intestinal PO_4 absorption and avoid PO_4-induced diarrhea. The dose of oral PO_4 should be divided 4 times a day and gradually increased from 15 to 50 to 100 mg of PO_4 per kilogram per day. The authors monitor peak serum PO_4 about 1 hour after the oral dose and adjust the PO_4 dose to bring the peak serum PO_4 concentration into the low normal range.
- Oral PO_4 must be accompanied by calcitriol 25 to 50 ng/kg/d divided twice a day (about 40–80 ng/kg/d of 1-hydroxycholecalciferol [alfacalcidol]), sufficient to keep intact PTH levels within the normal range. With successful therapy, normal rates of linear growth can be expected.
- If urine calcium/creatinine levels are consistently elevated, this may reflect excessive PO_4/calcitriol therapy and predispose to medullary nephrocalcinosis. Although medullary nephrocalcinosis does not seem to compromise renal function in childhood, it may be prudent to reduce the doses of PO_4 and calcitriol (in parallel) when this occurs.

Interestingly, secondary hyperparathyroidism can also be offset by oral cinacalcet (a calcimimetic) in XLH.[83–86] This permits lowering doses of calcitriol to maintain normal intactPTH levels and decreasing the oral PO_4 dose needed by reducing PTH-induced phosphaturia.

When oral therapy is started late or adherence is poor, skeletal deformities may become severe enough to require orthopedic intervention. In this case, surgery should be performed after a 3- to 6-month period of intense therapy to achieve good metabolic control and lower alkaline phosphatase levels. Close postoperative monitoring is equally important to maintain axial leg alignment. Whether the addition of D-mimetics (eg, paricalcitol) improves outcomes, especially in patients with XLH and secondary hyperparathyroidism, requires further studies[87–89] Recombinant human growth hormone has been used to stimulate growth in children with XLH, but the effect on final adult height seems to be modest. Although elevated levels of FGF23 are associated with left ventricular hypertrophy in chronic kidney disease, the heart is generally not affected in XLH.[37]

X-linked hypophosphatemia in adolescence During early to midadolescence, adherence to prescribed dosing may be suboptimal. The growth spurt at this time may further alter calcium/PO_4 homeostasis. This period is a period of risk for the development of tertiary hyperparathyroidism. The pathogenesis of this phenomenon is unknown, but several observations are pertinent:

- Mild secondary hyperparathyroidism is evident in some affected patients before any oral PO_4 therapy.
- The PHEX gene is not expressed in the kidney but is strongly expressed in parathyroid tissue, implying a role in normal PTH gland biology.
- Excessive oral PO_4, if not accompanied by sufficient calcitriol, transiently increases intact PTH levels in serum. It is conceivable that repeated stimulation also drives chief cell proliferation with its attendant risk of mutation in the genes that regulate cell cycle and risk of a benign adenoma.
  Tertiary hyperparathyroidism occurs in the second decade of life in a minority (20%–30%) of patients with XLH and with higher frequency in some families more than in others.
  It is recognized by the onset of gradually increasing total serum calcium levels with inappropriate serum iPTH. Often, a single benign parathyroid adenoma may be identified by a combination of technetium-99 m sestamibi (sesta

methoxyisobutylisonitrile) single-photon emission computed tomography imaging, and neck ultrasound. Hypercalcemia induces a shift from mild medullary nephrocalcinosis (associated with therapy) to a broader pattern of cortical nephrocalcinosis. When hypercalcemia is severe, there may be progressive loss of GFR, leading to end-stage renal failure. Predictably, the characteristic FGF23-driven phosphaturia recurs in renal allografts. To avert the consequences of sustained hypercalcemia, cinacalcet may be used temporarily to suppress serum calcium for months at a time. However, this strategy does not seem to cause involution of the offending benign adenoma, so subtotal parathyroidectomy with or without subcutaneous autotransplantation of any normal-appearing resected tissue is eventually required in most cases. Intraoperative measurement of serum iPTH is important to ascertain whether the offending tissue has been removed. Postoperative bone hunger may require calcium supplementation.

- Adolescents are at risk for dental abscesses due to defective dentin formation. Careful dental care to prevent caries is important. As linear growth comes to an end during adolescence, the primary rationale for oral PO_4/calcitriol therapy changes and some physicians reduce the intensity of therapy. Many patients are asymptomatic despite marked hypophosphatemia when therapy is stopped. However, others report mild bone pain and weakness without minimal calcitriol and PO_4 supplementation. Furthermore, there are observations in adult patients (discussed later) suggesting ongoing benefit in regard to dental and joint symptoms. In view of the well-known problems of medication adherence in adolescents, it seems reasonable to decrease the dose and dosing frequency in this period. It is prudent to restart full therapy, should patients sustain a traumatic injury and bone fracture or if a woman becomes pregnant (whether or not the fetus is affected). Because breast milk PO_4 is low in untreated female patients with XLH, unaffected offspring should have oral PO_4 supplementation with evaporated milk by bottle during the breastfeeding period.

Adulthood Although early calcitriol/PO_4 therapy minimizes joint deformities and improves final height, adult height remains about 2 SD less than the normal range.[79] Treated patients show better bone mineralization, but adult bone contains fewer trabeculae and considerable trabecular inhomogeneity.[90] Dual-energy x-ray absorptiometry studies must be analyzed with caution, because periarticular calcifications may falsely elevate bone mineral density estimates. Adults with XLH exhibit fibrochondrocyte hyperplasia in tendons and ligaments, causing them to thicken and calcify.[91] Most patients have multiple calcified entheses and report discomfort and limitation of movements in facet joints, particularly in the shoulders, lower back, and neck.[82] Occasionally, this can lead to foraminal stenosis that compresses nerve roots. Calcification of vertebral entheses is less common in patients who were treated with calcitriol and PO_4 during childhood.[92] The extent of enthesopathies correlates with decreased quality of life scores in adults with XLH.[93] Adults with XLH exhibit defects in both dentin and acellular cementum layers, increasing the risk of dental abscesses and tooth detachment.[94] Continued calcitriol/ PO_4 therapy in adulthood reduces the risk of severe dental complications.[95]

Alternative treatment approaches Based on the improved understanding of the central role of FGF23 in XLH and other hypophosphatemias, treatment with specifically designed inhibitors is a rationale and promising approach.[37,62,96–102] A recent publication describes the results of an open-label treatment trial with burosumab, a subcutaneously injected monoclonal antibody in 5- to 12-year-old children with XLH. The antibody led to improved TRP, serum PO_4 concentrations, linear growth, and clinical parameters.[103] A 24-week analysis of a double-blind, placebo-controlled randomized controlled trial in adult patients testing the same anti-FGF23 monoclonal antibody revealed better healing of fractures and improved biochemical markers of bone formation and resorption.[104] Other ongoing pediatric trials are listed on the Clinical Trials Web site (https://clinicaltrials.gov).

Autosomal dominant hypophosphatemia

Autosomal dominant hypophosphatemia (ADH) is caused by activating missense mutations of arginine residues at (R) 176 or 179 in *FGF23* that render the protein resistant to cleavage by FGF23-targeting converting enzymes and leads to high serum concentrations of intact FGF23 (see **Fig. 4**).[18,28,37] The penetrance of this comparably rare form of hypophosphatemia is variable. Clinical and laboratory findings can be similar to those in XLH, especially in patients with severe renal PO_4 wasting early in childhood.[28,105] A low serum iron concentration is associated with increased FGF23 expression and more severe disease manifestations.[106]

Treatment of ADH includes PO_4 supplements and calcitriol, similar to the treatment of XLH. Patients should be screened for iron deficiency. If present, appropriate iron therapy may normalize tubular PO_4 reabsorption and allow discontinuation of calcitriol and PO_4 supplement.

Autosomal recessive hypophosphatemia

Autosomal recessive forms of hypophosphatemia have been linked to inactivating mutations in several genes (**Table 2**). Patients present during childhood with clinical, laboratory, and radiological findings resembling those seen in patients with XLH and ADHR. The first variety, ARHR1, is caused by mutations in *Dentin Matrix Protein-1 (DMP1)*. DMP1 mutation leads to increased FGF23 production and impaired osteocyte maturation and skeletal mineralization (see **Fig. 1**).[104,107,108]

ARHR2 results from an inactivating mutation of the gene encoding ectonucleotide pyrophosphatase/phosphodiesterase-1 (*ENPP1*), which regulates matrix vesicle pathway and pyrophosphate-mediated bone mineralization.[58,109] Mutations of this gene have been linked to idiopathic infantile arterial calcification, ossification of the posterior longitudinal ligament of the spine, and insulin resistance.[110,111]

Hypophosphatemic rickets with hyperparathyroidism

This form of hypophosphatemia is caused by a de novo translocation with a breakpoint on chromosome 13q13.1, close to the Klotho gene, which leads to high plasma levels of αKlotho, the FGFR coreceptor for FGF23. Patients with this chromosomal abnormality also have increased FGF23 levels, in keeping with the importance of αKlotho in the regulation of serum PO_4, FGF23 expression, and PTH secretion.[41,58,112]

Fibrous dysplasia/McCune-Albright syndrome

Fibrous dysplasia/McCune-Albright syndrome (FD/MAS) is due to somatic (noninherited, mosaic) activating mutations in the GNAS gene in bone, endocrine glands, and skin.[113,114] The gene encodes the α-subunit of the guanine nucleotide-binding, stimulatory G-protein ($G_S\alpha$).[18,28,113] Its mutation causes osteoblastic differentiation, increased bone absorption, and fibrosis,[115] which replaces bone marrow and bone by fibrous tissue.

The phenotype is highly variable. Patients with FD/MAS develop fibro-osseous masses, café-au-lait spots, precocious puberty, and other endocrine disorders due to hypersecretion of various hormonal molecules. Additional features are

Table 2
Hypophosphatemia disorders with increased fibroblast growth factor 23 activity

Disease MIM Phenotype #	Genetic Variants (Gene Products)	MIM Gene* Chromosomal Location	Tissue Expression	Effects and Biological Consequences	Clinical Importance	Comments
XLH(R) X-linked hypophosphatemia/ hypophosphatemic rickets #307800	PHEX Loss-of-function mutation X-linked (dominant)	*300550 Xp22.2-p.22.1	Mainly bone/teeth (ectoenzyme); also skin, muscle, brain	Biological action incompletely understood (FGF23 is not a PHEX substrate) ↑ FGF23 mRNA in osteocytes and ↑ iFGF23 protein levels	Hyperphosphaturia Hypophosphatemia Normocalcemia Inappropriately low or normal calcitriol Rickets/osteomalacia	Most common form of inherited rickets ~1 per 20,000 Full penetrance, onset from birth
ADHR Autosomal dominant hypophosphatemic rickets #193100	FGF23 Gain of function mutation AD	*605380 12p13.32	Bone (mouse brain)	Resistance to cleavage (mutation in RXXR motif [Arg residues at positions 176 of 179]); stabilization (and elevation) of intact circulating (active) FGF23 levels	Hyperphosphaturia, hypophosphatemia Normocalcemia Inappropriately low or normal 1,25(OH)$_2$D$_3$ Rickets/osteomalacia	Incomplete penetrance, with variable onset Iron deficiency increases iFGF23 in patients with ADHR
ARHR1 Autosomal recessive hypophosphatemia (hypophosphatemic rickets) type 1 #241520	DMP1 Loss-of-function mutation AR	*600980 4q22.1	Mineralized tissue (osteoblast, osteocyte), also heart, kidney	Hydroxyapatite nucleation (?) Defective osteocyte maturation ↑ iFGF23 production in osteocytes Mechanism unclear	Hyperphosphaturia, hypophosphatemia Inappropriately normal 1,25(OH)$_2$D$_3$ Rickets, osteomalacia	—

(continued on next page)

Table 2
(continued)

Disease MIM Phenotype #	Genetic Variants (Gene Products)	MIM Gene* Chromosomal Location	Tissue Expression	Effects and Biological Consequences	Clinical Importance	Comments
ARHR2 Autosomal recessive hypophosphatemia (hypophosphatemic rickets) type 2 #613312	ENPP1 Loss-of-function mutation AR	*173335 6q23.2	Chondrocytes, renal tubules, parathyroid, placenta, others	Ectonucleotide pyrophosphatase/phosphodiesterase-1 converts P_i into PP_i inhibiting skeletal mineralization It may be involved in control of FGF23 production ↑ iFGF23	Hyperphosphaturia, hypophosphatemia, rickets, osteomalacia Ectopic calcification (aorta, kidney), hyperostosis. Idiopathic infantile arterial calcification (IIAC)	Rare (prevalence unknown)
ARHR3 Autosomal recessive hypophosphatemia (hypophosphatemic rickets) type 3 Otosclerotic bone dysplasia Raine syndrome #259775	FAM20C DMP4 Loss-of-function mutation AR	*611061 7p22.3	Mineralized tissue, others	Casein kinase (recognizes S-X-E motif) Loss of FAM20c may reduce functional DMP1 and lead to partial stabilization of FGF23 (resistance to physiologic furin-mediated cleavage) ↑ iFGF23	Hyperphosphaturia, hypophosphatemia, rickets/osteomalacia Tooth defects Craniofacial malformation & osteosclerosis of skull and long bones	—

Disorder	Gene/inheritance	Locus/OMIM	Tissue	Mechanism	Clinical features	Frequency
HRHPT Hypophosphatemic rickets and hyperparathyroidism #612089	αKL (αKlotho) de novo balanced chromosome 9:13 translocation; fusion of APRIN and αKL genes AD	Ch 13q13.1	Renal PTEC, renal artery, aorta, parathyroid, brain, others	↑ circulating Klotho in plasma ↑ FGF23 Enhanced FSG23-stimulated FGF receptor activation → inhibition of NaPi-IIa and NaPi-IIc cotransporters	Hyperphosphaturia Hypophosphatemia Hypercalcemia Heterotopic calcifications	Extremely rare
FD/MAS Fibrous dysplasia and McCune-Albright syndrome #174800	GNAS1 Gain-of-function (α-subunit, stimulating G-protein, G_s) Mosaic (postzygotic)	*139320 20q13.32	Mutated GNAS1 in fibrous skeletal lesions	Excess expression of FGF23 in focal FD tissues.[74] Mutation may halt differentiation of skeletal stem cells to mature osteoblasts	Fibrous skeletal lesions and solitary or multiple localized mineralization defects MAS: combined with café-au-lait spots, pubertas praecox, and/or thyrotoxicity	Rare
TIO Tumor-induced osteomalacia	9:13 translocation/ fusions (in some cases)	N/A	Tumorous tissue	Paraneoplastic PMT (phosphaturic mesenchymal tumor) with ↑ FGF23 production, Fibronectin/FGFR1 fusion protein, FGFR1 over expression	Hypophosphatemia Renal Pi wasting Osteomalacia	—

Abbreviations: AD, autosomal dominant; AR, autosomal recessive; FD, Fibrous dysplasia MAS, McCune–Albright syndrome; N/A, not applicable.

hyperthyroidism, pituitary gigantism (growth hormone), and Cushing syndrome (cortisol) due to adrenal hyperplasia, among others. The skeletal abnormalities are described as monostotic (Monostotic fibrous dysplasia, usually asymptomatic) or diffuse polyostotic changes polyostotic fibrous dysplasia that cause substantial morbidity or even death.[28,116]

Fibrous bony lesions are rich in FGF23-producing cells. Excess FGF23 causes PO_4 wasting in about one-half of patients.[18,117] Clinically important hypophosphatemia and rickets are more common in patients with MAS than in (P)FD.[18,118] The degree of (excess) FGF23 production has been attributed to alterations in FGF23 processing in FD lesions[119] and seems to correlate with the extent of FD.[117]

Therapeutic interventions for patients with FD are mainly surgical, that is, correction/stabilization of fractures and deformities. Medical treatment with (antiresorptive) bisphosphonates has been successfully tried.[118]

Hypophosphatemia Disorders with Normal or Suppressed Fibroblast Growth Factor 23 Activity (Inherited Intrarenal Phosphate Transport Defects)

Hypophosphatemia, hypercalcemia, and nephrocalcinosis

A homozygous mutation in SLC34A1 (NaPi-IIa), identified in a kindred in Israel (see **Table 1**; **Table 3**), was associated with hypophosphatemia, rickets, frequent fractures, and stunted growth.[120,121] The patients had hypercalciuria associated with increased $1,25(OH)_2D$ levels and features of (partial) renal Fanconi syndrome and mild-moderate chronic kidney disease in adulthood (Fanconi renotubular syndrome-2 [FRTS2]).[121] Subsequently, 4 more cases were reported from Argentina and Turkey (without Fanconi features) and an additional infant from the original kindred in Israel.[122,123]

Schlingmann and colleagues[47] recently described homozygous mutations in SLC34A1 in 4 infants from 3 Turkish families with parental consanguinity. In an extension study, 12 of 126 children with sporadic idiopathic infantile hypercalcemia were found to have biallelic (autosomal recessive) mutations of the renal PO_4 transporter (all negative for CYP24A1 [24-hydroxylase] variants). In addition to PO_4 wasting, the patients showed inappropriately high $1,25 (OH)_2D$ serum concentrations with corresponding hypercalcemia and hypercalciuria and suppressed intact PTH and FGF23 levels (see **Table 3**; **Table 4**).

Larger deletions, including SLC34A1, can occur as part of Sotos syndrome (associated with hypophosphatemia).[19,124]

Heterozygous variants in SLC34A1 were found among 2 of 20 patients with hypophosphatemia, demineralized bone, and nephrolithiasis, associated with a decreased threshold for PO_4 reabsorption.[18,125] However, the initial interpretation of the described condition (NPHLOP1) as autosomal dominant remains controversial[6,126] (see **Table 3**).

Hereditary hypophosphatemic rickets with hypercalciuria

Initially described in a Bedouin kindred,[127] hereditary hypophosphatemic rickets with hypercalciuria is characterized by hypophosphatemia and rickets due to tubular PO_4 wasting. It is caused by homozygous or compound heterozygous loss-of-function mutations in SLC34A3 (NaPi-IIc)[18,128,129] (see **Table 3**). Consequently, serum $1,25(OH)_2D$ is high and PTH and FGF23 are reduced, resulting in increased calcium absorption in the gut and secondary hypercalciuria, medullary nephrocalcinosis, and urolithiasis (see **Table 4**).[18,127–130]

Persons carrying one mutated allele are generally healthy and have a normal PO_4 balance but may have hypercalciuria and an increased risk of nephrocalcinosis and kidney stones.[19,128,131]

Table 3

Hypophosphatemia and hypophosphatemic rickets: hypophosphatemia disorders with normal or suppressed fibroblast growth factor 23 activity[a]

Disease MIM Phenotype #	Genetic Variant Gene Product Inheritance	MIM Gene* Chromosomal Location	Tissue Expression	Effects and Biological Consequences	Comments/References
Overlapping syndrome of hypophosphatemia, hypercalcemia, and nephrocalcinosis (HHN) NPHLOP1# 612286[b] Nephrolithiasis and osteoporosis associated with hypophosphatemia[125] FRTS2# 613388[c] Fanconi renotubular syndrome-2[120–123] HCINF2 or IH# 616963 Infantile hypercalcemia-2[47]	SLC34A1 (solute carrier family 34, member 1) NaPi-IIa (sodium/PO$_4$ cotransporter) AR[b,d]	*182309 5q35.3	Kidney (PTEC)	Renal Pi wasting, hypophosphatemia ↓ FGF23, ↑ 1,25(OH)$_2$D Hypercalcemia, hypercalciuria Nephrocalcinosis/stones Rickets, skeletal fractures	Clinical phenotype may improve in adulthood[19]
Hereditary hypophosphatemic rickets with hypercalciuria #241530	SLC34A3 (solute carrier family 34, member 3) NaPi-IIc (sodium/PO$_4$ cotransporter) Loss-of-function mutation AR	*609826 9q34.3	Kidney (PTEC)	Renal Pi wasting Hypophosphatemia ↑ 1,25(OH)$_2$D hypercalciuria suppressed PTH ↑ intestinal Ca^{++} absorption Nephrocalcinosis, stones	Rickets are common; clinical symptoms seem to persist into adulthood[19]

Abbreviation: PTEC, proximal tubular epithelial cells.

[a] See footnote to **Table 1**.

[b] Initially described as autosomal dominant,[125] but the role of the reported *SLC34A1* variant is controversial.[6]

[c] Few patients with mild to moderate chronic kidney disease in adulthood and modified biochemical profile.[121]

[d] Larger deletions, including the SLC34A1 gene, can occur as part of Sotos syndrome.[19,124]

Table 4
Biochemical abnormalities in patients with hypophosphatemic rickets

Disease MIM Phenotype #	Genetic Variants	FGF23	Serum PO$_4$	Serum Calcium	25(OH)D$_3$	1,25(OH)$_2$D$_3$	PTH	Urine Calcium
XLH X-linked dominant hypophosphatemia/rickets# 307800	PHEX	↑ or inappropriately N	↓	N or ↓	N	↓ or inappropriately N	N or ↑	N
ADHR AD hypophosphatemic rickets# 193100	FGF23 Activating mutation	↑ or inappropriately N	↓	N or ↓	N	↓ or inappropriately N	N	N
ARHR AR hypophosphatemic rickets Type 1# 241520 Type 2# 613312	DMP1 ENPP1	↑ or inappropriately N	↓	N	N	↓ or inappropriately N	N	N or ↓
HRHPT Hypophosphatemic rickets and hyperparathyroidism 612089	Balanced Chr 9:13 FN1-FGFR1 translocation/fusion	↑	↓	↑	N	N	↑	N

FD/MAS FD and MAS #174800	GNAS1	↑[a]	N or ↓	N	N or ↓	—	N
HHN Hypophosphatemia, hypercalcemia, and nephrocalcinosis NPHLOP1# 612286 FRTS2# 613388 HCINF2# 616963	SLC3A1 (NPT2a) NaPi-IIa	↓ or N	↑ or N	N or ↓	↓ (in children) ↑ (HCINF2)	↓ or N	↑ (in children) N (in adults)
Hereditary hypophosphatemic rickets with hypercalciuria #241530	SLC34A3 (NPT2c) NaPi-IIc	↓ or N	↓	N	↑	↓ or N	↑
TIO Tumor-induced osteomalacia	Chr 9:13 FN1-FGFR1 translocation/fusion (in some)	N or ↑	↓	N	N or ↓	N or ↑	—
Nutritional (vitamin D deficient) rickets	—	↓ or N	↓	↓↑	↓	↑	→

Abbreviations: see Footnote to **Table 1**.
[a] High FGF23 levels due to high number of FGF23-producing cells in fibrous bone lesions.
Data from Ref.[2,11,18,19,121,123,137,138]

Hypophosphatemia due to Acquired Defects in Phosphate Handling

Tumor-induced osteomalacia

Tumor-induced osteomalacia is a paraneoplastic disorder caused by the secretion of phosphatonins (phosphaturic hormones), including FGF23 (see **Table 2**), which leads to tubular P wasting and hypophosphatemia, osteomalacia, and vitamin D abnormalities.[132] Plasma PTH, PTH-related protein, and calcium concentrations are normal (see **Table 4**).

SUMMARY

Hypophosphatemic rickets, most due to the X-linked dominant form caused by pathogenic variants of the *PHEX* gene, continues to pose therapeutic challenges with important consequences for growth and bone development, high risk of fractions and poor bone healing, dental problems, and nephrolithiasis or nephrocalcinosis.

Conventional treatment consists of PO_4 supplement and pharmacologically dosed calcitriol carefully monitoring for clinical efficacy and treatment-emergent adverse effects. Genetic testing is encouraged, especially in sporadic cases. FGF23 measurement, although currently not routinely offered, has implications for the differential diagnosis of hypophosphatemia syndromes and, potentially, treatment monitoring. Newer therapeutic modalities focus on calcium sensing receptor modulation (cinacalcet) and biological molecules targeting FGF23 or its receptors (in clinical studies). The first trial results with biological agents are now becoming available and must be compared with the known, long-term effects of conventional treatments.

ACKNOWLEDGMENTS

We thank Giuseppe Pascale for help in the design of the figures.

REFERENCES

1. Winters RW, Graham JB, Williams TF, et al. A genetic study of familial hypophosphatemia and vitamin D resistant rickets with a review of the literature. Medicine (Baltimore) 1958;37(2):97–142.
2. Haffner D, Waldegger S. Disorders of phosphorus metabolism. In: Geary D, Schaefer F, editors. Pediatric kidney disease. Springer Berlin Heidelberg; 2016. p. 953–72.
3. Beck-Nielsen SS, Brixen K, Gram J, et al. Mutational analysis of PHEX, FGF23, DMP1, SLC34A3 and CLCN5 in patients with hypophosphatemic rickets. J Hum Genet 2012;57(7):453–8.
4. Consortium TH. A gene (PEX) with homologies to endopeptidases is mutated in patients with X-linked hypophosphatemic rickets. The HYP Consortium. Nat Genet 1995;11(2):130–6.
5. Gattineni J, Baum M. Genetic disorders of phosphate regulation. Pediatr Nephrol 2012;27(9):1477–87.
6. Wagner CA, Hernando N, Forster IC, et al. The SLC34 family of sodium-dependent phosphate transporters. Pflugers Arch 2014;466(1):139–53.
7. Pavone V, Testa G, Gioitta Iachino S, et al. Hypophosphatemic rickets: etiology, clinical features and treatment. Eur J Orthop Surg Traumatol 2015;25(2):221–6.
8. Bon N, Couasnay G, Bourgine A, et al. Phosphate (Pi)-regulated heterodimerization of the high-affinity sodium-dependent Pi transporters PiT1/Slc20a1 and PiT2/Slc20a2 underlies extracellular Pi sensing independently of Pi uptake. J Biol Chem 2018;293(6):2102–14.

9. Clinkenbeard EL, White KE. Heritable and acquired disorders of phosphate metabolism: etiologies involving FGF23 and current therapeutics. Bone 2017; 102:31–9.

10. Lee DB, Walling MW, Brautbar N. Intestinal phosphate absorption: influence of vitamin D and non-vitamin D factors. Am J Physiol 1986;250(3 Pt 1):G369–73.

11. Goldsweig BK, Carpenter TO. Hypophosphatemic rickets: lessons from disrupted FGF23 control of phosphorus homeostasis. Curr Osteoporos Rep 2015; 13(2):88–97.

12. Blaine J, Chonchol M, Levi M. Renal control of calcium, phosphate, and magnesium homeostasis. Clin J Am Soc Nephrol 2015;10(7):1257–72.

13. Bindels RJM, Hoenderop JGJ, Biber J. Transport of calcium, magnesium, and phosphate. In: Taal MS, Chertow GM, Marsden PA, et al, editors. Brenner & Rector's the kidney, vol. 1. Philadelphia: Elsevier; 2012. p. 226–51.

14. Bijvoet OL. Relation of plasma phosphate concentration to renal tubular reabsorption of phosphate. Clin Sci 1969;37(1):23–36.

15. Forster IC, Hernando N, Biber J, et al. Proximal tubular handling of phosphate: a molecular perspective. Kidney Int 2006;70(9):1548–59.

16. Peraino RA, Suki WN. Phosphate transport by isolated rabbit cortical collecting tubule. Am J Physiol 1980;238(5):F358–62.

17. Villa-Bellosta R, Ravera S, Sorribas V, et al. The Na+-Pi cotransporter PiT-2 (SLC20A2) is expressed in the apical membrane of rat renal proximal tubules and regulated by dietary Pi. Am J Physiol Renal Physiol 2009;296(4):F691–9.

18. Wagner CA, Rubio-Aliaga I, Biber J, et al. Genetic diseases of renal phosphate handling. Nephrol Dial Transplant 2014;29(Suppl 4):iv45–54.

19. Wagner CA, Rubio-Aliaga I, Hernando N. Renal phosphate handling and inherited disorders of phosphate reabsorption: an update. Pediatr Nephrol 2017. https://doi.org/10.1007/s00467-017-3873-3.

20. Levi M, Lotscher M, Sorribas V, et al. Cellular mechanisms of acute and chronic adaptation of rat renal P(i) transporter to alterations in dietary P(i). Am J Physiol 1994;267(5 Pt 2):F900–8.

21. Forster IC, Hernando N, Biber J, et al. Phosphate transporters of the SLC20 and SLC34 families. Mol Aspects Med 2013;34(2–3):386–95.

22. Inden M, Iriyama M, Zennami M, et al. The type III transporters (PiT-1 and PiT-2) are the major sodium-dependent phosphate transporters in the mice and human brains. Brain Res 2016;1637:128–36.

23. Yamada S, Wallingford MC, Borgeia S, et al. Loss of PiT-2 results in abnormal bone development and decreased bone mineral density and length in mice. Biochem Biophys Res Commun 2018;495(1):553–9.

24. Wang C, Li Y, Shi L, et al. Mutations in SLC20A2 link familial idiopathic basal ganglia calcification with phosphate homeostasis. Nat Genet 2012;44(3):254–6.

25. Biber J, Hernando N, Forster I, et al. Regulation of phosphate transport in proximal tubules. Pflugers Arch 2009;458(1):39–52.

26. Shimada T, Hasegawa H, Yamazaki Y, et al. FGF-23 is a potent regulator of vitamin D metabolism and phosphate homeostasis. J Bone Miner Res 2004; 19(3):429–35.

27. Deliot N, Hernando N, Horst-Liu Z, et al. Parathyroid hormone treatment induces dissociation of type IIa Na+-P(i) cotransporter-Na+/H+ exchanger regulatory factor-1 complexes. Am J Physiol Cell Physiol 2005;289(1):C159–67.

28. Gonciulea AR, Jan De Beur SM. Fibroblast growth factor 23-mediated bone disease. Endocrinol Metab Clin North Am 2017;46(1):19–39.

29. Feng JQ, Ye L, Schiavi S. Do osteocytes contribute to phosphate homeostasis? Curr Opin Nephrol Hypertens 2009;18(4):285–91.

30. Consortium A. Autosomal dominant hypophosphataemic rickets is associated with mutations in FGF23. Nat Genet 2000;26(3):345–8.

31. Fukumoto S, Martin TJ. Bone as an endocrine organ. Trends Endocrinol Metab 2009;20(5):230–6.

32. Weber TJ, Liu S, Indridason OS, et al. Serum FGF23 levels in normal and disordered phosphorus homeostasis. J Bone Miner Res 2003;18(7):1227–34.

33. Mirams M, Robinson BG, Mason RS, et al. Bone as a source of FGF23: regulation by phosphate? Bone 2004;35(5):1192–9.

34. Collins MT, Lindsay JR, Jain A, et al. Fibroblast growth factor-23 is regulated by 1alpha,25-dihydroxyvitamin D. J Bone Miner Res 2005;20(11):1944–50.

35. Liu S, Quarles LD. How fibroblast growth factor 23 works. J Am Soc Nephrol 2007;18(6):1637–47.

36. Berndt T, Kumar R. Phosphatonins and the regulation of phosphate homeostasis. Annu Rev Physiol 2007;69:341–59.

37. Kinoshita Y, Fukumoto S. X-linked hypophosphatemia and FGF23-related hypophosphatemic diseases: prospect for new treatment. Endocr Rev 2018;39(3): 274–91.

38. Shimizu Y, Tada Y, Yamauchi M, et al. Hypophosphatemia induced by intravenous administration of saccharated ferric oxide: another form of FGF23-related hypophosphatemia. Bone 2009;45(4):814–6.

39. Farrow EG, Yu X, Summers LJ, et al. Iron deficiency drives an autosomal dominant hypophosphatemic rickets (ADHR) phenotype in fibroblast growth factor-23 (Fgf23) knock-in mice. Proc Natl Acad Sci U S A 2011;108(46):E1146–55.

40. Kuro-o M, Matsumura Y, Aizawa H, et al. Mutation of the mouse klotho gene leads to a syndrome resembling ageing. Nature 1997;390(6655):45–51.

41. Erben RG. alpha-Klotho's effects on mineral homeostasis are fibroblast growth factor-23 dependent. Curr Opin Nephrol Hypertens 2018;27(4):229–35.

42. Chen G, Liu Y, Goetz R, et al. alpha-Klotho is a non-enzymatic molecular scaffold for FGF23 hormone signalling. Nature 2018;553(7689):461–6.

43. Olauson H, Mencke R, Hillebrands JL, et al. Tissue expression and source of circulating alphaKlotho. Bone 2017;100:19–35.

44. Kurosu H, Ogawa Y, Miyoshi M, et al. Regulation of fibroblast growth factor-23 signaling by klotho. J Biol Chem 2006;281(10):6120–3.

45. Urakawa I, Yamazaki Y, Shimada T, et al. Klotho converts canonical FGF receptor into a specific receptor for FGF23. Nature 2006;444(7120):770–4.

46. Erben RG, Andrukhova O. FGF23 regulation of renal tubular solute transport. Curr Opin Nephrol Hypertens 2015;24(5):450–6.

47. Schlingmann KP, Ruminska J, Kaufmann M, et al. Autosomal-recessive mutations in SLC34A1 encoding sodium-phosphate cotransporter 2A cause idiopathic infantile hypercalcemia. J Am Soc Nephrol 2016;27(2):604–14.

48. Imura A, Tsuji Y, Murata M, et al. alpha-Klotho as a regulator of calcium homeostasis. Science 2007;316(5831):1615–8.

49. Hoenderop JG, Nilius B, Bindels RJ. Molecular mechanism of active Ca2+ reabsorption in the distal nephron. Annu Rev Physiol 2002;64:529–49.

50. Chang Q, Hoefs S, van der Kemp AW, et al. The beta-glucuronidase klotho hydrolyzes and activates the TRPV5 channel. Science 2005;310(5747):490–3.

51. Dalton GD, Xie J, An SW, et al. New insights into the mechanism of action of soluble klotho. Front Endocrinol (Lausanne) 2017;8:323.

52. Guo R, Quarles LD. Cloning and sequencing of human PEX from a bone cDNA library: evidence for its developmental stage-specific regulation in osteoblasts. J Bone Miner Res 1997;12(7):1009–17.

53. Beck L, Tenenhouse HS, Meyer RA, et al. Renal expression of Na+-phosphate cotransporter mRNA and protein: effect of the Gy mutation and low phosphate diet. Pflugers Arch 1996;431(6):936–41.

54. Tenenhouse HS. X-linked hypophosphataemia: a homologous disorder in humans and mice. Nephrol Dial Transplant 1999;14(2):333–41.

55. Rowe PS. The chicken or the egg: PHEX, FGF23 and SIBLINGs unscrambled. Cell Biochem Funct 2012;30(5):355–75.

56. Salmon B, Bardet C, Khaddam M, et al. MEPE-derived ASARM peptide inhibits odontogenic differentiation of dental pulp stem cells and impairs mineralization in tooth models of X-linked hypophosphatemia. PLoS One 2013;8(2):e56749.

57. Bergwitz C, Juppner H. Regulation of phosphate homeostasis by PTH, vitamin D, and FGF23. Annu Rev Med 2010;61:91–104.

58. Rowe PS. A unified model for bone-renal mineral and energy metabolism. Curr Opin Pharmacol 2015;22:64–71.

59. Chesher D, Oddy M, Darbar U, et al. Outcome of adult patients with X-linked hypophosphatemia caused by PHEX gene mutations. J Inherit Metab Dis 2018;41(5):865–76.

60. Kumar R, Thompson JR. The regulation of parathyroid hormone secretion and synthesis. J Am Soc Nephrol 2011;22(2):216–24.

61. Riccardi D, Kemp PJ. The calcium-sensing receptor beyond extracellular calcium homeostasis: conception, development, adult physiology, and disease. Annu Rev Physiol 2012;74:271–97.

62. Fuente R, Gil-Pena H, Claramunt-Taberner D, et al. X-linked hypophosphatemia and growth. Rev Endocr Metab Disord 2017;18(1):107–15.

63. Kogawa M, Findlay DM, Anderson PH, et al. Osteoclastic metabolism of 25(OH)-vitamin D3: a potential mechanism for optimization of bone resorption. Endocrinology 2010;151(10):4613–25.

64. Bacic D, Lehir M, Biber J, et al. The renal Na+/phosphate cotransporter NaPi-IIa is internalized via the receptor-mediated endocytic route in response to parathyroid hormone. Kidney Int 2006;69(3):495–503.

65. Bourgeois S, Capuano P, Stange G, et al. The phosphate transporter NaPi-IIa determines the rapid renal adaptation to dietary phosphate intake in mouse irrespective of persistently high FGF23 levels. Pflugers Arch 2013;465(11):1557–72.

66. Beck-Nielsen SS, Brusgaard K, Rasmussen LM, et al. Phenotype presentation of hypophosphatemic rickets in adults. Calcif Tissue Int 2010;87(2):108–19.

67. Zivicnjak M, Schnabel D, Billing H, et al. Age-related stature and linear body segments in children with X-linked hypophosphatemic rickets. Pediatr Nephrol 2011;26(2):223–31.

68. Albano G, Moor M, Dolder S, et al. Sodium-dependent phosphate transporters in osteoclast differentiation and function. PLoS One 2015;10(4):e0125104.

69. Barbieri AM, Chiodini I, Ragni E, et al. Suppressive effects of tenofovir disoproxil fumarate, an antiretroviral prodrug, on mineralization and type II and type III sodium-dependent phosphate transporters expression in primary human osteoblasts. J Cell Biochem 2018;119(6):4855–66.

70. Hunziker EB. Mechanism of longitudinal bone growth and its regulation by growth plate chondrocytes. Microsc Res Tech 1994;28(6):505–19.

71. Miao D, Bai X, Panda DK, et al. Cartilage abnormalities are associated with abnormal Phex expression and with altered matrix protein and MMP-9 localization in Hyp mice. Bone 2004;34(4):638–47.

72. Liu S, Zhou J, Tang W, et al. Pathogenic role of Fgf23 in Hyp mice. Am J Physiol Endocrinol Metab 2006;291(1):E38–49.

73. Gonzalez Ballesteros LF, Ma NS, Gordon RJ, et al. Unexpected widespread hypophosphatemia and bone disease associated with elemental formula use in infants and children. Bone 2017;97:287–92.

74. Kobayashi K, Imanishi Y, Koshiyama H, et al. Expression of FGF23 is correlated with serum phosphate level in isolated fibrous dysplasia. Life Sci 2006;78(20):2295–301.

75. Eicher EM, Southard JL, Scriver CR, et al. Hypophosphatemia: mouse model for human familial hypophosphatemic (vitamin D-resistant) rickets. Proc Natl Acad Sci U S A 1976;73(12):4667–71.

76. Collins JF, Bulus N, Ghishan FK. Sodium-phosphate transporter adaptation to dietary phosphate deprivation in normal and hypophosphatemic mice. Am J Physiol 1995;268(6 Pt 1):G917–24.

77. Ruppe MD. X-Linked hypophosphatemia. In: Adam MP, Ardinger HH, Pagon RA, et al., editors. GeneReviews® [Internet]. Seattle (WA): University of Washington, Seattle; 1993-2018.2012 Feb 9 [updated 2017 Apr 13].

78. Beck-Nielsen SS, Brock-Jacobsen B, Gram J, et al. Incidence and prevalence of nutritional and hereditary rickets in southern Denmark. Eur J Endocrinol 2009;160(3):491–7.

79. Cagnoli M, Richter R, Bohm P, et al. Spontaneous growth and effect of early therapy with calcitriol and phosphate in X-linked hypophosphatemic rickets. Pediatr Endocrinol Rev 2017;15(Suppl 1):119–22.

80. Barth JH, Jones RG, Payne RB. Calculation of renal tubular reabsorption of phosphate: the algorithm performs better than the nomogram. Ann Clin Biochem 2000;37(Pt 1):79–81.

81. Stark H, Eisenstein B, Tieder M, et al. Direct measurement of TP/GFR: a simple and reliable parameter of renal phosphate handling. Nephron 1986;44(2):125–8.

82. Carpenter TO, Imel EA, Holm IA, et al. A clinician's guide to X-linked hypophosphatemia. J Bone Miner Res 2011;26(7):1381–8.

83. Alon US, Levy-Olomucki R, Moore WV, et al. Calcimimetics as an adjuvant treatment for familial hypophosphatemic rickets. Clin J Am Soc Nephrol 2008;3(3):658–64.

84. Raeder H, Shaw N, Netelenbos C, et al. A case of X-linked hypophosphatemic rickets: complications and the therapeutic use of cinacalcet. Eur J Endocrinol 2008;159(Suppl 1):S101–5.

85. Yavropoulou MP, Kotsa K, Gotzamani Psarrakou A, et al. Cinacalcet in hyperparathyroidism secondary to X-linked hypophosphatemic rickets: case report and brief literature review. Hormones (Athens) 2010;9(3):274–8.

86. Srivastava T, Alon US. Cinacalcet as adjunctive therapy for hereditary 1,25-dihydroxyvitamin D-resistant rickets. J Bone Miner Res 2013;28(5):992–6.

87. Carpenter TO, Imel EA, Ruppe MD, et al. Randomized trial of the anti-FGF23 antibody KRN23 in X-linked hypophosphatemia. J Clin Invest 2014;124(4):1587–97.

88. Shroff R, Wan M, Nagler EV, et al. Clinical practice recommendations for treatment with active vitamin D analogues in children with chronic kidney disease Stages 2-5 and on dialysis. Nephrol Dial Transplant 2017;32(7):1114–27.

89. Kalantar-Zadeh K, Shah A, Duong U, et al. Kidney bone disease and mortality in CKD: revisiting the role of vitamin D, calcimimetics, alkaline phosphatase, and minerals. Kidney Int Suppl 2010;(117):S10–21.

90. Colares Neto GP, Pereira RM, Alvarenga JC, et al. Evaluation of bone mineral density and microarchitectural parameters by DXA and HR-pQCT in 37 children and adults with X-linked hypophosphatemic rickets. Osteoporos Int 2017;28(5):1685–92.

91. Riccio AR, Entezami P, Giuffrida A, et al. Minimally Invasive surgical management of thoracic ossification of the ligamentum flavum associated with X-linked hypophosphatemia. World Neurosurg 2016;94:580.e5-10.

92. Zhang X, Imel EA, Ruppe MD, et al. Pharmacokinetics and pharmacodynamics of a human monoclonal anti-FGF23 antibody (KRN23) in the first multiple ascending-dose trial treating adults with X-linked hypophosphatemia. J Clin Pharmacol 2016;56(2):176–85.

93. Che H, Roux C, Etcheto A, et al. Impaired quality of life in adults with X-linked hypophosphatemia and skeletal symptoms. Eur J Endocrinol 2016;174(3): 325–33.

94. Biosse Duplan M, Coyac BR, Bardet C, et al. Phosphate and vitamin D prevent periodontitis in X-linked hypophosphatemia. J Dent Res 2017;96(4):388–95.

95. Connor J, Olear EA, Insogna KL, et al. Conventional therapy in adults with X-linked hypophosphatemia: effects on enthesopathy and dental disease. J Clin Endocrinol Metab 2015;100(10):3625–32.

96. Aono Y, Yamazaki Y, Yasutake J, et al. Therapeutic effects of anti-FGF23 antibodies in hypophosphatemic rickets/osteomalacia. J Bone Miner Res 2009; 24(11):1879–88.

97. Wöhrle S, Henninger C, Bonny O, et al. Pharmacological inhibition of fibroblast growth factor (FGF) receptor signaling ameliorates FGF23-mediated hypophosphatemic rickets. J Bone Miner Res 2013;28(4):899–911.

98. Imel EA, Zhang X, Ruppe MD, et al. Prolonged correction of serum phosphorus in adults with X-linked hypophosphatemia using monthly doses of KRN23. J Clin Endocrinol Metab 2015;100(7):2565–73.

99. Du E, Xiao L, Hurley MM. FGF23 neutralizing antibody ameliorates hypophosphatemia and impaired FGF receptor signaling in kidneys of HMWFGF2 transgenic mice. J Cell Physiol 2017;232(3):610–6.

100. Yamazaki Y, Tamada T, Kasai N, et al. Anti-FGF23 neutralizing antibodies show the physiological role and structural features of FGF23. J Bone Miner Res 2008; 23(9):1509–18.

101. Aono Y, Hasegawa H, Yamazaki Y, et al. Anti-FGF-23 neutralizing antibodies ameliorate muscle weakness and decreased spontaneous movement of Hyp mice. J Bone Miner Res 2011;26(4):803–10.

102. Fukumoto S. Targeting fibroblast growth factor 23 signaling with antibodies and inhibitors, is there a rationale? Front Endocrinol (Lausanne) 2018;9:48.

103. Carpenter TO, Whyte MP, Imel EA, et al. Burosumab therapy in children with X-linked hypophosphatemia. N Engl J Med 2018;378(21):1987–98.

104. Insogna KL, Briot K, Imel EA, et al. A randomized, double-blind, placebo-controlled, phase 3 trial evaluating the efficacy of burosumab, an anti-FGF23 antibody, in adults with X-linked hypophosphatemia: week 24 primary analysis. J Bone Miner Res 2018;33(8):1383–93.

105. Econs MJ, McEnery PT. Autosomal dominant hypophosphatemic rickets/osteomalacia: clinical characterization of a novel renal phosphate-wasting disorder. J Clin Endocrinol Metab 1997;82(2):674–81.

106. Imel EA, Peacock M, Gray AK, et al. Iron modifies plasma FGF23 differently in autosomal dominant hypophosphatemic rickets and healthy humans. J Clin Endocrinol Metab 2011;96(11):3541–9.

107. Lorenz-Depiereux B, Bastepe M, Benet-Pages A, et al. DMP1 mutations in autosomal recessive hypophosphatemia implicate a bone matrix protein in the regulation of phosphate homeostasis. Nat Genet 2006;38(11):1248–50.

108. Feng JQ, Ward LM, Liu S, et al. Loss of DMP1 causes rickets and osteomalacia and identifies a role for osteocytes in mineral metabolism. Nat Genet 2006; 38(11):1310–5.

109. Millan JL. The role of phosphatases in the initiation of skeletal mineralization. Calcif Tissue Int 2013;93(4):299–306.

110. Rutsch F, Ruf N, Vaingankar S, et al. Mutations in ENPP1 are associated with 'idiopathic' infantile arterial calcification. Nat Genet 2003;34(4):379–81.

111. Saito T, Shimizu Y, Hori M, et al. A patient with hypophosphatemic rickets and ossification of posterior longitudinal ligament caused by a novel homozygous mutation in ENPP1 gene. Bone 2011;49(4):913–6.

112. Brownstein CA, Adler F, Nelson-Williams C, et al. A translocation causing increased alpha-klotho level results in hypophosphatemic rickets and hyperparathyroidism. Proc Natl Acad Sci U S A 2008;105(9):3455–60.

113. Weinstein LS, Shenker A, Gejman PV, et al. Activating mutations of the stimulatory G protein in the McCune-Albright syndrome. N Engl J Med 1991;325(24): 1688–95.

114. Boyce AM, Turner A, Watts L, et al. Improving patient outcomes in fibrous dysplasia/McCune-Albright syndrome: an international multidisciplinary workshop to inform an international partnership. Arch Osteoporos 2017;12(1):21.

115. Chapurlat RD, Orcel P. Fibrous dysplasia of bone and McCune-Albright syndrome. Best Pract Res Clin Rheumatol 2008;22(1):55–69.

116. Bianco P, Robey P. Diseases of bone and the stromal cell lineage. J Bone Miner Res 1999;14(3):336–41.

117. Riminucci M, Collins MT, Fedarko NS, et al. FGF-23 in fibrous dysplasia of bone and its relationship to renal phosphate wasting. J Clin Invest 2003;112(5): 683–92.

118. Majoor BCJ, Andela CD, Bruggemann J, et al. Determinants of impaired quality of life in patients with fibrous dysplasia. Orphanet J Rare Dis 2017;12(1):80.

119. Bhattacharyya N, Wiench M, Dumitrescu C, et al. Mechanism of FGF23 processing in fibrous dysplasia. J Bone Miner Res 2012;27(5):1132–41.

120. Tieder M, Arie R, Modai D, et al. Elevated serum 1,25-dihydroxyvitamin D concentrations in siblings with primary Fanconi's syndrome. N Engl J Med 1988; 319(13):845–9.

121. Magen D, Berger L, Coady MJ, et al. A loss-of-function mutation in NaPi-IIa and renal Fanconi's syndrome. N Engl J Med 2010;362(12):1102–9.

122. Rajagopal A, Braslavsky D, Lu JT, et al. Exome sequencing identifies a novel homozygous mutation in the phosphate transporter SLC34A1 in hypophosphatemia and nephrocalcinosis. J Clin Endocrinol Metab 2014;99(11):E2451–6.

123. Demir K, Yildiz M, Bahat H, et al. Clinical heterogeneity and phenotypic expansion of NaPi-IIa-associated disease. J Clin Endocrinol Metab 2017;102(12): 4604–14.

124. Kenny J, Lees MM, Drury S, et al. Sotos syndrome, infantile hypercalcemia, and nephrocalcinosis: a contiguous gene syndrome. Pediatr Nephrol 2011;26(8): 1331–4.

125. Prie D, Huart V, Bakouh N, et al. Nephrolithiasis and osteoporosis associated with hypophosphatemia caused by mutations in the type 2a sodium-phosphate cotransporter. N Engl J Med 2002;347(13):983–91.

126. Magen D, Zelikovic I, Skorecki K. Genetic disorders of renal phosphate transport. N Engl J Med 2010;363(18):1774 [author reply: 1774–5].
127. Tieder M, Modai D, Samuel R, et al. Hereditary hypophosphatemic rickets with hypercalciuria. N Engl J Med 1985;312(10):611–7.
128. Bergwitz C, Roslin NM, Tieder M, et al. SLC34A3 mutations in patients with hereditary hypophosphatemic rickets with hypercalciuria predict a key role for the sodium-phosphate cotransporter NaPi-IIc in maintaining phosphate homeostasis. Am J Hum Genet 2006;78(2):179–92.
129. Lorenz-Depiereux B, Benet-Pages A, Eckstein G, et al. Hereditary hypophosphatemic rickets with hypercalciuria is caused by mutations in the sodium-phosphate cotransporter gene SLC34A3. Am J Hum Genet 2006;78(2):193–201.
130. Tieder M, Modai D, Shaked U, et al. "Idiopathic" hypercalciuria and hereditary hypophosphatemic rickets. Two phenotypical expressions of a common genetic defect. N Engl J Med 1987;316(3):125–9.
131. Dasgupta D, Wee MJ, Reyes M, et al. Mutations in SLC34A3/NPT2c are associated with kidney stones and nephrocalcinosis. J Am Soc Nephrol 2014;25(10):2366–75.
132. Imel EA, Econs MJ. Fibroblast growth factor 23: roles in health and disease. J Am Soc Nephrol 2005;16(9):2565–75.
133. Yu Y, Sanderson SR, Reyes M, et al. Novel NaPi-IIc mutations causing HHRH and idiopathic hypercalciuria in several unrelated families: long-term follow-up in one kindred. Bone 2012;50(5):1100–6.
134. Ramos EM, Carecchio M, Lemos R, et al. Primary brain calcification: an international study reporting novel variants and associated phenotypes. Eur J Hum Genet 2018;26(10):1462–77.
135. Amatschek S, Haller M, Oberbauer R. Renal phosphate handling in human–what can we learn from hereditary hypophosphataemias? Eur J Clin Invest 2010;40(6):552–60.
136. Sneddon WB, Ruiz GW, Gallo LI, et al. Convergent signaling pathways regulate parathyroid hormone and fibroblast growth factor-23 action on NPT2A-mediated phosphate transport. J Biol Chem 2016;291(36):18632–42.
137. Baroncelli GI, Toschi B, Bertelloni S. Hypophosphatemic rickets. Curr Opin Endocrinol Diabetes Obes 2012;19(6):460–7.
138. Minisola S, Peacock M, Fukumoto S, et al. Tumour-induced osteomalacia. Nat Rev Dis Primers 2017;3:17044.

Syndrome of Inappropriate Antidiuresis

Michael L. Moritz, MD

KEYWORDS

- SIAD • Hyponatremia • Arginine vasopressin (AVP) • Cerebral salt wasting
- Encephalopathy • Urea • V2 antagonists • Saline

KEY POINTS

- Virtually all acutely ill hospitalized patients are at risk for developing syndrome of inappropriate antidiuresis (SIAD) due to disease states associated with elevated arginine vasopressin (AVP) production.
- Hypotonic intravenous fluids should be avoided in patients at risk for SIAD to prevent hospital-acquired hyponatremia.
- Hypouricemia and an elevated fractional excretion of urate are the most specific biochemical features of SIAD.
- Symptomatic hyponatremia is a medical emergency that should be treated with hypertonic saline.
- Oral urea and vasopressin 2 antagonists are effective therapies to treat SIAD when conservative measures have failed.

INTRODUCTION

Hyponatremia (serum sodium <135 mEq/L) is one of the most frequently encountered electrolyte abnormalities in children. A common cause of hyponatremia in hospitalized children is the syndrome of inappropriate antidiuresis (SIAD). SIAD refers to euvolemic states of hypotonic hyponatremia caused by impaired free water excretion resulting from nonphysiologic stimuli for arginine vasopressin (AVP) production in the absence of renal or endocrine dysfunction. SIAD is essentially a diagnosis of exclusion. The causes of SIAD are numerous and expanding. It can be broadly classified as a result of tumors, pulmonary or central nervous system (CNS) disorders, medications, or other causes, such as infection, inflammation, and the postoperative state. When

Disclosure Statement: There no relationships with a commercial company that have direct financial interest in subject matter or materials discussed in the article or with a company making a competing product.
Pediatric Nephrology, Pediatric Dialysis, Division of Nephrology, Department of Pediatrics, UPMC Children's Hospital of Pittsburgh, The University of Pittsburgh School of Medicine, 4401 Penn Avenue, Pittsburgh, PA 15224, USA
E-mail address: Michael.Moritz@CHP.edu

Pediatr Clin N Am 66 (2019) 209–226
https://doi.org/10.1016/j.pcl.2018.09.005
0031-3955/19/© 2018 Elsevier Inc. All rights reserved.

pediatric.theclinics.com

euvolemic hyponatremia is caused by nonhemodynamic physiologic stimuli, such as pain, stress, nausea, and vomiting, this is referred to as an SIAD-like state. Postoperative hyponatremia and exercise-associated hyponatremia would be SIAD-like states, because many of the stimuli for AVP production are physiologic. SIAD can be difficult to diagnose because volume status is hard to assess accurately, and there are no specific biochemical tests for diagnosing SIAD. The presence of hypouricemia with an elevated fractional excretion of urate (FEUrate) is highly suggestive of SIAD after other potential causes of hyponatremia have been excluded. Hyponatremia from SIAD can result in potentially life-threatening encephalopathy, and overcorrection can similarly result in neurologic complications, which makes treatment challenging. New evidence suggests that even mild and seemingly asymptomatic hyponatremia can have deleterious consequences, which underscores the need for the prevention and treatment of hyponatremia. Most acutely ill hospitalized children are at risk for developing hyponatremia due to AVP excess. Hypotonic maintenance intravenous solutions should be avoided in favor of isotonic solutions in order to prevent hospital-acquired hyponatremia. The primary treatment of SIAD is correcting the underlying disorder. There are numerous treatment options for hyponatremia, with each having certain advantages and disadvantages.

This review discusses the pathogenesis, epidemiology, evaluation, clinical consequences, prevention, and treatment of SIAD.

PATHOGENESIS OF HYPONATREMIA

The body's primary defense against developing hyponatremia is the kidney's ability to generate dilute urine and excrete free water. Rarely is excess ingestion of free water alone the cause of hyponatremia, as an adult with normal renal function can typically excrete more than 15 L of free water per day. It is also rare to develop hyponatremia from excess urinary sodium losses in the absence of free water ingestion. In order for hyponatremia to develop, it typically requires a relative excess of free water intake in conjunction with an underlying condition that impairs urinary free water excretion

---

Box 1
Disorders in impaired renal water excretion

1. Effective circulating volume depletion
   a. Gastrointestinal losses: vomiting, diarrhea
   b. Skin losses: cystic fibrosis
   c. Renal losses: salt-wasting nephropathy, diuretics, cerebral salt wasting, hypoaldosteronism
   d. Edematous states: heart failure, cirrhosis, nephrosis, hypoalbuminemia
   e. Decreased peripheral vascular resistance: sepsis, hypothyroidism

2. Thiazide diuretics

3. Renal failure
   a. Acute
   b. Chronic

4. Nonhypovolemic states of antidiuretic hormone excess
   a. Syndrome of inappropriate of antidiuresis
   b. Nausea, emesis, pain, stress
   c. Postoperative state
   d. Cortisol deficiency

5. Nephrogenic syndrome of inappropriate antidiuresis

(**Box 1**). Renal water handling is primarily under the control of AVP, which is produced in the hypothalamus and released from the posterior pituitary.[1] AVP release impairs water diuresis by increasing the permeability to water in the collecting tubule. There are numerous hemodynamic and nonhemodynamic stimuli for AVP release, and this places almost all acutely ill patients at risk for hyponatremia (**Fig. 1**).[2] The body will attempt to preserve the extracellular volume (ECV) at the expense of the serum sodium, and therefore, a hemodynamic stimulus for AVP production will override any inhibitory hypo-osmolar effect of hyponatremia.[3]

PATHOGENESIS OF SYNDROME OF INAPPROPRIATE ANTIDIURESIS

SIAD was first reported in 1957 by Schwartz, Bartter and colleagues[4] in 2 patients with bronchogenic carcinoma and hyponatremia of unexplained cause. These 2 patients displayed clinical features similar to that of human subjects who had received

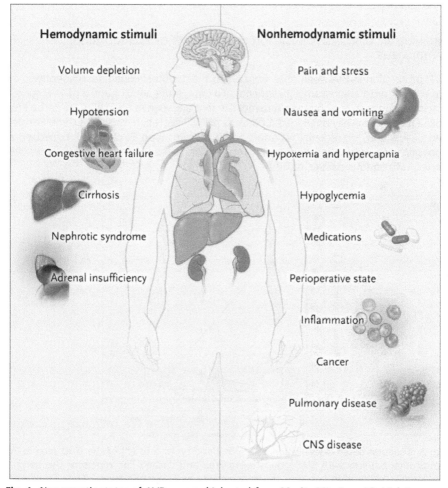

Fig. 1. Nonosmotic states of AVP excess. (*Adapted from* Moritz ML, Ayus JC. Maintenance intravenous fluids in acutely ill patients. N Engl J Med 2015;373:1350–60; Copyright © (2015) Massachusetts Medical Society; with permission.)

prolonged administration of a posterior pituitary extract, then called pitressin, which produced an antidiuresis.[5] Schwartz and Bartter[6] postulated that there was inappropriate secretion of an antidiuretic hormone. It was later realized that this antidiuretic hormone was in fact AVP.

Human and animal studies have been done to determine the cause of hyponatremia in SIAD, as the fall in serum sodium is not fully explained by free water retention alone.[7–9] The prevailing view is that the fall in serum sodium is due to a combination of free water retention and urinary solute excretion.[10] AVP excess increases water permeability in the collecting duct leading to water retention and subclinical volume expansion, with an increase in total body water of approximately 7% to 10%.[11] This volume expansion triggers hemodynamic regulatory mechanisms to maintain plasma volume at the expense of sodium, in part due to a pressure-natriuresis and the release of natriuretic peptides.[12] Patients with chronic SIAD do not usually have a urine osmolality exceeding 600 mOsm/kg, due to a compensatory mechanism called vasopressin escape, whereby water excretion will increase over time with a decrease in urine osmolality.[5,13–16]

ARGININE VASOPRESSIN REGULATION IN SYNDROME OF INAPPROPRIATE ANTIDIURESIS

AVP production in SIAD can arise from either the hypothalamus/neurohypophysis or the ectopic production from a malignancy. To date, there are 5 patterns of AVP secretion in response to the changes in osmolality that are seen in SIAD (**Fig. 2**). Zerbe and colleagues[17,18] initially described 4 patterns of AVP secretion, types A–D, and Fenske and colleagues[19,20] recently reported a fifth pattern, type E, classified based on a copeptin level. Interestingly, these 5 types are not disease specific and have been reported with various causes of SIAD.

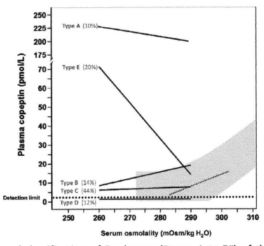

Fig. 2. Copeptin-based classification of 5 subtypes ("types A to E") of the SIAD seen in 50 consecutive patients with SIAD. The shaded area and dashed line represent the normal physiologic relationship between serum osmolality and copeptin levels. (*From* Fenske W, Sandner B, Christ-Crain M. A copeptin-based classification of the osmoregulatory defects in the syndrome of inappropriate antidiuresis. Best Pract Res Clin Endocrinol Metab 2016;30:219–33; with permission.)

In type A, AVP production is erratic, constantly elevated, and not influenced by serum osmolality. It is seen in patients with and without malignancies and is not necessarily due to ectopic production. In types B and E, AVP production behaves as if there is a hemodynamic stimulus for AVP, although overt volume depletion is not present.[19,20] It has been postulated that types B and E might represent a primary renal salt wasting (RSW) disorder, such as cerebral salt wasting (CSW) syndrome or an abnormal baroreceptor response.[19,21] In type C, the AVP response curve is normal, but occurs at a lower osmolar set point. Type C is referred to as resetting of the osmostats. In type D, AVP serum concentrations are not measurable. Some, but not all, of these patients have nephrogenic syndrome of inappropriate antidiuresis (NSIAD). In NSIAD, there is a gain-of-function mutation of the AVP receptor 2 (AVPR2) that causes constitutive activation of the receptor at the same location as the loss-of-function mutation seen in X-linked congenital nephrogenic diabetes insipidus.[22] NSIAD is a rare yet important cause of unexplained chronic euvolemic hyponatremia in infants. Not all patients with type D SIAD are found to have AVPR2 mutations though. There are reports of patients with type D SIAD with transient hyponatremia from medications or from malignancies that responded to vasopressin 2 antagonists (vaptans).[23,24] The A, B, C, D, E–type SIAD classification system is not typically used in clinical practice. This classification system demonstrates that SIAD is a heterogenous condition that can vary in both presentation and response to therapy.

CEREBRAL SALT WASTING SYNDROME

Another hyponatremic condition that is virtually indistinguishable from SIAD is CSW. CSW is a less common condition that is primarily but not exclusively associated with CNS disease. Maesaka and colleagues[25] have therefore suggested that RSW syndrome is a more appropriate term than CSW. CSW would be best described as a syndrome of inappropriate natriuresis.[21] In CSW, there is inappropriate and excessive release of natriuretic peptides leading to a primary natriuresis and volume depletion. The volume depletion stimulates a secondary neurohormonal response, with an increase in the renin angiotensin system and in AVP production. Signs of volume depletion are not always present, and there are no biochemistries that have consistently been used to distinguish CSW from SIAD at the time of presentation.[25] Natriuretic peptides are known to inhibit the renin angiotensin system and the secretion and action of AVP, and to increase glomerular filtration rate.[26] This complex mechanism can lead to biochemical features that are indistinguishable from those of SIAD, with a normal blood urea nitrogen and low uric acid, as well as normal plasma renin, aldosterone, and AVP levels in the setting of volume depletion. Patients with CSW typically have higher urinary volume and sodium excretion then those with SIAD.[27] CSW can occur in the absence of hyponatremia, and some cases can be mild.[28] CSW is primarily seen in neurosurgical patients and in particular adults with subarachnoid hemorrhage. There have been 4 prospective studies in adult neurosurgical patients whereby ECV was assessed by the gold-standard method of radioisotope dilution.[29–32] In these studies, more than 50% of the patients had decreased ECV, supporting a diagnosis of CSW rather than SIAD. There are numerous case reports of CSW occurring in children.[33] Large studies suggest that CSW may be more common than SIAD in children with CNS disease, particularly with tuberculosis meningitis[34,35] or brain tumors.[36]

EPIDEMIOLOGY OF SYNDROME OF INAPPROPRIATE ANTIDIURESIS

SIAD is one of the most common causes of hyponatremia in hospitalized children.[37] The causes of SIAD are so numerous that virtually every hospitalized patient should be considered to be at risk of developing it (**Box 2**). SIAD is most often the result of CNS disorders, pulmonary disorders, malignancies, and medications.[38] Many common childhood disorders are associated with SIAD, such as pneumonia,[39] bronchiolitis,[40] asthma,[41] positive pressure ventilation,[42] CNS infections,[43] and head trauma.[44] Elevated AVP serum concentration and hyponatremia are associated with febrile illnesses,[45] inflammation,[46,47] and infections.[48] Numerous classes of medication are associated with SIAD, including anticonvulsants, antidepressants, antipsychotics, opioids, chemotherapeutics, proton pump inhibitors, nonsteroidals, and recreational drugs.[49] The most common medications associated with SIAD in children are the anticonvulsant medications carbemazepine and oxcarbazepine,[50] and the chemotherapeutic medications vincristine[51] and cyclophosphamide.[52] Common physiologic stimuli for AVP release that can lead to an SIAD-like state are nausea, vomiting, pain, stress, hypoxia, and hypoglycemia.[53] Postoperative hyponatremia is frequently associated with an SIAD-like state due to numerous stimuli for AVP production, including pain, stress, nausea, vomiting, opioids, and positive pressure ventilation.[54,55] Exercise-associated hyponatremia is an important cause of symptomatic hyponatremia in the outpatient setting and has occurred in children and collegiate athletes.[56–58]

EVALUATION OF HYPONATREMIA AND DIAGNOSIS OF SYNDROME OF INAPPROPRIATE ANTIDIURESIS

The first step in the evaluation of hyponatremia is to confirm that hyponatremia is associated with hypo-osmolality (**Fig. 3**). Under certain circumstances, hyponatremia can be associated with either a normal serum osmolality, pseudohyponatremia, or an elevated osmolality, translocational hypernatremia. Pseudohyponatremia in children would be from severe hyperproteinemia, such as from intravenous immunoglobulin, or severe hyperlipidemia. Translocational hyponatremia would be from hyperglycemia, hypertonic radiocontrast, or mannitol.[59] If hyponatremia is associated with hypo-osmolality (true hyponatremia), the next step is to measure the urine osmolality to determine if there is an impaired ability to excrete free water. SIAD is essentially a diagnosis of exclusion. Before SIAD can be diagnosed, diseases causing decreased effective circulating volume, renal impairment, adrenal insufficiency, and hypothyroidism must be excluded.[6] Cortisol deficiency in particular should be ruled out because it can be clinically indistinguishable from SIAD and can manifest in times of stress.[60] Glucocorticoid hormones exert an inhibitory effect on AVP synthesis, which is the reason patients with glucocorticoid deficiency have markedly elevated AVP serum concentrations that are rapidly reversed by physiologic hydrocortisone replacement.[61] A serum cortisol concentration in the normal range does not rule out adrenal insufficiency as the cause of hyponatremia, as the appropriate adrenal response to hyponatremia would be to increase cortisol production.[60] An adrenocorticotropic hormone stimulation test should be considered if the cortisol serum concentration is not appropriately elevated in the setting of hyponatremia. Hypothyroidism can also resemble SIAD in infants.[62] Pseudohypoaldosteronism type 1, either primary from a genetic mutation or secondary from a urinary tract infection or obstruction, should be ruled out in infants with unexplained and refractory hyponatremia.[63]

The hallmarks of SIAD are mild volume expansion with low to normal plasma concentrations of creatinine, urea, uric acid, and potassium; impaired free water excretion with normal sodium excretion, which reflects sodium intake[13]; and hyponatremia that is relatively unresponsive to sodium administration in the absence of fluid restriction.

Box 2
Causes of syndrome of inappropriate antidiuresis

Central nervous system disorders
  Infection: meningitis, encephalitis
  Brain tumors
  Vascular abnormalities
  Psychosis
  Hydrocephalus
  Congenital malformations
  Postpituitary surgery
  Head trauma
  Subarachnoid hemorrhage
  Subdural hematoma
  Cerebrovascular accident
  Cavernous sinus thrombosis
  Stroke
  Guillain-Barrè syndrome
  Multiple sclerosis
  Amyotrophic lateral sclerosis
  Acute intermittent porphyria

Pulmonary disorders
  Pneumonia
  Tuberculosis
  Aspergillosis
  Asthma
  Bronchiolitis
  Cystic fibrosis
  Positive pressure ventilation
  Pneumothorax

Other causes
  Pain
  Stress
  Nausea/vomiting
  Postoperative
  Exercise-associated
  NSIAD
  Acquired immunodeficiency syndrome

Malignancies
  Carcinomas
  Bronchogenic
  Oat cell of the lung
  Stomach
  Duodenum
  Pancreas
  Prostate
  Ureter
  Bladder
  Thymoma
  Mesothelioma
  Endometrium
  Neuroblastoma
  Oropharynx
  Leukemias
  Lymphomas
  Sarcoma

Medications
  Vincristine
  Intravenous cytoxan

Ifosfamide
Carbamazepine
Oxcarbazepine
Sodium valproate
Lamitrigone
Opioids
Serotonin reuptake inhibitors
Tricyclic antidepressants
Nicotine
3,4-Methylenedioxymethamphetamine (ecstasy)
Nonsteroidal anti-inflammatory drugs
Proton pump inhibitors
Desmopressin

There are no urinary or plasma biomarkers that have a sufficiently high sensitivity and specificity as to diagnose SIAD independent of clinical assessment. Measurements of AVP or copeptin, a surrogate marker of vasopressin, have not proved useful in diagnosing SIAD.[64,65] The biochemical parameters most suggestive of SIAD in adults are a spot urine sodium concentration greater than 30 mEq/L, a fractional excretion of sodium greater than 0.5%, fractional excretion of urea greater than 55%, FEUrate greater than 11%, and plasma uric acid less than 4 mg/dL (see **Fig. 3**).[66] The specificity and sensitivity of these biomarkers have not been evaluated in children. The urinary biomarker most specific for diagnosing SIAD is an elevated FEUrate.[65,67] An FEUrate is unlikely to be elevated with diuretic use or adrenal insufficiency, whereas urinary sodium biochemistries may be. Maesaka[28] has proposed a FEUrate algorithm for the evaluation of hyponatremia.[68,69] An intriguing aspect of the algorithm is the ability to distinguish CSW and reset osmostat from other subtypes of SIAD. An elevated FEUrate is not usually present in reset osmostat, and the elevated FEUrate normalizes following the correction of serum sodium in SIAD, whereas the FEUrate remains persistently elevated following the correction of serum sodium in CSW. The urate algorithm has not been validated in large groups of patients, and the sensitivity and specificity are unknown. These parameters cannot be used in infants and children with renal disease because they are known to have higher FEUrates.[70]

CLINICAL CONSEQUENCES OF HYPONATREMIA

There is evidence to suggest that even mild and seemingly asymptomatic hyponatremia has deleterious consequences.[71] Hyponatremia is an independent risk factor for mortality in adults with SIAD.[72] Mild and chronic hyponatremia can result in subtle neurologic impairment leading to falls and associated bone fractures in the elderly, with increased bone fragility resulting from bone demineralization.[73–77] Hyponatremia represents a significant health care burden and results in increased medical costs and hospital stays.[78] There is emerging evidence that hyponatremia may alter the immune response and could explain why there is an increased rate of infections in hyponatremic patients.[79,80]

The most serious complication of hyponatremia is hyponatremic encephalopathy, which is a medical emergency that can be fatal or can lead to irreversible brain injury if inadequately treated.[81] The primary symptoms of hyponatremia are those of cerebral edema. The author and colleagues have reviewed this topic in detail elsewhere.[82,83] The most consistent symptoms are nonspecific and can be easily

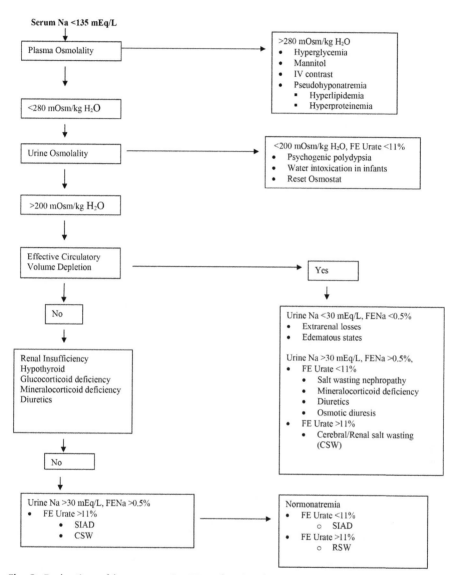

Fig. 3. Evaluation of hyponatremia. FENa, fractional excretion of sodium; FE Urate, fractional excretion of urate; IV, intravenous.

overlooked: headache, nausea, vomiting, and generalized weakness. Advanced symptoms include seizures, respiratory arrest, noncardiogenic pulmonary edema, and decorticate posturing.[83] Children are at particularly high risk for developing hyponatremic encephalopathy because they have a relatively larger brain to intracranial volume compared with adults.[84,85] The average serum sodium in children with hyponatremic encephalopathy is 120 mEq/L,[86,87] significantly higher than that seen in adults: 111 mEq/L.[54,88] More than 50% of children with serum sodium less than 125 mEq/L will develop hyponatremic encephalopathy.[82] Other risk factors for hyponatremic encephalopathy in children are hypoxemia and underlying CNS disease, both of which impair brain cell volume regulation.[83,89] Most children reported to have hyponatremic encephalopathy were otherwise healthy. They had received hypotonic fluids in the setting of SIAD, and multiple deaths have been reported.[82,83,90]

Prevention of Hospital-Acquired Hyponatremia

Hospital-acquired hyponatremia is a largely preventable condition and is not an inevitable consequence of elevated AVP serum concentrations.[55,91,92] Virtually all acutely ill hospitalized children are at risk for developing hyponatremia due to the numerous physiologic stimuli for AVP production and to the disease states associated with SIAD (see **Box 2**, **Fig. 1**).[93] The most important factor contributing to the development of hyponatremia is the administration of hypotonic fluids. A necessary requirement for the development of hyponatremia in SIAD is a source of free water, because hyponatremia cannot develop in the absence of fluid intake. The prevailing practice in pediatrics has been to administer hypotonic maintenance fluids (eg, 5% dextrose in a solution of 0.18%–0.45% saline) to acutely ill patients.[2,94,95] Numerous studies have demonstrated that hypotonic fluids are associated with a high incidence of hospital-acquired hyponatremia, in both surgical and nonsurgical patients and in the intensive care unit and general pediatric ward.[96–99] In 2003, the author's group recommended that acutely ill patients at risk for developing hyponatremia be administered isotonic maintenance fluids when indicated (5% dextrose solution of 0.9% saline) in order to prevent hospital-acquired hyponatremia.[100] Since that time, there have been more than 20 prospective trials in almost 3000 patients demonstrating that isotonic fluids decrease the incidence of hyponatremia 3- to 6-fold in comparison with hypotonic fluids.[101–103] Hypotonic maintenance fluids should be avoided in patients at risk for developing hyponatremia from disease states associated with SIAD. This group of patients includes those in the perioperative state, those receiving hydration for cancer chemotherapy, the critically ill, and those with bronchiolitis, pneumonia, or CNS disease. Practice guidelines and patient safety alerts have cautioned against using hypotonic fluids in these high-risk patients, because numerous preventable deaths have been reported as a result of the administration of hypotonic fluids.[104,105]

Treatment of Hyponatremic Encephalopathy

Hyponatremic encephalopathy is a medical emergency that requires immediate therapy with 3% sodium chloride (3% NaCl, 513 mEq/L). The author's group has reviewed the treatment and safe limits for correction in detail elsewhere.[83,106,107] Fluid restriction, isotonic saline, and vaptans have no role as initial therapy for hyponatremic encephalopathy because they are either ineffective, will not consistently increase the sodium by a sufficient degree, or do not have a rapid enough onset of action.[108] SIAD is a saline-resistant state, and the response to 3% NaCl will vary based on the severity of SIAD; therefore no equation will accurately predict the response to therapy. The consensus treatment of hyponatremic encephalopathy is to give repeated boluses of 3% NaCl (2 mL/kg, maximum 150 mL) in order to acutely raise the serum sodium by approximately 5 mEq/L (**Box 3**).[109] This approach should be used for both mild and severe symptoms and both acute and chronic hyponatremia. Three percent NaCl has proven to be safe and effective in treating hyponatremic encephalopathy in both children and adults.[86,110] If used properly, there is very little risk of overcorrection or developing cerebral demyelination in SIAD, as a spontaneous free-water diuresis is unlikely to occur due to elevated AVP.

Box 3
Treatment of symptomatic hyponatremia

1. 2 mL/kg bolus of 3% NaCl over 10 min. Maximum 150 mL

2. Repeat bolus 1 to 2 times as needed until symptoms improve. Goal: 5 to 6 mEq/L increase in serum sodium (SNa) in first 1 to 2 h

3. Recheck SNa following second or third bolus or every 2 h

4. Hyponatremic encephalopathy is unlikely if no clinical improvement following an acute increase in serum sodium of 5 to 6 mEq/L

5. Stop further therapy with 3% NaCl boluses when patient is either:
   a. Symptom free: awake, alert, responding to commands, resolution of headache and nausea
   b. Acute increase in sodium of 10 mEq/L in if first 5 h

6. Correction in first 48 h should:
   a. Not to exceed 15 to 20 mEq/L
   b. Avoid normonatremia or hypernatremia

Treatment of Asymptomatic Syndrome of Inappropriate Antidiuresis

SIAD is usually of short duration and resolves with treatment of the underlying disorder and discontinuation of the offending medication. Fluid restriction is the cornerstone of therapy, but is a slow method of correction and is frequently ineffective.[108] Fluid restriction in an adult is generally considered to be less than 1000 mL/d, which would translate to less than 600 mL/m²/d in a child.[111] This degree of fluid restriction is particularly difficult in infants, whereby most nutrition is from liquids. Normal saline (Na 154 mEq/L) is generally ineffective in correcting hyponatremia in SIAD and can in fact aggravate hyponatremia if the urine osmolality is greater than 500 mOsm/kg.[112,113] Loop diuretics may be helpful in managing hyponatremia, because they impair urinary concentration and increase urine electrolyte free water clearance.[114] For children with chronic asymptomatic hyponatremia from SIAD who do not respond to fluid restriction, the next step would be to increase the oral sodium intake or give oral urea in order to increase the renal solute load, thereby inducing an osmotic diuresis. Oral urea has proven to be successful in treating chronic hyponatremia in both children and adults who did not respond to conservative measures.[115,116] A once-daily dose of 15 to 30 g of urea in an adult appears to be effective and well tolerated. A commercially available lemon-flavored urea powder drink (Ure-Na be Nephcentric LLC) is now available in the United States.

Vaptans represent a relatively new class of medication for the management of SIAD.[117] These agents are a nonpeptide vasopressin V2 receptor antagonist that selectively antagonizes the antidiuretic effect of AVP and results in a urinary free water diuresis (aquaresis) without increasing loss of electrolytes. There have been numerous placebo-controlled trials that have demonstrated the safety and efficacy of these drugs for the treatment of hyponatremia associated with SIAD in adults.[118,119] Vaptans have also been used successfully in children.[120] Vaptans produce an aquaresis within 1 to 2 hours of administration, which abates within 12 to 24 hours. When used to treat hyponatremia, vaptans result in an approximately 5 to 7 mEq/L increase in serum sodium within the first 24 hours of administration, but the effect is highly variable.[119] The most common side effects of vaptans are increased thirst, polyuria, and dry mouth. There are currently 2 vaptans that are Food and Drug Administration approved in the United States, Tolvaptan, which is available in an oral formulation, and Conivaptan, which is available in an intravenous preparation. There are safety concerns with vaptans because they have been associated with alanine aminotransferase elevation and severe hepatotoxicity with long-term use, and serious overcorrection of hyponatremia has been reported.[121,122] Overcorrection is of particular concern in neurologically impaired or critically ill children with restricted access to water. These agents are inhibitors of cytochrome P450 and should not be used in conjunction with other drugs known to be metabolized by this pathway. At the present time, vaptans cannot be recommended as a first-line agent in the management of SIAD, because they are expensive, are not always necessary, and present safety concerns.[109] Vaptans do appear to be a suitable second-line agent for short-term use in patients with SIAD after conservative measures have failed.

SUMMARY

SIAD is a common cause of both outpatient and hospital-acquired hyponatremia due to numerous medications and disease states associated with AVP excess. SIAD is a diagnosis of exclusion and other possible causes of hyponatremia must be excluded. Hypotonic fluid should be avoided in patients at risk for SIAD in order to prevent hospital-acquired hyponatremia. Hyponatremic encephalopathy is the most serious complication and requires emergent therapy with 3% NaCl.

ACKNOWLEDGMENTS

The author would like to thank Karen Branstetter for her editorial assistance.

REFERENCES

1. Knepper MA, Kwon TH, Nielsen S. Molecular physiology of water balance. N Engl J Med 2015;372:1349–58.
2. Moritz ML, Ayus JC. Maintenance intravenous fluids in acutely ill patients. N Engl J Med 2015;373:1350–60.
3. Dunn FL, Brennan TJ, Nelson AE, et al. The role of blood osmolality and volume in regulating vasopressin secretion in the rat. J Clin Invest 1973;52:3212–9.
4. Schwartz WB, Bennet W, Curelop S, et al. A syndrome of renal sodium loss and hyponatremia probably resulting from inappropriate secretion of antidiuretic hormone. Am J Med 1957;23:529–42.
5. Leaf A, Bartter FC, Santos RF, et al. Evidence in man that urinary electrolyte loss induced by pitressin is a function of water retention. J Clin Invest 1953; 32:868–78.
6. Bartter FC, Schwartz WB. The syndrome of inappropriate secretion of antidiuretic hormone. Am J Med 1967;42:790–806.
7. Jaenike JR, Waterhouse C. The renal response to sustained administration of vasopressin and water in man. J Clin Endocrinol Metab 1961;21:231–42.
8. Verbalis JG. An experimental model of syndrome of inappropriate antidiuretic hormone secretion in the rat. Am J Physiol 1984;247:E540–53.
9. Southgate HJ, Burke BJ, Walters G. Body space measurements in the hyponatraemia of carcinoma of the bronchus: evidence for the chronic 'sick cell' syndrome? Ann Clin Biochem 1992;29(Pt 1):90–5.
10. Adler SM, Verbalis JG. Disorders of body water homeostasis in critical illness. Endocrinol Metab Clin North Am 2006;35:873–94, xi.
11. Verbalis JG. Pathogenesis of hyponatremia in an experimental model of the syndrome of inappropriate antidiuresis. Am J Physiol 1994;267:R1617–25.

12. Padfield PL, Brown JJ, Lever AF, et al. Blood pressure in acute and chronic vasopressin excess: studies of malignant hypertension and the syndrome of inappropriate antidiuretic hormone secretion. N Engl J Med 1981;304:1067–70.
13. Cooke CR, Turin MD, Walker WG. The syndrome of inappropriate antidiuretic hormone secretion (SIADH): pathophysiologic mechanisms in solute and volume regulation. Medicine (Baltimore) 1979;58:240–51.
14. Ecelbarger CA, Chou CL, Lee AJ, et al. Escape from vasopressin-induced antidiuresis: role of vasopressin resistance of the collecting duct. Am J Physiol 1998;274:F1161–6.
15. Ecelbarger CA, Nielsen S, Olson BR, et al. Role of renal aquaporins in escape from vasopressin-induced antidiuresis in rat. J Clin Invest 1997;99:1852–63.
16. Tian Y, Sandberg K, Murase T, et al. Vasopressin V2 receptor binding is down-regulated during renal escape from vasopressin-induced antidiuresis. Endocrinology 2000;141:307–14.
17. Robertson GL. Regulation of arginine vasopressin in the syndrome of inappropriate antidiuresis. Am J Med 2006;119:S36–42.
18. Zerbe R, Stropes L, Rebertson G. Annu Rev Med 1980;31:315–27.
19. Fenske WK, Christ-Crain M, Horning A, et al. A copeptin-based classification of the osmoregulatory defects in the syndrome of inappropriate antidiuresis. J Am Soc Nephrol 2014;25:2376–83.
20. Fenske W, Sandner B, Christ-Crain M. A copeptin-based classification of the osmoregulatory defects in the syndrome of inappropriate antidiuresis. Best Pract Res Clin Endocrinol Metab 2016;30:219–33.
21. Moritz ML. Syndrome of inappropriate antidiuresis and cerebral salt wasting syndrome: are they different and does it matter? Pediatr Nephrol 2012;27(5):689–93.
22. Feldman BJ, Rosenthal SM, Vargas GA, et al. Nephrogenic syndrome of inappropriate antidiuresis. N Engl J Med 2005;352:1884–90.
23. Kettritz R, Bichet DG, Luft FC. Transient nephrogenic syndrome of inappropriate antidiuresis. Clin Kidney J 2013;6:439–40.
24. Sekiya N, Awazu M. A case of nephrogenic syndrome of inappropriate antidiuresis caused by carbamazepine. CEN Case Rep 2018;7(1):66–8.
25. Maesaka JK, Imbriano LJ, Ali NM, et al. Is it cerebral or renal salt wasting? Kidney Int 2009;76:934–8.
26. Levin ER, Gardner DG, Samson WK. Natriuretic peptides. N Engl J Med 1998;339:321–8.
27. Arieff AI, Gabbai R, Goldfine ID. Cerebral salt-wasting syndrome: diagnosis by urine sodium excretion. Am J Med Sci 2017;354:350–4.
28. Maesaka JK, Miyawaki N, Palaia T, et al. Renal salt wasting without cerebral disease: diagnostic value of urate determinations in hyponatremia. Kidney Int 2007;71:822–6.
29. Nelson PB, Seif SM, Maroon JC, et al. Hyponatremia in intracranial disease: perhaps not the syndrome of inappropriate secretion of antidiuretic hormone (SIADH). J Neurosurg 1981;55:938–41.
30. Wijdicks EF, Vermeulen M, ten Haaf JA, et al. Volume depletion and natriuresis in patients with a ruptured intracranial aneurysm. Ann Neurol 1985;18:211–6.
31. Sivakumar V, Rajshekhar V, Chandy MJ. Management of neurosurgical patients with hyponatremia and natriuresis. Neurosurgery 1994;34:269–74 [discussion: 74].

32. Audibert G, Steinmann G, de Talance N, et al. Endocrine response after severe subarachnoid hemorrhage related to sodium and blood volume regulation. Anesth Analg 2009;108:1922–8.

33. Jimenez R, Casado-Flores J, Nieto M, et al. Cerebral salt wasting syndrome in children with acute central nervous system injury. Pediatr Neurol 2006;35:261–3.

34. Misra UK, Kalita J, Bhoi SK, et al. A study of hyponatremia in tuberculous meningitis. J Neurol Sci 2016;367:152–7.

35. Inamdar P, Masavkar S, Shanbag P. Hyponatremia in children with tuberculous meningitis: a hospital-based cohort study. J Pediatr neurosciences 2016;11: 182–7.

36. Hardesty DA, Kilbaugh TJ, Storm PB. Cerebral salt wasting syndrome in postoperative pediatric brain tumor patients. Neurocrit Care 2012;17:382–7.

37. Wattad A, Chiang ML, Hill LL. Hyponatremia in hospitalized children. Clin Pediatr (Phila) 1992;31:153–7.

38. Zerbe R, Stropes L, Robertson G. Vasopressin function in the syndrome of inappropriate antidiuresis. Annu Rev Med 1980;31:315–27.

39. Dhawan A, Narang A, Singhi S. Hyponatraemia and the inappropriate ADH syndrome in pneumonia. Ann Trop Paediatr 1992;12:455–62.

40. Poddar U, Singhi S, Ganguli NK, et al. Water electrolyte homeostasis in acute bronchiolitis. Indian Pediatr 1995;32:59–65.

41. Shimura N, Arisaka O. Urinary arginine vasopressin in asthma: consideration of fluid therapy. Acta Paediatr Jpn 1990;32:197–200.

42. Boemke W, Krebs MO, Djalali K, et al. Renal nerves are not involved in sodium and water retention during mechanical ventilation in awake dogs. Anesthesiology 1998;89:942–53.

43. Cotton MF, Donald PR, Schoeman JF, et al. Raised intracranial pressure, the syndrome of inappropriate antidiuretic hormone secretion, and arginine vasopressin in tuberculous meningitis. Childs Nerv Syst 1993;9:10–5 [discussion: 5–6].

44. Padilla G, Leake JA, Castro R, et al. Vasopressin levels and pediatric head trauma. Pediatrics 1989;83:700–5.

45. Hasegawa H, Okubo S, Ikezumi Y, et al. Hyponatremia due to an excess of arginine vasopressin is common in children with febrile disease. Pediatr Nephrol 2009;24:507–11.

46. Swart RM, Hoorn EJ, Betjes MG, et al. Hyponatremia and inflammation: the emerging role of interleukin-6 in osmoregulation. Nephron Physiol 2011;118: 45–51.

47. Mavani GP, DeVita MV, Michelis MF. A review of the nonpressor and nonantidiuretic actions of the hormone vasopressin. Front Med 2015;2:19.

48. Liamis G, Milionis HJ, Elisaf M. Hyponatremia in patients with infectious diseases. J Infect 2011;63:327–35.

49. Shepshelovich D, Schechter A, Calvarysky B, et al. Medication-induced SIADH: distribution and characterization according to medication class. Br J Clin Pharmacol 2017;83:1801–7.

50. Holtmann M, Krause M, Opp J, et al. Oxcarbazepine-induced hyponatremia and the regulation of serum sodium after replacing carbamazepine with oxcarbazepine in children. Neuropediatrics 2002;33:298–300.

51. Janczar S, Zalewska-Szewczyk B, Mlynarski W. Severe hyponatremia in a single-center series of 84 homogenously treated children with acute lymphoblastic leukemia. J Pediatr Hematol Oncol 2017;39:e54–8.

52. Salido M, Macarron P, Hernandez-Garcia C, et al. Water intoxication induced by low-dose cyclophosphamide in two patients with systemic lupus erythematosus. Lupus 2003;12:636–9.
53. Danziger J, Zeidel ML. Osmotic homeostasis. Clin J Am Soc Nephrol 2015; 10(5):852–62.
54. Ayus JC, Wheeler JM, Arieff AI. Postoperative hyponatremic encephalopathy in menstruant women. Ann Intern Med 1992;117:891–7.
55. Kanda K, Nozu K, Kaito H, et al. The relationship between arginine vasopressin levels and hyponatremia following a percutaneous renal biopsy in children receiving hypotonic or isotonic intravenous fluids. Pediatr Nephrol 2011;26: 99–104.
56. Hew-Butler T, Rosner MH, Fowkes-Godek S, et al. Statement of the third international exercise-associated hyponatremia consensus development conference, Carlsbad, California, 2015. Clin J Sport Med 2015;25:303–20.
57. Moritz ML, Lauridson JR. Fatal hyponatremic encephalopathy as a result of child abuse from forced exercise. Am J Forensic Med Pathol 2016;37:7–8.
58. Changstrom B, Brill J, Hecht S. Severe exercise-associated hyponatremia in a collegiate American football player. Curr Sports Med Rep 2017;16:343–5.
59. Fortgens P, Pillay TS. Pseudohyponatremia revisited: a modern-day pitfall. Arch Pathol Lab Med 2011;135:516–9.
60. Liamis G, Milionis HJ, Elisaf M. Endocrine disorders: causes of hyponatremia not to neglect. Ann Med 2011;43:179–87.
61. Kim JK, Summer SN, Wood WM, et al. Role of glucocorticoid hormones in arginine vasopressin gene regulation. Biochem Biophys Res Commun 2001;289: 1252–6.
62. Agathis NT, Libman IM, Moritz ML. Hyponatremia due to Severe Primary Hypothyroidism in an Infant. Front Pediatr 2015;3:96.
63. Amin N, Alvi NS, Barth JH, et al. Pseudohypoaldosteronism type 1: clinical features and management in infancy. Endocrinol Diabetes Metab case Rep 2013; 2013:130010.
64. Fenske W, Stork S, Blechschmidt A, et al. Copeptin in the differential diagnosis of hyponatremia. J Clin Endocrinol Metab 2009;94:123–9.
65. Nigro N, Winzeler B, Suter-Widmer I, et al. Evaluation of copeptin and commonly used laboratory parameters for the differential diagnosis of profound hyponatraemia in hospitalized patients: 'The Co-MED Study'. Clin Endocrinol (Oxf) 2017;86:456–62.
66. Decaux G, Musch W. Clinical laboratory evaluation of the syndrome of inappropriate secretion of antidiuretic hormone. Clin J Am Soc Nephrol 2008;3:1175–84.
67. Fenske W, Stork S, Koschker AC, et al. Value of fractional uric acid excretion in differential diagnosis of hyponatremic patients on diuretics. J Clin Endocrinol Metab 2008;93:2991–7.
68. Imbriano LJ, Ilamathi E, Ali NM, et al. Normal fractional urate excretion identifies hyponatremic patients with reset osmostat. J Nephrol 2012;25:833–8.
69. Imbriano LJ, Mattana J, Drakakis J, et al. Identifying different causes of hyponatremia with fractional excretion of uric acid. Am J Med Sci 2016;352:385–90.
70. Stiburkova B, Bleyer AJ. Changes in serum urate and urate excretion with age. Adv Chronic Kidney Dis 2012;19:372–6.
71. Hoorn EJ, Zietse R. Hyponatremia and mortality: moving beyond associations. Am J Kidney Dis 2013;62:139–49.

72. Cuesta M, Garrahy A, Slattery D, et al. Mortality rates are lower in SIAD, than in hypervolaemic or hypovolaemic hyponatraemia: Results of a prospective observational study. Clin Endocrinol (Oxf) 2017;87:400–6.

73. Renneboog B, Musch W, Vandemergel X, et al. Mild chronic hyponatremia is associated with falls, unsteadiness, and attention deficits. Am J Med 2006; 119:71.e1-8.

74. Ayus JC, Moritz ML. Bone disease as a new complication of hyponatremia: moving beyond brain injury. Clin J Am Soc Nephrol 2010;5:167–8.

75. Kinsella S, Moran S, Sullivan MO, et al. Hyponatremia independent of osteoporosis is associated with fracture occurrence. Clin J Am Soc Nephrol 2010;5: 275–80.

76. Verbalis JG, Barsony J, Sugimura Y, et al. Hyponatremia-induced osteoporosis. J Bone Miner Res 2010;25:554–63.

77. Ayus JC, Negri AL, Kalantar-Zadeh K, et al. Is chronic hyponatremia a novel risk factor for hip fracture in the elderly? Nephrol Dial Transplant 2012;27: 3725–31.

78. Amin A, Deitelzweig S, Christian R, et al. Evaluation of incremental healthcare resource burden and readmission rates associated with hospitalized hyponatremic patients in the US. J Hosp Med 2012;7:634–9.

79. van der Meer JW, Netea MG. A salty taste to autoimmunity. N Engl J Med 2013; 368:2520–1.

80. Mandai S, Kuwahara M, Kasagi Y, et al. Lower serum sodium level predicts higher risk of infection-related hospitalization in maintenance hemodialysis patients: an observational cohort study. BMC Nephrol 2013;14:276.

81. Moritz ML, Ayus JC. The pathophysiology and treatment of hyponatraemic encephalopathy: an update. Nephrol Dial Transplant 2003;18:2486–91.

82. Moritz ML, Ayus JC. Preventing neurological complications from dysnatremias in children. Pediatr Nephrol 2005;20:1687–700.

83. Moritz ML, Ayus JC. New aspects in the pathogenesis, prevention, and treatment of hyponatremic encephalopathy in children. Pediatr Nephrol 2010;25: 1225–38.

84. Arieff AI, Ayus JC, Fraser CL. Hyponatraemia and death or permanent brain damage in healthy children. BMJ 1992;304:1218–22.

85. Arieff AI, Kozniewska E, Roberts TP, et al. Age, gender, and vasopressin affect survival and brain adaptation in rats with metabolic encephalopathy. Am J Physiol 1995;268:R1143–52.

86. Sarnaik AP, Meert K, Hackbarth R, et al. Management of hyponatremic seizures in children with hypertonic saline: a safe and effective strategy. Crit Care Med 1991;19:758–62.

87. Bruce RC, Kliegman RM. Hyponatremic seizures secondary to oral water intoxication in infancy: association with commercial bottled drinking water. Pediatrics 1997;100:E4.

88. Ayus JC, Arieff AI. Chronic hyponatremic encephalopathy in postmenopausal women: association of therapies with morbidity and mortality. JAMA 1999;281: 2299–304.

89. Ayus JC, Achinger SG, Arieff A. Brain cell volume regulation in hyponatremia: role of sex, age, vasopressin, and hypoxia. Am J Physiol Renal Physiol 2008; 295:F619–24.

90. Halberthal M, Halperin ML, Bohn D. Lesson of the week: Acute hyponatraemia in children admitted to hospital: retrospective analysis of factors contributing to its development and resolution. BMJ 2001;322:780–2.

91. Khan I, Zimmerman B, Brophy P, et al. Masking of syndrome of inappropriate antidiuretic hormone secretion: the isonatremic syndrome. J Pediatr 2014;165: 722–6.
92. Neville KA, Sandeman DJ, Rubinstein A, et al. Prevention of hyponatremia during maintenance intravenous fluid administration: a prospective randomized study of fluid type versus fluid rate. J Pediatr 2010;156:313–9.e1-2.
93. Moritz ML, Ayus JC. Intravenous fluid management for the acutely ill child. Curr Opin Pediatr 2011;23:186–93.
94. Holliday MA, Segar WE. The maintenance need for water in parenteral fluid therapy. Pediatrics 1957;19:823–32.
95. Freeman MA, Ayus JC, Moritz ML. Maintenance intravenous fluid prescribing practices among paediatric residents. Acta Paediatr 2012;101:e465–8.
96. Carandang F, Anglemyer A, Longhurst CA, et al. Association between maintenance fluid tonicity and hospital-acquired hyponatremia. J Pediatr 2013;163: 1646–51.
97. Choong K, Arora S, Cheng J, et al. Hyponatremia in children following surgery- a randomized controlled trial of hypotonic versus isotonic maintenance fluids. Pediatrics 2011;128:857–66.
98. Rey C, Los-Arcos M, Hernandez A, et al. Hypotonic versus isotonic maintenance fluids in critically ill children: a multicenter prospective randomized study. Acta Paediatr 2011;100:1138–43.
99. Shukla S, Basu S, Moritz ML. Use of hypotonic maintenance intravenous fluids and hospital-acquired hyponatremia remain common in children admitted to a general pediatric ward. Front Pediatr 2016;4:90.
100. Moritz ML, Ayus JC. Prevention of hospital-acquired hyponatremia: a case for using isotonic saline. Pediatrics 2003;111:227–30.
101. McNab S, Duke T, South M, et al. 140 mmol/L of sodium versus 77 mmol/L of sodium in maintenance intravenous fluid therapy for children in hospital (PIMS): a randomised controlled double-blind trial. Lancet 2015;385:1190–7.
102. Foster BA, Tom D, Hill V. Hypotonic versus isotonic fluids in hospitalized children: a systematic review and meta-analysis. J Pediatr 2014;165(1):163–9.e2.
103. Fuchs J, Adams ST, Byerley J. Current issues in intravenous fluid use in hospitalized children. Rev Recent Clin Trials 2017;12:284–9.
104. (UK) NCGC. IV fluids in children: intravenous fluid therapy in children and young people in hospital. London: National Institute for Health and Care Excellence (UK); 2015.
105. Koczmara C, Wade AW, Skippen P, et al. Hospital-acquired acute hyponatremia and reports of pediatric deaths. Dynamics 2010;21:21–6.
106. Moritz ML, Ayus JC. 100 cc 3% sodium chloride bolus: a novel treatment for hyponatremic encephalopathy. Metab Brain Dis 2010;25:91–6.
107. Moritz ML, Ayus JC. Management of hyponatremia in various clinical situations. Curr Treat Options Neurol 2014;16:310.
108. Verbalis JG, Greenberg A, Burst V, et al. Diagnosing and treating the syndrome of inappropriate antidiuretic hormone secretion. Am J Med 2016;129:537.e9-23.
109. Spasovski G, Vanholder R, Allolio B, et al. Clinical practice guideline on diagnosis and treatment of hyponatraemia. Nephrol Dial Transplant 2014;29(Suppl 2):i1–39.
110. Ayus JC, Caputo D, Bazerque F, et al. Treatment of hyponatremic encephalopathy with a 3% sodium chloride protocol: a case series. Am J Kidney Dis 2015; 65:435–42.

111. Winzeler B, Lengsfeld S, Nigro N, et al. Predictors of nonresponse to fluid restriction in hyponatraemia due to the syndrome of inappropriate antidiuresis. J Intern Med 2016;280:609–17.
112. Musch W, Decaux G. Treating the syndrome of inappropriate ADH secretion with isotonic saline. Qjm 1998;91:749–53.
113. Greenberg A, Verbalis JG, Amin AN, et al. Current treatment practice and outcomes. Report of the hyponatremia registry. Kidney Int 2015;88(1):167–77.
114. Decaux G. Treatment of the syndrome of inappropriate secretion of antidiuretic hormone by long loop diuretics. Nephron 1983;35:82–8.
115. Soupart A, Coffernils M, Couturier B, et al. Efficacy and tolerance of urea compared with vaptans for long-term treatment of patients with SIADH. Clin J Am Soc Nephrol 2012;7:742–7.
116. Chehade H, Rosato L, Girardin E, et al. Inappropriate antidiuretic hormone secretion: long-term successful urea treatment. Acta Paediatr 2012;101:e39–42.
117. Berl T. Vasopressin antagonists. N Engl J Med 2015;372:2207–16.
118. Schrier RW, Gross P, Gheorghiade M, et al. Tolvaptan, a selective oral vasopressin V2-receptor antagonist, for hyponatremia. N Engl J Med 2006;355:2099–112.
119. Berl T, Quittnat-Pelletier F, Verbalis JG, et al. Oral tolvaptan is safe and effective in chronic hyponatremia. J Am Soc Nephrol 2010;21:705–12.
120. Tuli G, Tessaris D, De Sanctis L, et al. Tolvaptan utilization in children with chronic hyponatremia due to inappropriate antidiuretic hormone secretion (SIADH). Three case reports and review of the literature. J Clin Res Pediatr Endocrinol 2017;9:288–92.
121. Torres VE, Chapman AB, Devuyst O, et al. Tolvaptan in patients with autosomal dominant polycystic kidney disease. N Engl J Med 2012;367:2407–18.
122. Malhotra I, Gopinath S, Janga KC, et al. Unpredictable nature of tolvaptan in treatment of hypervolemic hyponatremia: case review on role of vaptans. Case Rep Endocrinol 2014;2014:807054.

Nephrogenic Diabetes Insipidus

Catherine Kavanagh, MD, Natalie S. Uy, MD*

KEYWORDS

- Nephrogenic diabetes insipidus • Polyuria • Vasopressin • Polydipsia • Aquaporin

KEY POINTS

- Nephrogenic diabetes insipidus (NDI) is due to failure of the kidneys to respond to vasopressin, resulting in increased excretion of dilute urine.
- NDI can be congenital (AVPR2 or AQP2 mutations) or acquired.
- Low-solute diet, thiazide ± amiloride diuretics, and prostaglandin inhibitors are currently the mainstay of NDI treatment.
- Novel therapies for NDI, including molecular chaperones, are under investigation in animal models, but there are limited data in clinical studies.

Nephrogenic diabetes insipidus (NDI), the clinical triad of polyuria, polydipsia, and hypernatremia,[1] results from the physiologic inability to concentrate urine due to failure of the kidneys to respond to antidiuretic hormone (ADH; and also named arginine vasopressin or AVP), resulting in increased excretion of dilute urine. This review focuses on the diagnosis of NDI, the various causes, treatment options, and future perspectives.

PATHOPHYSIOLOGY

Vasopressin is produced by the paraventricular and supraoptic nuclei of the hypothalamus and is then secreted from the posterior pituitary gland, in response to elevations in plasma osmolality or hypovolemia. The osmotic threshold for ADH or vasopressin release is a plasma osmolality of about 280 to 290 mOsmol/kg[2]. Above this threshold, there is a progressive increase in vasopressin secretion.

The target of vasopressin is the V2 receptors (V2R) located at the basolateral membrane of the principal cells of the collecting duct, which is the site of renal water handling for regulation of approximately 10% of the glomerular filtrate. Once bound, intracellular production of cyclic adenosine monophosphatase (cAMP) increases,

Disclosure Statement: There are no financial conflicts of interests to disclose.
Department of Pediatric Nephrology, Columbia University Medical Center, 3959 Broadway, CHN 1115, New York, NY 10032, USA
* Corresponding author.
E-mail address: nsu1@columbia.edu

activating cAMP-dependent protein kinase. This activation leads to phosphorylation and trafficking of the aquaporin channel (AQP2), followed by insertion of AQP2 along the apical cell membrane of the collecting duct, thereby allowing water to enter the cell (**Fig. 1**).[2]

NDI is caused by renal insensitivity to vasopressin, resulting in large volumes of dilute urine with secondary polydipsia. Primary and secondary forms of NDI exist. Congenital defects are more common at the site of the V2R than the AQP2 channel. Acquired NDI is associated with electrolyte abnormalities, obstructive uropathy, and numerous drugs, most commonly lithium[3,4] (**Table 1**).

DIAGNOSIS
History

NDI must be high on the differential for an infant with frequent wet and heavy diapers. Children with NDI display marked thirst especially for cold water. Infants are often found drinking bathwater or sucking on wet washcloths and may even refuse food and milk or formula in preference of water. Patients with primary NDI will usually present in the first year of life, mostly boys, with failure to thrive and vomiting. In contrast, acquired NDI is much more common in adults than primary NDI.

The definition of polyuria is age specific, and several cutoffs have been defined based on age (**Table 2**): greater than 150 mL/kg/d for neonates, 100 to 110 mL/kg/d in children up to age 2, and 40 to 50 mL/kg/d in older children.[5] However, children with NDI may present in a state of dehydration and may not have such high urine output.

Laboratory Evaluation

A first morning-specific gravity may be used to estimate the renal concentrating ability. First morning urine sample can be used as a screening test in some polyuric patients, because a concentrated first morning urine (urine specific gravity 1.030) excludes NDI.

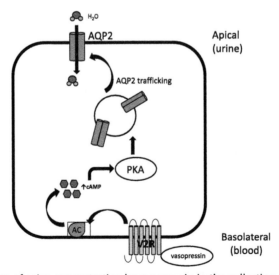

Fig. 1. Mechanism of urine concentration by vasopressin in the collecting duct. Vasopressin binds to V2R, which stimulates a signaling cascade that leads to the insertion of AQP2 channels in the apical side and allows water reabsorption. AC, adenylyl cyclase; PKA, protein kinase.

Table 1 Causes of nephrogenic diabetes insipidus	
Congenital	**Acquired**
X-linked NDI- Xq28 encoding AVPR2 (arginine vasopressin receptor 2) Autosomal recessive NDI- Ch12q13 encoding AQP2	Antimicrobials: foscarnet, aminoglycoside, methicillin, rifampin Electrolyte abnormalities: hypokalemia, hypercalcemia, hypercalciuria Renal parenchyma disorders, obstructive uropathy Other drugs: *lithium*, furosemide, colchicine, cisplatin, isophosphamide, vinblastine Systemic disorders: amyloidosis, sarcoidosis, sickle cell disease and trait, Sjögren syndrome

However, specific gravity may be elevated by the presence of proteinuria and glucosuria. Laboratory evaluation must also include serum osmolality and urine osmolality. As hypokalemia and hypercalcemia can be underlying causes for secondary NDI, serum chemistry is also necessary. Diabetes insipidus (DI) is associated with urine that is inappropriately dilute with a urine osmolality less than 300 mOsm/kg in the setting of a serum osmolality greater than 300 mOsm/kg.

A water-deprivation test can be used to establish the diagnosis of NDI if serum osmolality is less than 300 mOsm/kg. If serum osmolality is greater than 300 mOsm/kg in a child with polyuria, the water deprivation test is unnecessary and can potentially be harmful. In these cases, DDAVP (D-amino D-arginine vasopressin) test should be performed to differentiate between central and NDI.

The aim of the water deprivation test is to induce mild dehydration and challenge the kidney to preserve water. This test should be performed in a controlled environment with medical staff and access to frequent laboratory monitoring (**Fig. 2**).[4,6] The test must be stopped if the patient develops greater than 5% loss of body weight or develops any symptoms of hypovolemia. If urine osmolality is greater than 1000 mOsm/kg once or more than 600 mOsm/kg for 2 voids, then the test must be stopped because the patient does not have DI.[3] If the patient has serum osmolality greater than 300 mOsm/kg and urine osmolality is less than 600 mOsm/kg, the child meets criteria of DI and should be given DDAVP to differentiate between central and NDI. A urine osmolality less than 300 mOsm/kg after DDAVP is consistent with NDI.

GENETICS
AVPR2 Mutations

Most cases of primary NDI (90%) is the result of loss-of-function mutation to the V2R, which is encoded by the AVPR2 gene. The gene is located on chromosome region Xq28, and the mode of inheritance is X-linked recessive. Therefore, most patients with NDI are boys, but, as a result of skewed X-inactivation, girls can be affected

Table 2 Definition of polyuria based on age	
Age	**Urine Output, mL/kg/d**
Neonates	>150
Children up to 2 y old	100–110
Older than 2 y	40–50

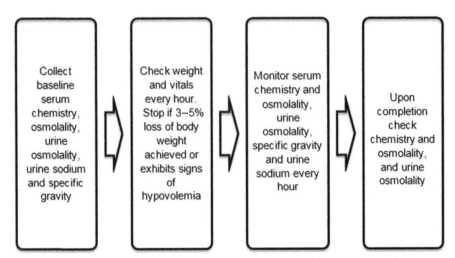

Fig. 2. Water deprivation test. Duration of test: 7 hours in children; 4 hours in infants.

with variable degrees of polyuria and polydipsia. X-linked recessive NDI occurs in about one in 250,000 boys.

AQP2 Mutations

In approximately 10% of patients, congenital NDI is due to loss-of-function mutations in the AQP2 gene, located on chromosome 12. The mode of inheritance is usually autosomal recessive, although a few mutations have been described as autosomal dominant.

Acquired Nephrogenic Diabetes Insipidus

Secondary forms of NDI can be a result of primary disorders, which affect tubular function, such as nephronophthisis, Bartter syndrome, or apparent mineralocorticoid excess. Tubular dysfunction often results in hypokalemia and hypercalciuria, both of which can also be causes of NDI and associated with decreased AQP2 expression.[7] Hypercalciuria can affect the calcium-sensing receptor on the luminal side of the collecting duct and alter AQP2 trafficking, resulting in a urinary concentration defect.[8,9] Other electrolyte abnormalities that can result in NDI include hypercalcemia (Ca >11 mg/dL), and although the mechanism is not completely understood, this may also be associated with activation of the calcium-sensing receptor in the thick ascending limb of the loop of Henle (LOH), thereby reducing sodium reabsorption and calcium reabsorption in the LOH, impairing the medullary osmotic gradient needed for urinary concentration.[10]

Other secondary forms of NDI include obstructive uropathy, which results in downregulation of AQP2 expression. In unilateral obstruction, AQP2 reduction is seen only in the obstructed kidney in animal studies.[11] Downregulation of AQP2 expression can persist up to 30 days after relief of obstruction, which can explain the slow recovery from postobstructive diuresis.[11,12]

Numerous drugs can be responsible for acquired NDI, as listed in **Table 1**. Lithium treatment is the predominant cause of acquired NDI. Lithium enters the cell through epithelial sodium channels (ENaC) with limited transport out of the cells, causing accumulation of intracellular lithium. The exact mechanism of lithium toxicity is incompletely understood, but data suggest that lithium inhibits adenylyl cyclase in the collecting duct, causing downregulation of AQP2 and diminished water reabsorption.[13] In animal studies, chronic lithium treatment led to epithelial remodeling in the collecting duct and a reduction in principal cells.[14]

Partial Nephrogenic Diabetes Insipidus

Some patients with congenital NDI have a mild phenotype; they present after infancy with normal development, and with symptoms of polyuria or enuresis. Evaluation typically reveals intermediate urine osmolality after DDAVP administration (greater than plasma osmolality, but <800 mOsm/kg), suggestive of partial NDI. However, children less than 3 years of age may not be able to maximally concentrate their urine yet, and values between 500 and 800 mOsm/kg can be physiologic.

Patients with partial NDI typically carry mutations that result in partial function of either AVPR2 or AQP2. More recently, Mamenko and colleagues[15] identified a novel mutation in the STIM1 (stream interaction molecule) gene, and a novel physiologic mechanism via calcium signaling, which results in partial NDI. STIM1 encodes the endoplasmic reticulum (ER) calcium sensor that triggers store-operative calcium entry, which is the mechanism by which ER calcium depletion can lead to prolonged calcium influx to drive changes in cellular processes.[16] STIM1 mutation was associated with decreased intracellular calcium levels, and failure of vasopressin to induce a sustained intracellular calcium mobilization in the collecting ducts, resulting in decreased AQP2 abundance. Animals with STIM1 mutation developed polyuria, polydipsia, elevated serum osmolality, dilute urine, and elevated vasopressin levels.[15]

TREATMENT
General Aspects of Treatment

Treatment of a patient with NDI can be most difficult during infancy, when children are dependent on their caregivers for adequate hydration. Fluids should be offered every 2 hours; feeding per nasogastric or gastrostomy tube is often helpful overnight. When requiring intravenous fluids, hypotonic fluids (1/4 isotonic or 0.22%) are usually appropriate due to ongoing urinary losses of essentially pure water; replacement fluids with higher osmolality than urine osmolality will worsen hypernatremia. For example, in a patient with NDI that has a maximum urine osmolality of 100 mOsm/kg and receives 0.45% saline (which has an osmolality of 154 mOsm/kg = 77 mOsm sodium and 77 mOsm chloride), the patient will need to void 1.54 L of urine for each liter of 0.45% saline received to excrete the osmotic load. Therefore, in patients with NDI, the administration of fluids that are hypertonic as compared with urine (but hypotonic to plasma) can lead to hypernatremic dehydration. However, if there are increased salt losses (ie, diarrhea) or if hypotonic fluids are administered at a rate that is higher than the urine losses, hyponatremia could occur. Isotonic fluids should only be administered for acute intravascular volume expansion in hypovolemic shock, requiring normal saline boluses. Otherwise, 0.9% saline will result in excess sodium chloride administration and worsen hypernatremia.

Low-Solute Diet

Another important component in the treatment of patients with NDI is a reduction of osmotic load, which consists of dietary restriction of proteins and sodium, with the goal of reducing the amount of protein metabolites and sodium to be excreted by the kidney. When urine osmolality is fixed in patients with NDI, urine output is determined by osmotic load or solute excretion, and therefore, the use of a low-salt, low-protein diet can decrease urine output. In children, minimizing the osmotic load, while providing the recommended caloric and protein intake to enable normal growth and development, can be challenging. A typical Western diet contains an osmotic load of about 800 mOsm per day. An individual with a urine osmolality of 800 mOsm/kg only needs 1 L of water to excrete that load. However, a patient with NDI and a maximum urine osmolality of 100 mOsm/kg needs to void at least 8 L of water for excretion. In addition, 1 g of table salt (17 mmol of sodium) contains an osmotic load of 34 mOsm (17 mOsm sodium and 17 mOsm of chloride). In a patient with NDI and a urine osmolality of 100 mOsm/kg, each gram of table salt increases urine output by 340 mL. A recommended dietary intake for a child with NDI would be an osmotic load of 15 mOsm/kg/d. A child with NDI and fixed urine osmolality of 100 mOsm/kg will need a fluid intake of 150 mL/kg/d to excrete that solute load.

DIURETICS
Thiazides

The use of diuretics in polyuric disorders seems counterintuitive. Thiazides block the sodium-chloride cotransporter (NCC) in the distal convoluted tubule and thus increase sodium concentration and urine osmolality. This increase in salt losses decreases the intravascular volume further, increases an already activated renin-angiotensin-aldosterone system, and decreases the volume of glomerular filtrate. As a result, sodium and water reabsorption increases in the proximal tubule, thereby decreasing volume delivery to the distal nephron and decreasing amount of tubular fluid available to become urine. Thiazides are often the initial medication treatment of NDI, typically hydrochlorothiaze at 2 to 4 mg/kg/d divided in 2 doses. In conjunction with low-solute diet, thiazide diuretics can decrease urine output by as much as 70%.[17]

Amiloride

Hypokalemia is a common complication of thiazide administration, but supplementation with potassium salts increases the osmotic load. Therefore, the combination of thiazide with a potassium-sparing diuretic can be used, amiloride 0.1 to 0.3 mg/kg/d. Amiloride blocks the ENaC, decreasing sodium reabsorption and increasing urine osmolality. Amiloride is also beneficial with lithium-induced NDI, by blocking ENaC, through which lithium enters the cell.

PROSTAGLANDIN SYNTHESIS INHIBITORS

Inhibitors of prostaglandin synthesis, such as indomethacin (1–3 mg/kg/d in 3 to 4 divided doses), can be used in the treatment of NDI. The exact mechanism remains to be elucidated, but typically prostaglandin inhibitors minimize urinary losses by decreasing glomerular filtration rate (GFR), and renal function must be monitored closely. However, experiments in animals and humans suggest that indomethacin increases urine osmolality and reduces water diuresis without affecting GFR and may be independent of vasopressin.[18] Some evidence suggests that binding of prostaglandin E2 to basolateral prostaglandin receptors may inhibit adenylyl cyclase and the shuttling of AQP2 to the apical membrane,[18] thereby reducing water diuresis.[18,19]

Indomethacin can reduce urine output by 25% to 50% more than thiazides alone,[17] but use must be monitored carefully, especially when first initiated. Indomethacin, especially with concomitant use of thiazide, can cause rapid lowering of serum sodium and hyponatremic seizures.[20] Other side effects of indomethacin include abdominal pain or gastric bleeding, which can be reduced with the use of H2 blocker or proton pump inhibitor.

NOVEL TREATMENTS
Acetazolamide/Lithium-Induced Nephrogenic Diabetes Insipidus

Discontinuation of lithium therapy can resolve the symptoms of NDI, but this is usually not an option because the beneficial effects of lithium on the psychiatric condition outweigh the complications of NDI on quality of life. In addition to the treatment options previously discussed, recent studies suggest the potential use of acetazolamide for lithium-induced NDI. Thiazides, which inhibit the NCC and are derived from carbonic anhydrase, still reduced polyuria in mice lacking NCC with lithium-induced NDI, suggesting that an additional antidiuretic effect of thiazides may be due to carbonic anhydrase inhibition.[21] In an animal model of lithium-induced NDI, acetazolamide was as effective as thiazide/amiloride in reducing polyuria, increasing urine osmolality and increasing AQP2 abundance, but with fewer side effects. The thiazide/amiloride-treated mice developed hyponatremia, hyperkalemia, hypercalcemia, metabolic acidosis, and increased serum lithium concentrations, which were not observed in the acetazolamide-treated mice.[21,22] Reduction in polyuria after acetazolamide treatment was partially caused by a tubular-glomerular feedback response and reduced GFR. Case reports in adult patients with lithium-induced NDI have shown promising results with acetazolamide treatment: decreased urine output, increased urine osmolality without major side effects,[23] but further studies are still needed to assess the safety of acetazolamide, especially in patients with reduced GFR.

FUTURE PERSPECTIVES
Molecular Chaperones

Multiple novel therapies, including mutation-specific treatment, are being examined to improve NDI treatment. Most mutations identified in the AVPR2 gene lead to the improper folding of V2R with entrapment in the ER and preventing their function at the plasma membrane. Retention of V2R is dependent on ER calcium stores for optimal function. By inhibiting the sarcoplasmic calcium pump and depleting ER calcium stores, the mutated V2R can overcome entrapment, as demonstrated in vitro.[24] Other promising treatments that have been successful in vitro include the use of molecular chaperones, or AVPR2-receptor antagonists, that can bind to the mutated V2R, and induce proper folding of the receptor, leading to release from the ER.[24-26] The use of this receptor ligand, or pharmacologic chaperone, has been studied in small trials in vivo. Although the reduction in urine output and increase in urine osmolality were modest,[25] the potential use of a targeted, mutation-specific therapy for patients with congenital NDI appears promising.

REFERENCES

1. Bothra M, Jain V. Diabetes insipidus in pediatric patients. Indian J Pediatr 2014; 81(12):1285–6.
2. Nielsen S, Frokiaer J, Marples D, et al. Aquaporins in the kidney: from molecules to medicine. Physiol Rev 2002;82(1):205–44.
3. Dabrowski E, Kadakia R, Zimmerman D. Diabetes insipidus in infants and children. Best Pract Res Clin Endocrinol Metab 2016;30(2):317–28.
4. Saborio P, Tipton GA, Chan JC. Diabetes insipidus. Pediatr Rev 2000;21(4):122–9 [quiz: 129].
5. Leung AK, Robson WL, Halperin ML. Polyuria in childhood. Clin Pediatr (Phila) 1991;30(11):634–40.
6. Robertson GL. Diabetes insipidus: differential diagnosis and management. Best Pract Res Clin Endocrinol Metab 2016;30(2):205–18.

7. Hebert SC, Brown EM, Harris HW. Role of the Ca(2+)-sensing receptor in divalent mineral ion homeostasis. J Exp Biol 1997;200(Pt 2):295–302.

8. Sands JM, Naruse M, Baum M, et al. Apical extracellular calcium/polyvalent cation-sensing receptor regulates vasopressin-elicited water permeability in rat kidney inner medullary collecting duct. J Clin Invest 1997;99(6):1399–405.

9. Earm JH, Christensen BM, Frokiaer J, et al. Decreased aquaporin-2 expression and apical plasma membrane delivery in kidney collecting ducts of polyuric hypercalcemic rats. J Am Soc Nephrol 1998;9(12):2181–93.

10. Hebert SC. Extracellular calcium-sensing receptor: implications for calcium and magnesium handling in the kidney. Kidney Int 1996;50(6):2129–39.

11. Frokiaer J, Christensen BM, Marples D, et al. Downregulation of aquaporin-2 parallels changes in renal water excretion in unilateral ureteral obstruction. Am J Physiol 1997;273(2 Pt 2):F213–23.

12. Frokiaer J, Marples D, Knepper MA, et al. Bilateral ureteral obstruction downregulates expression of vasopressin-sensitive AQP-2 water channel in rat kidney. Am J Physiol 1996;270(4 Pt 2):F657–68.

13. Marples D, Christensen S, Christensen EI, et al. Lithium-induced downregulation of aquaporin-2 water channel expression in rat kidney medulla. J Clin Invest 1995;95(4):1838–45.

14. Christensen BM, Marples D, Kim YH, et al. Changes in cellular composition of kidney collecting duct cells in rats with lithium-induced NDI. Am J Physiol Cell Physiol 2004;286(4):C952–64.

15. Mamenko M, Dhande I, Tomilin V, et al. Defective store-operated calcium entry causes partial nephrogenic diabetes insipidus. J Am Soc Nephrol 2016;27(7):2035–48.

16. Hoth M, Penner R. Depletion of intracellular calcium stores activates a calcium current in mast cells. Nature 1992;355(6358):353–6.

17. Bouley R, Hasler U, Lu HA, et al. Bypassing vasopressin receptor signaling pathways in nephrogenic diabetes insipidus. Semin Nephrol 2008;28(3):266–78.

18. Stoff JS, Rosa RM, Silva P, et al. Indomethacin impairs water diuresis in the DI rat: role of prostaglandins independent of ADH. Am J Physiol 1981;241(3):F231–7.

19. Libber S, Harrison H, Spector D. Treatment of nephrogenic diabetes insipidus with prostaglandin synthesis inhibitors. J Pediatr 1986;108(2):305–11.

20. Boussemart T, Nsota J, Martin-Coignard D, et al. Nephrogenic diabetes insipidus: treat with caution. Pediatr Nephrol 2009;24(9):1761–3.

21. Sinke AP, Kortenoeven ML, de Groot T, et al. Hydrochlorothiazide attenuates lithium-induced nephrogenic diabetes insipidus independently of the sodium-chloride cotransporter. Am J Physiol Renal Physiol 2014;306(5):F525–33.

22. de Groot T, Sinke AP, Kortenoeven ML, et al. Acetazolamide attenuates lithium-induced nephrogenic diabetes insipidus. J Am Soc Nephrol 2016;27(7):2082–91.

23. Gordon CE, Vantzelfde S, Francis JM. Acetazolamide in lithium-induced nephrogenic diabetes insipidus. N Engl J Med 2016;375(20):2008–9.

24. Romisch K. A cure for traffic jams: small molecule chaperones in the endoplasmic reticulum. Traffic 2004;5(11):815–20.

25. Morello JP, Salahpour A, Laperriere A, et al. Pharmacological chaperones rescue cell-surface expression and function of misfolded V2 vasopressin receptor mutants. J Clin Invest 2000;105(7):887–95.

26. Bernier V, Morello JP, Zarruk A, et al. Pharmacologic chaperones as a potential treatment for X-linked nephrogenic diabetes insipidus. J Am Soc Nephrol 2006;17(1):232–43.

Hemolytic Uremic Syndrome

Ellen M. Cody, MD[a], Bradley P. Dixon, MD[b],*

KEYWORDS

- Hemolytic uremic syndrome • *Escherichia coli* • Shiga toxin • Pneumococcal HUS
- Atypical HUS • Cobalamin C

KEY POINTS

- Shiga toxin–associated hemolytic uremic syndrome (HUS) is responsible for approximately 90% of cases of HUS in children, and supportive care remains the backbone of therapy.
- With early fluid resuscitation in the enteritis phase, outcomes for Shiga toxin–associated HUS have improved; however, up to 25% of patients develop chronic kidney disease, hypertension, or proteinuria.
- *Streptococcus pneumoniae* is likely an underrepresented cause of HUS, responsible for about 5% of cases in children, most commonly in association with complicated pneumonia.
- Atypical HUS is due to genetic dysregulation of the alternative complement pathway or coagulation cascade, with outcomes significantly improved after the advent of the complement-targeted monoclonal antibody eculizumab.

INTRODUCTION

First described by Gasser and colleagues[1] in 1955, hemolytic uremic syndrome (HUS) is the clinical triad of thrombocytopenia, anemia, and acute kidney injury. It is classically associated with enterocolitis from Shiga toxin–producing *Escherichia coli* (STEC), which accounts for 85% to 95% of cases in children.[2,3] Approximately 5% of cases are associated with invasive infections by *Streptococcus pneumoniae*, which is known as *S pneumoniae*–HUS (SP-HUS). Genetic dysregulation of the alternative complement pathway or coagulation cascade, also known as atypical HUS (aHUS), accounts for 5% to 10%. In rare cases, it is associated with a hereditary disorder of cobalamin C metabolism.[3] Additional causes of HUS include drug exposure (**Box 1**); other systemic conditions, such as malignant hypertension, autoimmune diseases, malignancy, solid organ and hematopoietic stem-cell transplantation; and various other infections.[6]

Disclosure Statement: The authors have nothing to disclose.
[a] Department of Pediatrics, University of Colorado School of Medicine, 13123 East 16th Avenue, Box 158, Aurora, CO 80045, USA; [b] Departments of Pediatrics & Medicine, University of Colorado School of Medicine, 12631 E. 17th Avenue, Aurora, CO 80045, USA
* Corresponding author.
E-mail address: bradley.dixon@childrenscolorado.org

Pediatr Clin N Am 66 (2019) 235–246
https://doi.org/10.1016/j.pcl.2018.09.011
0031-3955/19/© 2018 Elsevier Inc. All rights reserved.

Box 1
Drugs implicated in hemolytic uremic syndrome

Calcineurin inhibitors: cyclosporine, tacrolimus

Quinine

Vascular endothelial growth factor inhibitors

Quetiapine

Drugs of abuse: cocaine, intravenous oxymorphone

Chemotherapeutics: mitomycin, gemcitabine

Antiplatelet agents: ticlopidine, clopidogrel

Data from Refs.[3–5]

Despite their varied causes and inciting pathogeneses, these different forms of HUS share the common features of creation of a prothrombotic and proinflammatory state on the endothelial cell surface,[3] with subsequent formation of fibrin and platelet thrombi in capillaries and arterioles, leading to the classic clinical triad.

SHIGA TOXIN–ASSOCIATED HEMOLYTIC UREMIC SYNDROME
Epidemiology and Pathomechanism

HUS associated with STEC (STEC-HUS) is classically a disease of children, with a peak incidence from 3 to 5 years of age. In the United States and Europe, the predominant pathogen is *E coli* O157:H7, whereas *Shigella dysenteriae* type 1 remains a predominant cause of disease in other countries.[5] The overall incidence of HUS is 1 to 2 cases per 100,000 per year, with most cases attributed to STEC-HUS.[3] In children presenting with *E coli* enterocolitis, approximately 15% will progress to the development of HUS, with younger age, leukocytosis, and female gender increasing the chances of progression.[2] Most Enterohemorrhagic *E coli* strains express the adhesin intimin, allowing Shiga toxin to enter the blood stream[7] and then bind globotriaosylceramide (Gb3) on endothelial cells, which is also present on renal tubular cells.[2,4] After undergoing endocytosis, the toxin causes ribosomal inactivation, leading to cell death. Shiga toxin also is proinflammatory and prothrombotic, inducing endothelial secretion of von Willebrand factor.[4] Finally, there is evidence that Shiga toxin itself induces complement activation,[8] based on high plasma concentrations of sC5b-9 and Bb in the acute phase of the illness, which rapidly return to normal during convalescence. Such activation is postulated to be due to alternative pathway dysregulation by the binding of Shiga toxin to Factor H in a concentration-dependent manner and disruption of its regulatory activity on the endothelial cell surface.[7]

Clinical Presentation

The typical prodrome for STEC-HUS consists of watery diarrhea after a 3 to 5 day incubation period following inoculation, with progression to bloody diarrhea and severe crampy abdominal pain, accompanied by nausea and vomiting.[2] Thrombocytopenia and acute kidney injury generally ensue as the gastrointestinal symptoms resolve,[4] typically within 2 to 14 days after onset of diarrhea.[9] Extrarenal manifestations are thought to occur due to multisystem thrombotic microangiopathy (TMA), with the most common life-threatening extrarenal manifestation being neurologic, with incidence estimates varying widely from 3% to 26%.[10,11] This neurologic injury may be potentiated by other factors associated with HUS, including massive cytokine release, hypertension, and hyponatremia.[10] Additional extrarenal manifestations include cardiovascular involvement (eg, myocardial infarction, congestive heart failure, and dilated cardiomyopathy), pulmonary hemorrhage, bowel necrosis and perforation, pancreatitis and resulting diabetes mellitus, and cholecystitis.[12]

Management

Despite this entity being recognized for more than 60 years, supportive care remains the primary management strategy for STEC-HUS. This involves meticulous fluid and electrolyte management after oligoanuric renal failure develops, packed red blood cell (pRBC) transfusion, and dialysis. Recent studies have demonstrated that early and cautious fluid resuscitation in the setting of enterocolitis before the development of HUS may improve renal and neurologic outcomes.[13–16]

Although early studies suggested a risk of progression to HUS with systemic antibiotic administration in the setting of enterocolitis with STEC, later studies have presented conflicting data.[2,9,17,18] Indeed, recent data emerging from the 2011 epidemic of STEC-HUS in Germany identified that with macrolide antibiotic administration there was no worsened disease activity; reduction of long-term E coli carriage[19]; and, ultimately, decreased incidence of seizures.[20]

Another intervention long thought to aggravate disease is platelet transfusions, particularly given the prominent role of platelets in the disease pathogenesis. However, this dogma has also been recently challenged because studies have found no difference in the duration of the requirement of dialysis access[21] or in aspects of disease severity, including requirement of dialysis, hypertension, extrarenal manifestations, or death, in patients receiving platelet transfusions.[22,23]

The use of therapeutic plasma exchange has long been debated in STEC-HUS although there have been no large randomized control trials to completely evaluate this therapy and it has not uniformly been found to improve outcomes.[24] Plasmapheresis was widely used used in the German outbreak, mainly for neurologic involvement of the disease and, after review, no definitive evidence supported its efficacy.[11,20] Per the American Society of Apheresis, plasmapheresis is a category III recommendation with neurologic involvement of STEC-HUS and a category IV recommendation in STEC-HUS without neurologic involvement.[25]

Given evidence of the facilitating role of the complement system in STEC-HUS, eculizumab (a humanized monoclonal antibody targeting the terminal complement pathway, used successfully in aHUS) has been used in a small series of subjects with severe neurologic involvement of STEC-HUS[26] and more extensively in the 2011 German O104:H4 epidemic.[27] However, despite its mechanistic plausibility, no definitive evidence has emerged from these studies showing short-term[20,28] or intermediate-term benefit[29] from the use of eculizumab.

Finally, multiple Shiga toxin–specific therapies have been applied in attempts to prevent systemic disease progression. However, to be most effective, such therapies would require administration to sequester the toxin before the onset of TMA. The earliest attempt to directly mitigate toxin using SYNSORB Pk, a silicon dioxide particle mimicking Gb3 to bind Shiga toxin in the gut, demonstrated no improvement in disease severity or clinical course.[30] More recent agents targeting Shiga toxin, including intravenous peptides and anti-Shiga toxin monoclonal antibodies, have shown to be protective in animal models of the disease[31,32] but with no published efficacy in humans. Most recently, immunoadsorption was used in the German outbreak for patients with severe neurologic complications, with reported rapid improvement,[33] although such evidence is largely anecdotal.

Prognosis

Acute mortality of STEC-HUS is estimated to be between 3% to 5%,[2,9] with the primary causes of death being neurologic,[34] cardiovascular, or intraabdominal catastrophe. Beyond the acute period of illness, long-term renal sequelae have been identified in approximately 25% of survivors from the acute phase of STEC-HUS,[35] including GFR below 80 mL/min/1.73 m^2, proteinuria, and hypertension. Prolonged anuria (typically greater than 2 weeks) portends worse renal outcomes, and patients rarely recover renal function if dialysis requirement exceeds 4 weeks.[12] There are few studies describing long-term outcomes of extra-renal organ involvement. In the largest published case series of neurologic involvement of STEC-HUS, such involvement led to death in 17% (usually in the acute phase), severe neurologic sequelae in 23% but complete recovery in 50%.[10]

STREPTOCOCCUS PNEUMONIAE HEMOLYTIC UREMIC SYNDROME
Epidemiology and Pathomechanism

Estimated to account for approximately 5% of all cases of HUS in children, and 38% to 43% of HUS not caused by Shiga toxin,[36] pneumococcal HUS or S pneumoniae-associated HUS (SP-HUS) has an annual incidence of approximately 0.06 per 100,000 children less than 18 years of age.[3] The incidence of HUS following invasive pneumococcal infections is estimated to be about 0.4% to 0.6%, most commonly occurring after pneumonia, particularly complicated by empyema, or meningitis.[37] With the introduction of the PCV7 vaccine, the annual incidence has remained the same but 19A has become the predominant associated strain. It is as yet unknown if PCV13, which includes strain 19A, will lead to a decrease in the incidence of SP-HUS. The mechanism of disease is hypothesized to involve removal of sialic acid from cell surfaces by a circulating neuraminidase produced by S pneumoniae, resulting in exposure of the Thomsen-Friedenreich cryptantigen (T-antigen). Preformed IgM antibodies against T-antigen react to RBCs, platelets, and endothelial cells, leading to aggregation in the microcirculation and TMA.[2] Other hypothesized mechanisms of disease include loss of cell surface binding sites of Factor H, a regulatory protein of the alternative complement pathway, by desialylation. Several pneumococcal serotypes (serotypes 2 and 3) have also demonstrated direct binding of Factor H by bacterially expressed proteins such as Hic and surface protein C, which may inhibit its action.[37]

Clinical Presentation

Symptoms usually develop 3 to 13 days after onset of pneumococcal disease, with most developing within 7 to 9 days which is slightly longer than the latency period of STEC-HUS.[36] Compared with STEC-HUS, children affected by SP-HUS are younger with more severe renal and/or hematological disease, require longer hospital stays, and more often experience ongoing renal insufficiency due to cortical necrosis.[2,36] Diagnosis of SP-HUS can be challenging, particularly given its frequent coexistence with disseminated intravascular coagulation (DIC). The direct Coombs test detects antibodies and complement that coat erythrocytes and has been shown to be positive in 90% of SP-HUS; however, there is no data on the rate of positive Coombs tests in pneumococcal infections without HUS.[36,37]

Management

Therapy for SP-HUS remains supportive with treatment of the underlying pneumococcal infection. Best supportive care is similar to that of STEC-HUS, with maintenance of electrolyte balance, adequate nutrition, and renal replacement therapy if required, although patients with SP-HUS more often require dialysis than those with STEC-HUS (75% vs 59%[37]). Due to concern that anti-T antigen antibodies may be present in blood products,[37,38] dextran washing of pRBCs before transfusion is recommended,[36] and plasma-containing blood products such as fresh frozen plasma (FFP) are frequently avoided. Given the hypothesized involvement of anti-T antigen antibodies, use of plasmapheresis specifically with albumin to remove the antibodies has been attempted,[38,39] but with limited systematic evidence that it may improve outcomes.[36,37] Due to evidence of complement activation,[40,41] eculizumab has been used to treat severe cases of SP-HUS, with improvement in platelet counts and subjective improvement in irritability.[40] However, randomized control trials are be needed to further evaluate its efficacy in streptococcal-mediated disease.

Prognosis

Outcomes of SP-HUS are worse than those associated with STEC-HUS, with an acute mortality of 12.3%, mainly in association with meningitis.[36,37] The long-term prognosis of SP-HUS is also worse, with 1 study finding 23% of survivors with chronic kidney disease (CKD), 28% with proteinuria, and 19% with hypertension,[37] with 26% to 40% overall affected compared with approximately 25% of subjects in STEC-HUS.[12,35] The greatest risk factor for the development of CKD are those patients requiring dialysis for greater than 20 days.[37] Additionally, more patients with SP-HUS require renal transplantation due to the severity of their disease.[42]

ATYPICAL HEMOLYTIC UREMIC SYNDROME
Epidemiology and Pathomechanism

aHUS, also termed complement-mediated TMA,[4] is responsible for approximately 5% to 10% of HUS seen in children. Overall incidence is estimated at 2 per 1,000,000 individuals in the United States, with 70% of children having their first episode before 2 years of age, and with equal frequency in boys and girls when onset is in childhood.[2,43] The disease is frequently sporadic despite heterozygous pathogenic variants in complement genes often identified in the patient and one of their healthy parents,[3] which suggests that genetic background creates a susceptibility to, but is insufficient to cause, disease. Penetrance of the disease is incomplete, with approximately 50% of family members who carry the mutation not manifesting with disease by age 45 years, across all disease-associated genes.[43]

There are 3 main mechanisms of complement dysregulation attributed to disease pathogenesis: loss of function mutations in complement regulatory proteins, such as Factor H, Factor I, Membrane Cofactor Protein (CD46), and thrombomodulin; gain of function mutations in effector proteins, such as Factor B or C3; and formation of neutralizing autoantibodies against Factor H.[44] However, up to 30% of patients have no demonstrable mutation in the known disease-associated genes.[5] The resulting complement dysregulation leads to increased C3b deposition on the endothelial cell surface, resulting in increased formation of the potent proinflammatory anaphylatoxin C5a and the lytic terminal complement complex C5b-9,[4] leading to endothelial injury and TMA.

The paradigm that aHUS is a disease exclusively of complement dysregulation has been challenged in recent years with the identification of mutations in proteins that regulate the coagulation system. This was first noted with thrombomodulin, which regulates both complement and coagulation,[45] and more recently with the identification of homozygous or compound heterozygous mutations in diacylglycerol kinase epsilon (DGKE), an intracellular regulatory kinase, in a cohort of patients all younger than 1 year of age with autosomal recessive inheritance and complete penetrance.[46]

Loss of function of the DGKE protein results in protein kinase C activation, ultimately causing upregulation of prothrombotic factors, such as von Willebrand factor, and downregulation of vascular endothelial growth factor, resulting in a shift to a prothrombotic state in the microvasculature.[46,47] Subsequently, other variants in coagulation-associated genes, such as plasminogen, have been identified in a subset of aHUS patients.[48]

Clinical Features

Approximately 80% of patients with aHUS present in a fulminant manner, usually with a triggering event such as an upper respiratory infection or viral gastroenteritis, making the distinction from STEC-HUS difficult.[2,43] The remaining 20% of patients can have a more indolent onset, with subclinical anemia, fluctuating thrombocytopenia, and preserved renal function at diagnosis.[43] Such patients may also have an insidious onset with nonspecific symptoms, such as malaise, fatigue, and anorexia, making diagnosis difficult.[5] Low serum levels of C3 with normal serum levels of C4 indicate alternative pathway activation[2] but are only observed in approximately one-third of patients at presentation. The renal manifestations of aHUS are variable across patients and can include acute kidney injury, nephrotic range proteinuria resulting from glomerular basement membrane damage, and malignant hypertension.[3] Extrarenal manifestations occur in approximately 20% of patients, with neurologic involvement being the most common, estimated at 10%, including irritability, drowsiness, seizures, diplopia, cortical blindness, hemiparesis or hemiplegia, stupor, or coma.[43] Additionally, myocardial infarction due to cardiac microangiopathy has been reported in about 3% of patients and likely explains cases of sudden death.[43] Pulmonary hemorrhage, ischemic colitis, pancreatitis, hepatocellular injury, and peripheral vascular disease have also been described.

Management

Plasma therapy, either through plasma infusion or plasma exchange, was historically the mainstay of management for aHUS, without definitive evidence that it directly targets the underlying disease or prevents progression to end-stage renal disease (ESRD).[49] With the advent of eculizumab, a monoclonal antibody that binds with high affinity to the complement protein C5 and blocks activation of the terminal complement pathway, the prognosis has significantly improved, with studies finding full recovery of renal and neurologic function.[50–54] The drug acts rapidly, with complement inhibition occurring within 1 hour of drug administration,[55] thus recommendations are that patients receive eculizumab within 24 hours of presentation with aHUS, particularly as evidence has shown that time-to-treatment is a significant factor in determining recovery of renal function.[49] Overall, the drug has a favorable safety profile, although patients are recommended to receive meningococcal vaccination and prophylaxis,[56] as well as prompt assessment for meningococcal disease in the setting of febrile illnesses. For Factor H autoantibody-mediated disease, there are established guidelines for plasma exchange in combination with immunosuppressive agents, particularly in a setting in which eculizumab is not available, although new evidence suggests that eculizumab is equally efficacious in inducing remission and preventing life-threatening complications.[3,56,57] A host of novel complement-targeted therapies with promise for the treatment of aHUS are under development, either providing additional means of targeting the terminal complement pathway or targeting other nodes in the alternative complement pathway.[58]

Kidney transplantation has met with greater success with decreased recurrence of aHUS post-transplant and graft loss in patients for whom the allograft will reconstitute a functional membrane bound or intracellular protein, such as with *MCP* or *DGKE*, as opposed to patients with variants in hepatically synthesized circulating factors, such as Factor H, C3, or Factor B, with a 50% to 100% risk of recurrence posttransplant.[3] However, sequential or combined liver-kidney transplantation has proven effective in restoring the expression of these circulating complement factors and remains a therapeutic option to effectively cure the disease in a subset of aHUS patients.[59] Specifically considering patients with aHUS due to *DGKE* mutations, there seems to be no clear benefit of eculizumab or plasma therapy because patients have demonstrated relapse while receiving these therapies.[3,46]

Prognosis

In the era before eculizumab, outcomes of aHUS were quite poor, with 79% of patients experiencing death or ESRD within 3 years of diagnosis,[55] and mutations in *CFH* resulting in the most severe outcomes.[60] Comparatively, patients with mutations in *MCP* had more favorable outcomes; however, these patients experienced frequent relapses and 25% progressed to ESRD at a median age of 18 years.[60] Patients with aHUS associated with mutations in *DGKE* usually progress to severe CKD and ESRD by age 20 to 25 years because optimal therapy has not yet been established.[46] With the advent of eculizumab, progression to ESRD from diagnosis seems to be attenuated.[51] However, there is ongoing debate about the optimal duration of eculizumab therapy for aHUS. Harboring a known pathogenic variant in a disease-associated gene seems to be the most important predictor of relapse after discontinuation of eculizumab, with patients harboring *CFH* variants having the highest risk and those without identified mutations the lowest risk; however, there is no clear consensus on how to withdraw or taper dosing.[61,62] The Kidney Diseases Improving Global Outcomes (KDIGO) initiative has proposed the use of a CH50 level of less than 10% of normal for monitoring of sufficient complement blockade on eculizumab therapy,[63] and studies are ongoing to decrease eculizumab infusion frequency using such testing, with early reports of success and no further TMA relapses.[64,65]

COBALAMIN C HEMOLYTIC UREMIC SYNDROME
Epidemiology and Pathomechanism

Cobalamin C hemolytic uremic syndrome is a form of HUS that is a rare autosomal recessive disorder of cobalamin (vitamin B12) metabolism that causes TMA and multiorgan dysfunction in infants, although there is 1 reported case with presentation in adulthood.[2,4] Its incidence is estimated at 1 in 100,000 live births[66] with more than 300 cases described.[67] The mutations are on the *MMACHC* gene encoding the methylmalonic aciduria and homocystinuria type C protein, leading to hyperhomocysteinemia, decreased plasma methionine levels, and methylmalonic aciduria. Although the exact mechanism by which this metabolic derangement causes disease is unclear,[66] hyperhomocysteinemia likely alters the antithrombotic properties of the vascular endothelium by disrupting nitric oxide-mediated inhibition of platelet aggregation and increasing expression of procoagulant factors from the endothelium.[68] More than 40 mutations in *MMACHC* have been identified; however, 1 mutation (271dupA) has accounted for 40% of all cases, primarily in Europe.[2]

CLINICAL FEATURES

The clinical presentations of cobalamin C deficiency vary considerably and are generally divided into early-onset and late-onset disease, with early-onset disease having a more severe phenotype.[66] Early-onset disease usually manifests within the first year of life and has multisystem involvement, presenting with feeding difficulties, failure to thrive, somnolence/lethargy, and hypotonia.[66] Patients with late-onset disease are rare and can present any time from childhood to adulthood, generally with milder symptoms, which may lead to misdiagnosis.[66] The renal complications are most commonly TMA but may also include tubulointerstitial nephritis and proximal renal tubular acidosis.[68] Excess homocysteine and methylmalonate in the urine is diagnostic of this condition.[2]

Management

The primary therapy for infants is supplementation with parenteral hydroxycobalamin. In 1 published adult case, the patient's TMA did not respond to eculizumab but did respond to hydroxycobalamin, betaine, and folinic acid.[4] It is unlikely that plasma exchange or infusion offer any additional therapeutic benefit.[68]

Prognosis

Mortality is high, making prompt diagnosis essential because patients with early-onset disease have a 25% mortality with an average survival of less than 10 months without therapy.[2,67] Renal dysfunction does occur, with CKD, hypertension, and proteinuria occurring in 40%. Neurologic sequelae are also quite common with developmental delay.[4] With treatment, the TMA, other hematological manifestations, feeding difficulties, and cardiac manifestations may improve and/or resolve; however, the neurologic and ophthalmologic problems tend to remain and continue to progress.[67]

REFERENCES

1. Gasser C, Gautier E, Steck A, et al. Hemolytic-uremic syndrome: bilateral necrosis of the renal cortex in acute acquired hemolytic anemia. Schweiz Med Wochenschr 1955;85(38–39):905–9 [in German].
2. Salvadori M, Bertoni E. Update on hemolytic uremic syndrome: diagnostic and therapeutic recommendations. World J Nephrol 2013;2(3):56–76.
3. Fakhouri F, Zuber J, Frémeaux-Bacchi V, et al. Haemolytic uraemic syndrome. Lancet 2017;390(10095):681–96.
4. George JN, Nester CM. Syndromes of thrombotic microangiopathy. N Engl J Med 2014;371(7):654–66.
5. Kottke-Marchant K. Diagnostic approach to microangiopathic hemolytic disorders. Int J Lab Hematol 2017;39(Suppl 1):69–75.
6. Chan JC, Eleff MG, Campbell RA. The hemolytic-uremic syndrome in nonrelated adopted siblings. J Pediatr 1969;75(6):1050–3.
7. Orth D, Khan AB, Naim A, et al. Shiga toxin activates complement and binds factor H: evidence for an active role of complement in hemolytic uremic syndrome. J Immunol 2009;182(10):6394–400.
8. Thurman JM, Marians R, Emlen W, et al. Alternative pathway of complement in children with diarrhea-associated hemolytic uremic syndrome. Clin J Am Soc Nephrol 2009;4(12):1920–4.
9. Safdar N, Said A, Gangnon RE, et al. Risk of hemolytic uremic syndrome after antibiotic treatment of Escherichia coli O157:H7 enteritis: a meta-analysis. JAMA 2002;288(8):996–1001.
10. Nathanson S, Kwon T, Elmaleh M, et al. Acute neurological involvement in diarrhea-associated hemolytic uremic syndrome. Clin J Am Soc Nephrol 2010; 5(7):1218–28.

11. Loos S, Ahlenstiel T, Kranz B, et al. An outbreak of Shiga toxin-producing *Escherichia coli* O104:H4 hemolytic uremic syndrome in Germany: presentation and short-term outcome in children. Clin Infect Dis 2012;55(6):753–9.

12. Spinale JM, Ruebner RL, Copelovitch L, et al. Long-term outcomes of Shiga toxin hemolytic uremic syndrome. Pediatr Nephrol 2013;28(11):2097–105.

13. Ake JA, Jelacic S, Ciol MA, et al. Relative nephroprotection during *Escherichia coli* O157:H7 infections: association with intravenous volume expansion. Pediatrics 2005;115(6):e673–80.

14. Hickey CA, Beattie TJ, Cowieson J, et al. Early volume expansion during diarrhea and relative nephroprotection during subsequent hemolytic uremic syndrome. Arch Pediatr Adolesc Med 2011;165(10):884–9.

15. Grisaru S, Xie J, Samuel S, et al. Associations between hydration status, intravenous fluid administration, and outcomes of patients infected with Shiga Toxin-producing *Escherichia coli*: a systematic review and meta-analysis. JAMA Pediatr 2017;171(1):68–76.

16. Ardissino G, Tel F, Possenti I, et al. Early volume expansion and outcomes of hemolytic uremic syndrome. Pediatrics 2016;137(1):345–52.

17. Wong CS, Jelacic S, Habeeb RL, et al. The risk of the hemolytic-uremic syndrome after antibiotic treatment of *Escherichia coli* O157:H7 infections. N Engl J Med 2000;342(26):1930–6.

18. Smith KE, Wilker PR, Reiter PL, et al. Antibiotic treatment of *Escherichia coli* O157 infection and the risk of hemolytic uremic syndrome, Minnesota. Pediatr Infect Dis J 2012;31(1):37–41.

19. Nitschke M, Sayk F, Härtel C, et al. Association between azithromycin therapy and duration of bacterial shedding among patients with Shiga toxin-producing enteroaggregative *Escherichia coli* O104:H4. JAMA 2012;307(10):1046–52.

20. Menne J, Nitschke M, Stingele R, et al. Validation of treatment strategies for enterohaemorrhagic *Escherichia coli* O104:H4 induced haemolytic uraemic syndrome: case-control study. BMJ 2012;345:e4565.

21. Weil BR, Andreoli SP, Billmire DF. Bleeding risk for surgical dialysis procedures in children with hemolytic uremic syndrome. Pediatr Nephrol 2010;25(9):1693–8.

22. Balestracci A, Martin SM, Toledo I, et al. Impact of platelet transfusions in children with post-diarrheal hemolytic uremic syndrome. Pediatr Nephrol 2013;28(6): 919–25.

23. Beneke J, Sartison A, Kielstein JT, et al. Clinical and laboratory consequences of platelet transfusion in Shiga toxin-mediated hemolytic uremic syndrome. Transfus Med Rev 2017;31(1):51–5.

24. Michael M, Elliott EJ, Ridley GF, et al. Interventions for haemolytic uraemic syndrome and thrombotic thrombocytopenic purpura. Cochrane Database Syst Rev 2009;(1):CD003595.

25. Schwartz J, Padmanabhan A, Aqui N, et al. Guidelines on the use of therapeutic apheresis in clinical practice-evidence-based approach from the writing committee of the American Society for Apheresis: the seventh special issue. J Clin Apher 2016;31(3):149–62.

26. Lapeyraque AL, Malina M, Fremeaux-Bacchi V, et al. Eculizumab in severe Shiga-toxin-associated HUS. N Engl J Med 2011;364(26):2561–3.

27. Kielstein JT, Beutel G, Fleig S, et al. Best supportive care and therapeutic plasma exchange with or without eculizumab in Shiga-toxin-producing *E. coli* O104:H4 induced haemolytic-uraemic syndrome: an analysis of the German STEC-HUS registry. Nephrol Dial Transplant 2012;27(10):3807–15.

28. Delmas Y, Vendrely B, Clouzeau B, et al. Outbreak of *Escherichia coli* O104:H4 haemolytic uraemic syndrome in France: outcome with eculizumab. Nephrol Dial Transplant 2014;29(3):565–72.

29. Loos S, Aulbert W, Hoppe B, et al. Intermediate follow-up of pediatric patients with hemolytic uremic syndrome during the 2011 outbreak caused by *E. coli* O104:H4. Clin Infect Dis 2017;64(12):1637–43.

30. Trachtman H, Cnaan A, Christen E, et al. Effect of an oral Shiga toxin-binding agent on diarrhea-associated hemolytic uremic syndrome in children: a randomized controlled trial. JAMA 2003;290(10):1337–44.

31. Melton-Celsa AR, O'Brien AD. New therapeutic developments against shiga toxin-producing *Escherichia coli*. Microbiol Spectr 2014;2(5):1–14.

32. Sheoran AS, Chapman-Bonofiglio S, Harvey BR, et al. Human antibody against shiga toxin 2 administered to piglets after the onset of diarrhea due to *Escherichia coli* O157:H7 prevents fatal systemic complications. Infect Immun 2005;73(8): 4607–13.

33. Greinacher A, Friesecke S, Abel P, et al. Treatment of severe neurological deficits with IgG depletion through immunoadsorption in patients with *Escherichia coli* O104:H4-associated haemolytic uraemic syndrome: a prospective trial. Lancet 2011;378(9797):1166–73.

34. Ardissino G, Daccò V, Testa S, et al. Hemoconcentration: a major risk factor for neurological involvement in hemolytic uremic syndrome. Pediatr Nephrol 2015; 30(2):345–52.

35. Garg AX, Suri RS, Barrowman N, et al. Long-term renal prognosis of diarrhea-associated hemolytic uremic syndrome: a systematic review, meta-analysis, and meta-regression. JAMA 2003;290(10):1360–70.

36. Copelovitch L, Kaplan BS. *Streptococcus pneumoniae*-associated hemolytic uremic syndrome. Pediatr Nephrol 2008;23(11):1951–6.

37. Spinale JM, Ruebner RL, Kaplan BS, et al. Update on *Streptococcus pneumoniae* associated hemolytic uremic syndrome. Curr Opin Pediatr 2013;25(2):203–8.

38. Hopkins CK, Yuan S, Lu Q, et al. A severe case of atypical hemolytic uremic syndrome associated with pneumococcal infection and T activation treated successfully with plasma exchange. Transfusion 2008;48(11):2448–52.

39. Weintraub L, Ahluwalia M, Dogra S, et al. Management of *Streptococcal pneumoniae*-induced hemolytic uremic syndrome: a case report. Clin Nephrol Case Stud 2014;2:9–17.

40. Gilbert RD, Nagra A, Haq MR. Does dysregulated complement activation contribute to haemolytic uraemic syndrome secondary to *Streptococcus pneumoniae*? Med Hypotheses 2013;81(3):400–3.

41. Szilagyi A, Kiss N, Bereczki C, et al. The role of complement in *Streptococcus pneumoniae*-associated haemolytic uraemic syndrome. Nephrol Dial Transplant 2013;28(9):2237–45.

42. Banerjee R, Hersh AL, Newland J, et al. *Streptococcus pneumoniae*-associated hemolytic uremic syndrome among children in North America. Pediatr Infect Dis J 2011;30(9):736–9.

43. Loirat C, Fremeaux-Bacchi V. Atypical hemolytic uremic syndrome. Orphanet J Rare Dis 2011;6:60.

44. Dixon BP, Gruppo RA. Atypical hemolytic uremic syndrome. Pediatr Clin North Am 2018;65(3):509–25.

45. Delvaeye M, Noris M, De Vriese A, et al. Thrombomodulin mutations in atypical hemolytic-uremic syndrome. N Engl J Med 2009;361(4):345–57.

46. Lemaire M, Frémeaux-Bacchi V, Schaefer F, et al. Recessive mutations in DGKE cause atypical hemolytic-uremic syndrome. Nat Genet 2013;45(5):531–6.
47. Bruneau S, Néel M, Roumenina LT, et al. Loss of DGKepsilon induces endothelial cell activation and death independently of complement activation. Blood 2015; 125(6):1038–46.
48. Bu F, Maga T, Meyer NC, et al. Comprehensive genetic analysis of complement and coagulation genes in atypical hemolytic uremic syndrome. J Am Soc Nephrol 2014;25(1):55–64.
49. Walle JV, Delmas Y, Ardissino G, et al. Improved renal recovery in patients with atypical hemolytic uremic syndrome following rapid initiation of eculizumab treatment. J Nephrol 2017;30(1):127–34.
50. Legendre CM, Licht C, Muus P, et al. Terminal complement inhibitor eculizumab in atypical hemolytic-uremic syndrome. N Engl J Med 2013;368(23):2169–81.
51. Licht C, Greenbaum LA, Muus P, et al. Efficacy and safety of eculizumab in atypical hemolytic uremic syndrome from 2-year extensions of phase 2 studies. Kidney Int 2015;87(5):1061–73.
52. Greenbaum LA, Fila M, Ardissino G, et al. Eculizumab is a safe and effective treatment in pediatric patients with atypical hemolytic uremic syndrome. Kidney Int 2016;89(3):701–11.
53. Fakhouri F, Hourmant M, Campistol JM, et al. Terminal complement inhibitor eculizumab in adult patients with atypical hemolytic uremic syndrome: a single-arm, open-label trial. Am J Kidney Dis 2016;68(1):84–93.
54. Avila A, Vizcaíno B, Molina P, et al. Remission of aHUS neurological damage with eculizumab. Clin Kidney J 2015;8(2):232–6.
55. Cofiell R, Kukreja A, Bedard K, et al. Eculizumab reduces complement activation, inflammation, endothelial damage, thrombosis, and renal injury markers in aHUS. Blood 2015;125(21):3253–62.
56. Loirat C, Fakhouri F, Ariceta G, et al. An international consensus approach to the management of atypical hemolytic uremic syndrome in children. Pediatr Nephrol 2016;31(1):15–39.
57. Diamante Chiodini B, Davin JC, Corazza F, et al. Eculizumab in anti-factor h antibodies associated with atypical hemolytic uremic syndrome. Pediatrics 2014; 133(6):e1764–8.
58. Ricklin D, Barratt-Due A, Mollnes TE. Complement in clinical medicine: Clinical trials, case reports and therapy monitoring. Mol Immunol 2017;89:10–21.
59. Saland J. Liver-kidney transplantation to cure atypical HUS: still an option post-eculizumab? Pediatr Nephrol 2014;29(3):329–32.
60. Noris M, Caprioli J, Bresin E, et al. Relative role of genetic complement abnormalities in sporadic and familial aHUS and their impact on clinical phenotype. Clin J Am Soc Nephrol 2010;5(10):1844–59.
61. Ardissino G, Possenti I, Tel F, et al. Discontinuation of eculizumab treatment in atypical hemolytic uremic syndrome: an update. Am J Kidney Dis 2015;66(1): 172–3.
62. Zhang K, Lu Y, Harley KT, et al. Atypical hemolytic uremic syndrome: a brief review. Hematol Rep 2017;9(2):7053.
63. Goodship TH, Cook HT, Fakhouri F, et al. Atypical hemolytic uremic syndrome and C3 glomerulopathy: conclusions from a "Kidney Disease: Improving Global Outcomes" (KDIGO) controversies conference. Kidney Int 2017;91(3):539–51.
64. Cugno M, Gualtierotti R, Possenti I, et al. Complement functional tests for monitoring eculizumab treatment in patients with atypical hemolytic uremic syndrome. J Thromb Haemost 2014;12(9):1440–8.

65. Ardissino G, Tel F, Sgarbanti M, et al. Complement functional tests for monitoring eculizumab treatment in patients with atypical hemolytic uremic syndrome: an update. Pediatr Nephrol 2018;33(3):457–61.

66. Martinelli D, Deodato F, Dionisi-Vici C. Cobalamin C defect: natural history, pathophysiology, and treatment. J Inherit Metab Dis 2011;34(1):127–35.

67. Fischer S, Huemer M, Baumgartner M, et al. Clinical presentation and outcome in a series of 88 patients with the cblC defect. J Inherit Metab Dis 2014;37(5): 831–40.

68. Sharma AP, Greenberg CR, Prasad AN, et al. Hemolytic uremic syndrome (HUS) secondary to cobalamin C (cblC) disorder. Pediatr Nephrol 2007;22(12): 2097–103.

Chronic Kidney Disease and Dietary Measures to Improve Outcomes

Oleh M. Akchurin, MD

KEYWORDS

- Chronic kidney disease • Pediatrics • Children • Stature • Growth • Development
- Nutrition • Renal diet

KEY POINTS

- Chronic kidney disease is an irreversible deterioration of renal function that may progress to end-stage renal disease.
- The goals of chronic kidney disease management in pediatric patients include slowing disease progression, prevention and treatment of complications, and optimizing growth, development, and quality of life.
- Nutritional management is critically important for the prevention of acute and chronic complications and optimization of physical and neurocognitive development in children with chronic kidney disease.
- Control of blood pressure, proteinuria, and metabolic acidosis in chronic kidney disease with dietary and pharmacologic measures may slow disease progression and postpone dialysis or kidney transplantation.
- Further research is required to clarify the role of dietary protein intake and control of dyslipidemia in the progression of pediatric chronic kidney disease.

INTRODUCTION AND OVERVIEW

Chronic kidney disease (CKD) can be defined as a sustained damage of the renal parenchyma leading to chronic deterioration of renal function that may gradually progress to end-stage renal disease (ESRD). ESRD remains uniformly fatal without renal replacement therapy (dialysis or kidney transplantation). The term CKD acknowledges that this condition exists on a continuum with differing degrees of renal impairment rather than a discrete state of renal insult (acute kidney injury). The term CKD has replaced previously used terms chronic renal insufficiency and chronic renal failure. Although kidney transplantation revolutionized the care of patients with ESRD, most

Disclosure Statement: Grant/Research support: Rohr Family Clinical Scholar Award (Weill Cornell Medicine). National Institute of Diabetes and Digestive and Kidney Diseases K08 DK114558.
Weill Cornell Medical College (Pediatric Nephrology), 525 E 68th Street, Box 176, New York, NY 10065, USA
E-mail address: Oma9005@med.cornell.edu

children with transplanted kidneys presently have various degrees of allograft injury or dysfunction (CKD of a transplanted kidney). Throughout their lifetime, individuals with pediatric-onset CKD may repeatedly transition between predialysis CKD, various dialysis modalities, and kidney transplants (**Fig. 1**). Kidney transplantation leads to better survival and quality of life than dialysis. However, complications and requirement for rigorous supportive care still significantly limit the quality of life of pediatric kidney transplant recipients.

Etiology

According to the 2017 United States Renal Data System annual data report, the leading causes of ESRD in children during 2011 to 2015, similar to earlier years, were congenital anomalies of the kidney and urinary tract (22%), primary glomerular diseases (21.8%), cystic/hereditary/congenital disorders (12.5%), and secondary glomerular diseases/vasculitidies (10.7%; **Fig. 2**). The most common individual diagnoses associated with pediatric ESRD included focal segmental glomerulosclerosis (11.6%), renal hypoplasia/dysplasia (10%), congenital obstructive uropathies (9.7%), and systemic lupus erythematosus (6.3%).[1] This distribution is very different from the CKD in adults, which in developed countries is most typically associated with diabetes mellitus or hypertension.[2,3]

KIDNEY DEVELOPMENT AND CHRONIC KIDNEY DISEASE

Prenatal factors play an important role in the development of CKD in many children. Although genetic background contributes to the development of congenital anomalies of the kidney and urinary tract, epigenetic and maternal influences may play a role in nephron endowment and account for differences in the final nephron number. Each human kidney has on average 1 million nephrons, but there is a substantial variability (from 200,000 to 1,800,000 nephrons).[4] The majority of nephrons are formed during the third trimester of pregnancy,[5] and no newly forming nephrons can be found in fetal kidneys beyond the 36th week of gestation.[6] It seems that premature babies born before 36 weeks of gestation are able to form new nephrons postnatally, but this ability may be limited. Prematurity, low birth weight, and other prenatal factors diminishing nephron endowment were shown in retrospective studies to increase the risk of CKD later in life, even without associated overt renal anomalies,[7] thus supporting a concept of *fetal programming* of late-onset pediatric and adult CKD.[8]

However, more than one-half of the individuals who develop CKD in childhood are born with structurally and functionally abnormal kidneys and urinary tract. Regardless

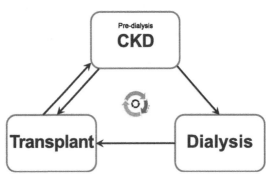

Fig. 1. Life cycle of children with chronic kidney disease.

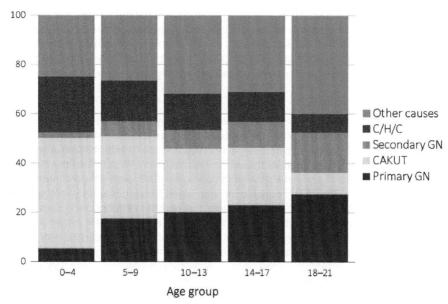

Fig. 2. Distribution of reported incident pediatric patients with end-stage renal disease (ESRD) by primary cause of ESRD, 2011 to 2015. C/H/C, cystic/hereditary/congenital diseases; CAKUT, congenital anomalies of the kidney and urinary tract; GN, glomerulonephritis. (*From* The United States Renal Data System, USRDS 2017 Annual Data Report. Available at: https://www.usrds.org/2017/view/Default.aspx. Accessed October 07, 2018.)

of the individual anatomic abnormality, prognosis largely depends on the number of functioning nephrons. Tubular dysfunction may predominate compared with glomerular impairment in the first years of life, manifesting as defective reabsorption of the filtered solutes, causing renal salt wasting. Survival of children with severe bilateral obstructive anomalies depends on their lung development, which requires factors present in amniotic fluid. Although fetal oliguria or anuria owing to urinary tract obstruction, usually bilateral, does not cause fetal uremia (as placenta provides the necessary clearance), it leads to oligohydramnios and pulmonary hypoplasia (Potter sequence).[9] The release of obstruction after birth may cause postobstructive diuresis and severe electrolyte abnormalities.[10]

Glomerular diseases tend to present later in childhood and to progress more rapidly.[11,12] In both early- and late-onset pediatric CKD, kidneys eventually become affected by tubulointerstitial fibrosis and exhibit nephron loss. This impairs the ability of the kidney to remove metabolic waste, including end-products of protein metabolism. Impaired renal clearance leads to accumulation of uremic toxins, the solutes that would normally be excreted by the kidneys but accumulate in patients with CKD and have adverse impact on biologic functions.[13] The European Uremic Toxin Work Group compiled a database that currently consists of more than 150 identified substances that were found at higher concentrations in the blood of patients with CKD as compared with normal individuals (http://www.uremic-toxins.org/). Uremic toxins are also produced by gut microbiota, particularly indoxyl sulfate and p-Cresyl sulfate.[14] Alterations in the gut microbiota in patients with CKD may increase production of these uremic toxins.[15]

Serum urea and creatinine are routinely used as markers of renal dysfunction, although they do not seem to be intrinsically toxic in CKD. Furthermore, the accumulation of uremic toxins only partially correlates with GFR in pediatric patients with CKD.[16] The term *azotemia* is used to denote the biochemical presence of uremic toxins, whereas the term *uremia* usually refers to the clinical manifestations of azotemia. Systemic manifestations of CKD are related not only to uremia, but also to the impaired homeostatic functions of the kidney (**Fig. 3**).

Clinical Evaluation of Renal Function and Chronic Kidney Disease Stages

The glomerular filtration rate (GFR) is a measure of kidney function. The GFR is defined as the amount of plasma filtered by the kidneys during a certain period of time (usually 1 minute). Given differences in circulating blood volume, the GFR in children is normalized by body surface area (units of measurement: mL/min/1.73 m^2). Healthy children younger than 2 years of age have physiologically lower GFR even when corrected for body surface area.[17] The GFR is equal to the sum of the filtration rates in all of the functioning nephrons; therefore, it correlates with the number of functioning nephrons. Healthy kidneys have substantial reserve to maintain adequate GFR under various physiologic conditions. Although providing a tremendous biologic benefit, functional nephron excess complicates clinical evaluation of the early CKD stages. This happens in part because unaffected nephrons are able to provide compensation to the damaged nephrons.[18] Hypertrophy of the remaining nephrons may occur, resulting in partial restoration of GFR. Therefore, there is no linear correlation between nephron loss and the loss of the GFR.

The GFR can be measured indirectly using clearance of substances that are freely filtered in the glomeruli but not secreted or reabsorbed by the tubules, such as inulin. Inulin clearance require intravenous inulin infusion, repeated blood sampling and urine collection, which makes it impractical in clinical settings. Creatinine clearance can also be used to assess the GFR; however, tubules are able to secrete creatinine, which is one of the limitations of creatinine clearance as a measure of the GFR. Tubular creatinine secretion increases with a decreased GFR. Therefore, creatinine clearance can overestimate the GFR in children with CKD. Other limitations of serum creatinine as a marker of kidney function include its dependence on muscle mass and physical activity. Many physiologic substances and drugs interfere with creatinine assays, which can lead to falsely high or low serum creatinine values.[19,20] Serum cystatin C is one of the most widely used alternative biomarkers to estimate GFR. Cystatin C, unlike creatinine, is produced by all nucleated cells, and is not dependent on muscle

Functions of the kidney

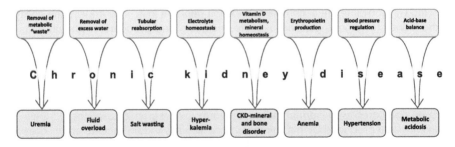

Manifestations and complications of CKD

Fig. 3. Impairment of different kidney functions in chronic kidney disease (CKD) leads to distinct manifestations and complications of CKD.

mass. Various formulas have been developed to estimate GFR based on serum markers and other variables (**Box 1**).[21]

The Kidney Disease: Improving Global Outcomes (KDIGO) 2012 Clinical Practice Guideline for Evaluation and Management of Chronic Kidney Disease recommends stratifying CKD in children older than 2 years based on the GFR into 5 stages (**Table 1**). For a GFR of greater than 60 mL/min/1.73 m^2, the evidence of irreversible kidney damage is required to make a diagnosis of CKD, for example, fixed proteinuria, or characteristic renal imaging, or histology. KDIGO criteria require the duration of renal insufficiency at least 3 months (except in babies <3 months of age) to make a diagnosis of CKD.

Presentation and Screening

The majority of children with CKD have congenital anomalies of the kidney and urinary tract, which may be detected on the prenatal ultrasound examination. A lack of prenatal care may delay the diagnosis in these children. If not diagnosed in early childhood, children with nonglomerular CKD may present later with polyuria, growth impairment, or an accidental finding of elevated serum creatinine, blood urea nitrogen or abnormal imaging (eg, multiple renal cysts noted during abdominal ultrasound examination performed for a nonrenal indication). Importantly, many children remain asymptomatic for years, sometimes until they reach ESRD. It is currently rare in developed countries for children to have symptoms of chronic uremia at presentation (anorexia, vomiting, fatigue, cognitive dysfunction, and confusion). Classic findings of uremic pericarditis or

---

Box 1
Formulas for estimation of the glomerular filtration rate in children

Original Schwartz (1976): $eGFR = k \times \dfrac{body\ length(cm)}{plasma\ creatinine(mg/dL)}$
where k = 0.33 (preterm infant); k = 0.45 (full term); k = 0.55 (children and adolescent females); k = 0.7 (adolescent males)

Counahan-Barratt: $eGFR = 0.43 \times \dfrac{body\ length(cm)}{plasma\ creatinine(mg/dL)}$

"Bedside" Schwartz (CKiD$_{Cr}$): $eGFR = 0.413 \times \dfrac{body\ length(cm)}{plasma\ creatinine(mg/dL)}$

$CKiD_{Cys-C}$: $eGFR = 70.69 \times [cystatin\ C\ (mg/L)]^{-0.931}$

$CKiD_{Cr-Cys-C}$: $eGFR = 39.8 \times \left(\dfrac{body\ length(m)}{serum\ creatinine(mg/dL)}\right)^{0.456} \times \left(\dfrac{1.8}{cystatin\ C(mg/L)}\right)^{0.418}$

$\times \left(\dfrac{30}{BUN(mg/dL)}\right)^{0.079} \times 1.076^{sex} \times \left(\dfrac{height(m)}{1.4}\right)^{0.179}$

where sex = 1 for male and 0 for female

High-risk populations with reduced muscle mass
- Oncology patients
- Hematopoietic stem cell transplant recipients
- Spina bifida/muscular dystrophy
- Spinal cord injury

Cystatin C–based formulas are especially useful in children with reduced muscle mass.
Abbreviations: BUN, blood urea nitrogen; eGFR, estimated glomerular filtration rate.
From Mian AN, Schwartz GJ. Measurement and estimation of glomerular filtration rate in children. Adv Chronic Kidney Dis 2017;24(6):352; with permission.

Table 1
Chronic kidney disease (CKD) staging based on the glomerular filtration rate (GFR)

CKD Stage/GFR Category	GFR (mL/min/1.73 m^2)	Terms
G1	$\geq$90	Normal or high
G2	60–89	Mildly decreased
G3a	45–59	Mildly to moderately decreased
G3b	30–44	Moderately to severely decreased
G4	15–29	Severely decreased
G5	<15	Kidney failure

If no evidence of kidney damage, neither GFR category G1 nor G2 fulfill the criteria for CKD.
From Levin A, Stevens PE, Bilous RW, et al. Kidney Disease: Improving Global Outcomes (KDIGO) CKD Work Group. KDIGO 2012 clinical practice guideline for the evaluation and management of chronic kidney disease. Kidney Int Suppl 2013;3(1):14; with permission.

uremic pruritus are currently also rare in children presenting with CKD. Children with glomerular CKD may present with more specific renal signs and symptoms, such as edema and elevated blood pressure, or may have an accidental finding of proteinuria.

The subtle and insidious onset of CKD prompted a consideration of *CKD screening*. The American Academy of Pediatrics currently does not recommend universal CKD screening with urinalyses in healthy children, owing to concerns of its cost ineffectiveness.[22] However, targeted screening is appropriate in selected high-risk populations (**Box 2**)[23,24] and should include quantification of urine protein based on a first morning void urine sample with or without urinalysis and accurate blood pressure measurement.

Box 2
Conditions associated with increased risk of chronic kidney disease in children

- Low birth weight/prematurity
- History of acute kidney injury
- Obesity
- Diabetes
- Hypertension
- History of glomerulopathies, including SLE, HSP, HUS
- Sickle cell disease
- CAKUT, congenital or acquired single kidney
- Recurrent UTIs
- Congenital heart disease
- Family history of chronic kidney disease

Chronic kidney disease screening is required in these categories of children (see text for details).
Abbreviations: CAKUT, congenital anomalies of kidney and urinary tract; HSP, Henoch-Schoenlein purpura; HUS, hemolytic uremic syndrome; SLE, systemic lupus erythematosus; UTI, urinary tract infections.

MANIFESTATIONS AND COMPLICATIONS OF CHRONIC KIDNEY DISEASE, THEIR DIETARY AND PHARMACOLOGIC MANAGEMENT
Chronic Kidney Disease–Mineral and Bone Disorder

CKD is frequently associated with disorders of mineral and bone metabolism, which can manifest as one or all of the following interrelated abnormalities.

- Disturbances of calcium, phosphorus, parathyroid hormone (PTH), fibroblast growth factor 23 (FGF23), and vitamin D metabolism.
- Alterations of bone turnover, mineralization, elongation and strength.
- Extraskeletal calcification.

The kidney is the only site of conversion of 25(OH)-vitamin D to the highly active 1,25(OH)$_2$ form (see **Fig. 3**). Recent data reveal a much more complex role of the kidney in mineral and bone metabolism than previously appreciated. The pathogenesis of CKD-mineral and bone disorder (MBD) remains far from being completely understood. However, it is well-established that subclinical changes in bone and mineral biomarkers can be detected very early in the course of CKD (at stage 2), before the decrease in calcitriol levels.[25,26] One of these early events is elevation of FGF23, a phosphatonin produced by osteocytes, which enhances renal phosphate excretion. The role of elevated FGF23 in early stages of CKD may be protective, because it likely helps to postpone the development of hyperphosphatemia. However, a gradual decrease in the number of functioning nephrons and deficiency of Klotho, an FGF23 co-receptor, eventually overwhelms the phosphaturic effect of FGF23. Moreover, FGF-23 worsens 1,25(OH)$_2$-vitamin D deficiency, by directly inhibiting 1α-hydroxylase gene expression via activation of the ERK1/2 signaling pathway.[27] Thus, it contributes to the early pathogenesis of secondary hyperparathyroidism, before the development of serum mineral abnormalities.[28] Hyperphosphatemia usually develops at stage 4 CKD, and stimulates parathyroid gland function, thus contributing to secondary hyperparathyroidism. The net effect of these systemic changes, coupled with current therapies, may paradoxically result either in excessive bone resorption or bone formation. However, even in cases of apparent increase in bone mass, bone strength still suffers because the deposited bone collagen fibers are immature.[29]

The current goals of CKD-MBD management are as follows.

- Correction of hyperphosphatemia (phosphate binders, low phosphorus diet).
- Avoiding positive calcium balance beyond what is needed by the growing child (limiting the dose of calcium-based phosphate binders, timely introduction of non–calcium-based phosphate binders) to prevent vascular calcifications.
- Correction of secondary hyperparathyroidism (calcitriol and vitamin D analogues), as necessary to achieve the previous 2 goals. Importantly, the optimal PTH levels in patients with CKD currently remain unknown. The latest KDIGO guidelines suggest that calcitriol and vitamin D analogues not be routinely used in adults with CKD not on dialysis, although they may be considered in children with CKD to maintain serum calcium level in the age-appropriate normal range.[30]

Improvement of bone quality and prevention of vascular calcifications would be the ultimate goals; however, no therapies are currently available to directly target renal osteodystrophy or vascular quality in children. Bisphosphonates and other osteoporosis medications can be considered in adult CKD patients with osteoporosis and/or high risk of fracture.[30]

Dietary management

Dietary management of CKD-MBD includes dietary phosphorus restriction in cases of hyperphosphatemia or hyperparathyroidism. Conventional hemodialysis does not provide adequate phosphate removal; therefore, dietary phosphorus control seem to be especially important in patients on dialysis. The KDOQI guidelines recommend limiting phosphorus intake to 100% of the daily recommended intake for age when PTH is elevated, and to 80% of the daily recommended intake for age when both PTH and serum phosphorus are elevated.[31]

Age-specific normative values should be used for the assessment of hyperphosphatemia, because serum phosphorus is physiologically higher in younger children and babies.[32] Breast milk is naturally low in phosphorus and is the preferred nutrition in babies with CKD. If breast milk is not available, a low-phosphorus renal formula should be used. Both breast milk and formulas can be additionally pretreated with sevelamer, a phosphate binder.[33] It is well-accepted that foods and beverages that are naturally high in phosphorus (**Box 3**) and those containing phosphorus additives should be avoided. Phosphorus additives contain nonorganic phosphorus which is absorbed more avidly than organic phosphorus. Phosphorus in animal foods is absorbed more easily than that in plant foods. Low-phosphorus healthy choices for children with CKD include fruits and vegetables, corn, and rice.

Dietary phosphorus restriction in patients with CKD has many practical challenges, and its effects are surprisingly not clear. The association between hyperphosphatemia and adverse outcomes is well-established in adults with CKD, and dietary phosphorus restriction led to improvement of renal function in animal models.[34] However, no well-designed trials have been conducted to demonstrate the effect of lowering serum phosphorus on clinically meaningful outcomes in patients with CKD. Furthermore, the direct effects of dietary phosphorus restriction on serum phosphorus in clinical settings are still not definitively established.[30] The conventional concept that correction of hyperphosphatemia and/or hyperparathyroidism in children with CKD should improve their growth is based on very small series.[35] Because dietary protein is the major source of dietary phosphorus, there is a concern that strict adherence to a low-phosphorus diet may contribute to protein–energy wasting. Therefore, a balanced consideration of the currently available evidence about clinical merits of phosphorus restricted diet coupled with the acknowledgment of its impact on patient-centered outcomes seems to be a reasonable approach to dietary counseling regarding phosphorus intake in CKD.

Box 3
High phosphorus food items that should be limited or avoided in chronic kidney disease

- Dark colas/sodas, chocolate drinks, cocoa
- Dairy products (cheese, milk, ice cream, yogurt)
- Organ meats, liver
- Oysters, sardines
- Dried beans and peas
- Nuts and nut butters
- Chocolate
- Bran cereals and oatmeal, whole grain products
- Egg yolks

Metabolic Acidosis of Chronic Kidney Disease

The kidneys play a major role in the maintenance of acid–base balance by means of hydrogen ion excretion, reabsorption of the filtered bicarbonate, and generation of new bicarbonate ions and other buffers. The kidneys excrete hydrogen ion through titratable acid and urinary ammonium. Renal ammonia genesis is the primary mechanism responsible for the regulation of hydrogen ion excretion. CKD can affect all components involved in renal regulation of acid–base balance leading to metabolic acidosis. Metabolic acidosis is especially common and develops earlier in the course of CKD in children with tubular dysfunctions, for example, those with renal dysplasia. For example, 18% of children with a GFR of greater than or equal to 50 mL/min/1.73 m^2 enrolled in the Chronic Kidney Disease in Children (CKiD) study had metabolic acidosis and were treated with alkaline therapy.[36] Children typically have normal anion gap (hyperchloremic) metabolic acidosis in early CKD, but may develop high anion gap metabolic acidosis in advanced CKD, once the ability of the kidney to excrete organic acids becomes limited. When circulating buffers are depleted, bone begins to buffer excess hydrogen ions, which leads to the release of calcium from bone. If left untreated, this process may contribute to osteopenia and growth impairment, and increase the risk of secondary hyperparathyroidism and CKD progression.[37] Advanced acidosis may contribute to hyperkalemia. Metabolic acidosis in CKD also adversely affects protein and muscle metabolism, stimulates inflammation, and enhances insulin resistance.[38] The correction of acidosis seems to attenuate CKD progression[39] and improve secondary hyperparathyroidism,[40] as well as nutritional status, muscle strength,[41] and quality of life in adults with CKD.[42]

Current guidelines by KDOQI and KDIGO recommend to maintain serum bicarbonate level in patients with CKD at or above 22 mEq/L (20 mEq/L for infants <2 years of age).[31,43]

Dietary management

Dietary management of metabolic acidosis in CKD consists of a reduction of H$^+$ intake by removing or limiting H$^+$-producing dietary components, and adding base-producing dietary components. A typical Western diet is acid producing, particularly owing to a substantial amount of animal protein, whereas fruits and vegetables are able to alkalinize the diet. However, in patients with advanced CKD, dietary content of fruits and vegetables and the kinds of fruits and vegetables consumed have to be carefully monitored to prevent hyperkalemia. Although dietary measures may be sufficient to prevent metabolic acidosis in early stages of CKD,[44,45] many patients also require additional pharmacologic alkali therapy, for example, citric acid/sodium citrate or sodium bicarbonate. Alkali should be administered at least 2 to 3 times a day. Gastrointestinal side effects are relatively common and are related in part to the release of CO_2 when $NaHCO_3$ comes in contact with gastric HCl. Close sodium intake monitoring is required to avoid volume expansion and hypertension. A novel sodium-free hydrochloric acid-binding agent, TRC101, showed promising efficacy and safety in adults with CKD.[46] Caution is necessary when using alkali in patients with hypocalcemia because rapidly increasing the pH in these patients may precipitate tetany. There is also a concern that long-term alkali therapy may promote vascular calcification.[47] Blood collection for metabolic evaluation in children with CKD should be done before the first daily alkali dose.[48]

Potassium Balance in Chronic Kidney Disease

Advanced CKD frequently leads to inadequate renal potassium excretion owing to loss of nephron mass, and thus a decrease in the number of collecting ducts to secrete K$^+$. Hyperkalemia is a well-recognized risk factor for arrhythmias and cardiac arrest,[49] and it predictably leads to higher mortality.[50,51] Other factors that may contribute to hyperkalemia in patients with CKD include high dietary potassium intake, a catabolic state with increased tissue breakdown, and inorganic metabolic acidosis. Hyperkalemia develops earlier in patients with diabetes, in part owing to the decreased mineralocorticoid activity/hyporeninemic hypoaldosteronism frequently seen in these patients.[52] Hyperkalemia is a side effect of some medications commonly used in CKD, including angiotensin-converting enzyme inhibitors and angiotensin receptor blockers, potassium-sparing diuretics, calcineurin inhibitors, and prostaglandin inhibitors (eg, nonsteroidal anti-inflammatory drugs). There is an adaptive increase in colonic potassium secretion in patients with advanced CKD and ESRD.[53] Because the amount of stool potassium correlates with wet stool weight, constipation is a concern in patients with CKD and hyperkalemia.[52] Traumatic blood collection and red blood cell hemolysis are the most common reasons for laboratory reports of elevated potassium in children. Interpretation of serum potassium in children should be based on the age-specific normative ranges; younger children and infants have a physiologically higher serum potassium.

Dietary management

The typical diet of a healthy adult American contains about 3500 to 4500 mg of potassium a day. A low potassium diet provides about 2000 mg of potassium a day. In children, KDOQI recommends restriction of potassium intake to 40 to 120 mg/kg/d for infants and younger children and 30 to 40 mg/kg/d for older children.[31] Breast milk is naturally low in potassium and is the best nutrition for babies with CKD. If breast milk is not available, renal low-potassium formulas should be used. If necessary, formulas may be pretreated with a potassium binder to further lower the potassium content. **Table 2** provides examples of high- and low-potassium foods. In addition, families should be educated about cooking techniques that can lower potassium content in meals, such as peeling, dicing, and presoaking potassium-rich vegetables, and discarding the broth.[54] Similar to phosphorus, it is currently not required to list potassium on the Nutrition Facts Label Panel in the United States.[55]

Sodium polystyrene sulfonate is a cation-exchange resin (potassium binder) that can be used orally or rectally to treat hyperkalemia. Approximately 100 mg (4 mEq) of sodium is released per 1 g of medication in exchange of potassium, which can lead to volume expansion. A rare but serious side effect of polystyrene sulfonate is colonic necrosis,[56] which limits its use in neonates, especially those already at risk for necrotizing enterocolitis. Patiromer (RLY5016) and zirconium cyclosilicate (ZS-9) are novel emergent oral agents for the treatment of chronic hyperkalemia.[57] Patiromer was

Table 2		
Examples of high- and low-potassium food items		
	High Potassium	**Relatively Low Potassium Alternatives**
Fruits	Orange and orange juice	Apple, apple juice, applesauce
	Banana	Blueberries, cranberries
	Cantaloupe, honeydew	Raspberries, strawberries
	Mango, papaya	Grapes and grape juice
	Nectarine	Mandarin oranges
	Raisins and other dried fruits	Pineapple and pineapple juice
Vegetables	Tomatoes and tomato products	Eggplant
	Potato (white and sweet)	Yellow squash and zucchini
	Pumpkin, butternut squash	Onions
		Cucumber
Other foods	Chocolate	Rice
	Salt substitutes	Pasta
	Nuts and seeds	Bread (not whole grains)

approved by the US Food and Drug Administration for the management of nonemergent hyperkalemia in adults; no information is currently available on its use in children.

Sodium Balance, Intravascular Volume, Hypertension, and Dyslipidemia in Children with Chronic Kidney Disease

Children with CKD may experience a spectrum of dysnatremias, ranging from deficit to excess. Children with obstructive uropathies and/or renal dysplasia may experience excessive urine sodium loss, requiring sodium supplementation. Some peritoneal dialysis patients have excessive sodium loss with ultrafiltration, which may also need to be replaced. It has been suggested that, without adequate repletion, chronic total body sodium deficit may contribute to growth impairment.[58] Children with nephrotic syndrome, glomerulonephritidies, and severely decreased GFR frequently retain sodium, leading to expansion of the extracellular volume and/or hypertension. Elevated office blood pressure was associated with faster GFR decline in children with CKD in the CKiD study.[11] The ESCAPE trial demonstrated that aggressive blood pressure control slows the progression of CKD.[59] Restriction of sodium intake was beneficial in a few studies in adult patients with CKD,[60,61] although more studies are needed to definitively determine the optimal sodium intake in children and adults with CKD.[62] Excessive salt restriction can bring its own risks, such as stimulation of the renin–aldosterone axis, catecholamine production, and dyslipidemia.[63] Recent studies suggested a U-shaped relationship between sodium intake and outcomes, including mortality, in the general population.[64,65] Thus, dietary sodium intake should be closely monitored and individually optimized in patients with CKD. Urine sodium (ideally based on a 24-hour collection) provides a good measure of dietary sodium intake and should complement dietary recall. KDOQI guidelines recommend 1500 to 2400 mg/d sodium intake for children who require sodium restriction.[31] However, based on the Food Frequency Questionnaire, the median daily sodium intake was 3089 mg in children with CKD from the CKiD study cohort, indicating that further efforts are needed for improvement of nutritional counseling.[66]

The high prevalence of other factors that have been associated with cardiovascular disease in adults have been documented in children with CKD, including dyslipidemia.[36,67] In the CKiD study cohort, 45% of children with moderate CKD had dyslipidemia; many of those children had nephrotic-range proteinuria.[68] However, it remains unknown if dyslipidemia in children with CKD contributes to cardiovascular morbidity and mortality. KDIGO recommends dietary measures and weight control as a first line of dyslipidemia treatment in children. Owing to very limited available data, the guidelines do not recommend the use of statins in children with CKD younger than 10 years. Boys older than 10 years and postmenarchal girls with severely elevated low-density lipoprotein cholesterol "who place a higher value on the potential for preventing cardiovascular events and are less concerned about adverse events from statin use might be candidates for statin use—especially those with multiple additional risk factors such as family history of premature coronary disease, diabetes, hypertension, smoking, and ESRD."[69]

Anemia and Iron Metabolism in Children with Chronic Kidney Disease

Anemia is a well-recognized complication of CKD, and a major determinant of quality of life and morbidity in patients with CKD.[70,71] Anemia complicates CKD in about 50% of children before they reach ESRD.[72] Erythropoietin, a hormone essential for erythropoiesis, is produced in the kidney, and erythropoietin axis is predictably disrupted in CKD (see **Fig. 3**). The introduction of erythropoiesis-stimulating agents (ESA) revolutionized care for patients with CKD and ESRD and resulted in a significant decrease of blood transfusions in the CKD population. However, wide ranges of ESA doses are required to improve anemia in different patients with CKD, and high doses of ESAs, unfortunately, are associated with increased mortality in adult patients with CKD. Thus, hemoglobin targets in adults with CKD receiving ESAs are currently set significantly lower than in the general population.[73] It remains controversial whether hemoglobin targets in children with CKD should be higher than those in adults with CKD, in part owing to concern that higher hemoglobin is needed to promote growth and cognitive development in children.[74]

Endogenous erythropoietin and ESAs are effective only when iron is readily available for erythropoiesis. Iron metabolism is disrupted in patients with CKD, particularly owing to elevated hepcidin,[75] a hepatic hormone that prevents iron egress from cells by binding to iron exporter, ferroportin. Hepcidin excess suppresses iron absorption and leads to iron sequestration in macrophages and hepatocytes, which leads to functional iron deficiency in CKD.[76] Therapeutic iron supplementation becomes necessary, but it further stimulates hepcidin,[77] which not only worsens anemia, but may contribute to growth impairment in juvenile CKD.[78] While it is currently unclear whether hepcidin excess precedes erythropoietin dysfunction in the course of CKD, the prevalence of iron therapy in children with mild to moderate CKD is much higher than the prevalence of ESA therapy.[79] There is a growing concern about iron overload and toxicity in CKD.[80,81] Indeed, increased iron content has been found in the liver and spleen of children with ESRD.[82]

It remains unclear whether iron status has an impact on the growth of children with CKD independent of anemia. Iron deficiency anemia can impair growth in children without CKD and iron supplementation improves the growth of these children.[83–85] Iron excess, however, can be as devastating as iron deficiency, mainly because free iron has a high potential for biologic toxicity. Specifically, iron excess negatively affects growth in children with transfusion-dependent thalassemia and hereditary iron overload disorders.[86] Furthermore, even mild iron excess during childhood may negatively affect growth and neurocognitive development of otherwise healthy children.[87–90] Therefore, although enteral or intravenous iron supplementation is currently essential in many children with CKD, especially those requiring ESA therapy, it should be used judiciously and with a close (at least every 3 months)[91] monitoring of iron status. Inflammation is a potent stimulation of hepcidin production, and reduction of inflammation in children with CKD has potential for the improvement of their iron status and anemia.[92]

Protein–Energy Metabolism and Nutritional Status in Children with Chronic Kidney Disease

Nutritional status in children with CKD may be affected by several factors, including loss of appetite (anorexia), altered gastrointestinal motility, malabsorption, intestinal dysbiosis, and uremic abnormalities of energy, protein, lipid, and carbohydrate metabolism. Assessment of nutritional status in children with CKD is complex (**Box 4**)[31,93] and should be ideally conducted jointly be a pediatric nephrologist and a pediatric dietitian experienced in the nutritional management of patients with CKD.[94] The term malnutrition refers to an inadequately low dietary intake, typically with adaptive increase in appetite and decrease in metabolic rate[95]; therefore, this term is usually not applicable to the alterations of nutritional status currently seen in children with CKD, especially in developed countries. Indeed, in the CKiD study, children with CKD consumed more protein and calories than recommended.[66] The majority of children with CKD in the United States have a normal body mass index when they reach ESRD, about 40% are overweight or obese, and only 10% to 15% are underweight, according to the United States Renal Data System.[1] Despite normal or elevated body mass index in most children with CKD in the United States, there is a

---

Box 4
Nutritional assessment in children with chronic kidney disease

I. Dietary assessment
  - Dietary recall
  - Food Frequency Questionnaire

II. Anthropometric assessment
  - Body weight, length, body mass index, head circumference
  - Waist circumference, skinfold thickness, somatogram, and frame size

III. Advanced assessment of body composition
  - Dual x-ray absorptiometry
  - Bioelectrical impedance analysis
  - MRI (proton density contrast weighting, Dixon-related fat–water-separation)

IV. Biochemical assessment
  - Serum albumin and prealbumin
  - Normalized protein equivalent of nitrogen appearance
  - Creatinine index (in patients on dialysis)

---

concern that some of these children may have a disproportion between lean and fat body mass, and relative loss of muscle mass, including the possibility of sarcopenic obesity. The International Society of Renal Nutrition has developed diagnostic criteria for protein-energy wasting.[96] Adaptation of these criteria to the pediatric population has been proposed based on the validation in the CKiD study cohort.[97]

Dietary management

The importance of protein metabolism in CKD has been recognized more than a century ago, particularly because the classical markers of uremia—blood urea nitrogen and creatinine—are both products of protein metabolism. In the predialysis era, dietary protein restriction has been a mainstay of CKD management, making it possible to decrease the values of blood urea nitrogen and serum creatinine. However, the Modification of Diet in Renal Disease Study, the largest to date randomized clinical trial to test the effect of protein restriction on CKD progression in adults was inconclusive.[98] Currently, protein restriction is usually not recommended in children with CKD. KDOQI recommends 100% to 140% of the daily recommended intake protein intake for ideal body weight in children with stage 3 CKD, and 100% to 120% in children with stages 4 to 5 CKD.[31] Dialysis is associated with additional protein losses, which need to be taken into account when calculating protein requirements for children on dialysis, as well as urine protein losses in children with the nephrotic syndrome. Certain vitamins may accumulate in advanced CKD owing to decreased excretion and should not be taken in excess.[99] Specific "renal" multivitamin preparations for patients with CKD are commercially available.

Statural Growth in Children with Chronic Kidney Disease

Growth impairment is a common problem in children with all stages of CKD. In the North American Pediatric Renal Trials and Collaborative Studies report, more than 35% of children had impaired growth at the time of enrollment.[100] In the era preceding the introduction of recombinant human growth hormone (rhGH) therapy, almost one-half of patients with childhood-onset ESRD had final adult heights below the 3rd percentile.[101] Growth impairment is one of the major factors affecting the quality of life in children with CKD.[102] Short children with CKD miss school more frequently and spend more time admitted in the hospital.[103] Furthermore, growth impairment is a poor predictor of survival in children with ESRD.[104] The risk of death increased by 14% for each unit of decrease of height z-score at the time of dialysis initiation in children from the United States Renal Data System.[105]

CKD seems to distinctly affect all phases of body growth.[58] As with any chronic disease, growth velocity is most affected during periods of rapid growth. Both prematurity and low birth weight/intrauterine growth restriction are common in children who subsequently develop CKD, and are the risk factors for poor growth outcomes, independent of renal function[106] (*fetal phase*). During the *infantile phase*, the adverse effects of CKD on growth may be most intense and are thought to be largely mediated by inadequate nutrition. The growth hormone (GH) axis becomes critical for growth in the *childhood phase*, and the gonadotropin-sexual hormones axis is frequently affected by CKD in the *pubertal phase*.

Disturbance of the GH/insulinlike growth factor (IGF)-1 axis plays an important role in most children at some point in the course of CKD.[107] In children with CKD, fasting serum GH levels are normal or elevated, suggesting GH insensitivity.[107] Indeed, GH receptor expression is decreased in the liver tissue of juvenile mice[78] and rats[108] with experimental CKD, leading to inadequate production of IGF-1. Furthermore, the levels of circulating IGF-binding proteins are increased in CKD,[109] decreasing the free, bioactive IGF-1.[110] Other factors that may contribute to growth impairment in children with CKD include alterations in nutritional status, metabolic acidosis, fluid and electrolyte abnormalities, CKD-MBD, and anemia. Although optimization of nutrition is important, sufficient or even excessive caloric and nutrient intake does not always prevent growth impairment in children with CKD.[111,112] Gastrostomy feeding seems to be superior to oral or nasogastric feeding in infants on peritoneal dialysis.[113] The relationship between anemia and growth in children with CKD remains incompletely understood.[58] Growth impairment is a hallmark of untreated chronic anemias of nonrenal origin. However, the correction of anemia with ESA in several multicenter clinical trials did not result in a catchup growth.[114,115] The effect of iron therapy on growth has not been investigated in CKD; however, preclinical data suggest that hepcidin blockade can be advantageous.[78]

rhGH has been FDA-approved for the treatment of short stature in children with CKD. Consensus guidelines for rhGH therapy in children with CKD are available.[116] However, the use of rhGH therapy in the United States seems to be low,[117] and many families are noncompliant with the rhGH treatment regimen.[79] A recent survey of pediatric nephrologists identified family refusal as the most common reason for rhGH underuse, usually owing to fear of injections.[94] Logistical challenges, including those related to insurance approval, were also reported to influence practice patterns of rhGH therapy in children with CKD in North America.[94] Evaluation of bone age is required in short children older than 12 years with CKD before rhGH therapy initiation. Importantly, fusion of the growth plates can be significantly delayed in adolescents with CKD, in part owing to delayed pubertal development.[58] Thus, in many cases rhGH may be offered even in older adolescents with CKD.[118] Although not sufficiently studied in children with CKD, rhGH therapy may potentially have additional benefits, beyond the improvement in linear growth, such as mobilization of adipose tissue, an increase in lean body mass, improvement in physical function,[116] stimulation of erythropoiesis, and lowering circulating hepcidin.[119]

SUMMARY

CKD is a sustained loss of kidney function involving many organ systems and metabolic pathways, which impairs the statural growth, physical, and neurocognitive development of affected children. Pediatric CKD is associated with poor quality of life, and high morbidity and mortality. Our understanding of the interventions that may slow disease progression and would lead to improvement of patient-centered outcomes, including quality of life, has advanced in recent years. Aggressive control of hypertension; correction of metabolic acidosis, water, and electrolyte abnormalities; and preventing episodes of acute on chronic kidney injury seem to constitute the most promising strategies. Nutritional management is a critically important component of care for children with CKD related to key outcomes. Effective dietary support requires coordinated team efforts of a pediatric nephrologist, pediatric renal dietitian, social worker, primary care provider, and the family. Timely introduction of transplant and/or dialysis services improves outcomes in most children with advanced CKD and ESRD. Further collaborative research is needed to resolve many outstanding controversies in the pathophysiology, diagnostic approaches, and management of pediatric CKD.

REFERENCES

1. United States Renal Data System. 2017 USRDS annual data report: Epidemiology of kidney disease in the United States. National Institutes of Health, National Institute of Diabetes and Digestive and Kidney Diseases, Bethesda, MD, 2017. Available at: https://www.usrds.org/faq.aspx.

2. Jha V, Garcia-Garcia G, Iseki K, et al. Chronic kidney disease: global dimension and perspectives. Lancet 2013;382(9888):260–72.

3. Hu J-R, Coresh J. The public health dimension of chronic kidney disease: what we have learnt over the past decade. Nephrol Dial Transplant 2017;32(suppl_2): ii113–20.

4. Hoy WE, Douglas-Denton RN, Hughson MD, et al. A stereological study of glomerular number and volume: preliminary findings in a multiracial study of kidneys at autopsy. Kidney Int 2003;63:S31–7.

5. Hinchliffe S, Sargent P, Howard C, et al. Human intrauterine renal growth expressed in absolute number of glomeruli assessed by the disector method and Cavalieri principle. Lab Invest 1991;64(6):777–84.

6. Osathanondh V, Potter E. Development of human kidney as shown by microdissection. III. Formation and interrelationship of collecting tubules and nephrons. Arch Pathol 1963;76:290–302.

7. Eriksson JG, Salonen MK, Kajantie E, et al. Prenatal growth and CKD in older adults: longitudinal findings from the Helsinki Birth Cohort Study, 1924-1944. Am J Kidney Dis 2018;71(1):20–6.

8. Luyckx VA, Brenner BM. Low birth weight, nephron number, and kidney disease. Kidney Int 2005;68:S68–77.

9. Pøtter EL. Bilateral renal agenesis. J Pediatr 1946;29(1):68–76.

10. Bülchmann G, Schuster T, Heger A, et al. Transient pseudohypoaldosteronism secondary to posterior urethral valves-a case report and review of the literature. Eur J Pediatr Surg 2001;11(04):277–9.

11. Warady BA, Abraham AG, Schwartz GJ, et al. Predictors of rapid progression of glomerular and nonglomerular kidney disease in children and adolescents: the Chronic Kidney Disease in Children (CKiD) cohort. Am J Kidney Dis 2015;65(6): 878–88.

12. Furth SL, Pierce C, Hui WF, et al. Estimating time to ESRD in children with CKD. Am J Kidney Dis 2018;71(6):783–92.

13. Duranton F, Cohen G, De Smet R, et al. Normal and pathologic concentrations of uremic toxins. J Am Soc Nephrol 2012;23(7):1258–70.

14. Yacoub R, Wyatt CM. Manipulating the gut microbiome to decrease uremic toxins. Kidney Int 2017;91(3):521–3.
15. Vaziri ND, Wong J, Pahl M, et al. Chronic kidney disease alters intestinal microbial flora. Kidney Int 2013;83(2):308–15.
16. Snauwaert E, Van Biesen W, Raes A, et al. Accumulation of uraemic toxins is reflected only partially by estimated GFR in paediatric patients with chronic kidney disease. Pediatr Nephrol 2017;33(2):315–23.
17. Schwartz GJ, Brion LP, Spitzer A. The use of plasma creatinine concentration for estimating glomerular filtration rate in infants, children, and adolescents. Pediatr Clin North Am 1987;34(3):571–90.
18. Schnaper HW. Remnant nephron physiology and the progression of chronic kidney disease. Pediatr Nephrol 2014;29(2):193–202.
19. Greenberg N, Roberts WL, Bachmann LM, et al. Specificity characteristics of 7 commercial creatinine measurement procedures by enzymatic and Jaffe method principles. Clin Chem 2012;58(2):391–401.
20. Weber J, Van Zanten A. Interferences in current methods for measurements of creatinine. Clin Chem 1991;37(5):695–700.
21. Mian AN, Schwartz GJ. Measurement and estimation of glomerular filtration rate in children. Adv Chronic Kidney Dis 2017;24(6):348–56.
22. Sekhar DL, Wang L, Hollenbeak CS, et al. A cost-effectiveness analysis of screening urine dipsticks in well-child care. Pediatrics 2010;125(4):660–3.
23. Massengill SF, Ferris M. Chronic kidney disease in children and adolescents. Pediatr Rev 2014;35(1):16–29.
24. Seo-Mayer PW. Focus on subspecialties: children at risk for chronic kidney disease benefit from targeted screening. AAP News 2015.
25. Sabbagh Y, Graciolli FG, O'Brien S, et al. Repression of osteocyte Wnt/β-catenin signaling is an early event in the progression of renal osteodystrophy. J Bone Miner Res 2012;27(8):1757–72.
26. Graciolli FG, Neves KR, Barreto F, et al. The complexity of chronic kidney disease–mineral and bone disorder across stages of chronic kidney disease. Kidney Int 2017;91(6):1436–46.
27. Perwad F, Zhang MY, Tenenhouse HS, et al. Fibroblast growth factor 23 impairs phosphorus and vitamin D metabolism in vivo and suppresses 25-hydroxyvitamin D-1α-hydroxylase expression in vitro. Am J Physiol Renal Physiol 2007; 293(5):F1577–83.
28. Gutierrez O, Isakova T, Rhee E, et al. Fibroblast growth factor-23 mitigates hyperphosphatemia but accentuates calcitriol deficiency in chronic kidney disease. J Am Soc Nephrol 2005;16(7):2205–15.
29. Malluche HH, Porter DS, Pienkowski D. Evaluating bone quality in patients with chronic kidney disease. Nat Rev Nephrol 2013;9(11):671.
30. Wheeler DC, Winkelmayer WC. KDIGO 2017 clinical practice guideline update for the diagnosis, evaluation, prevention, and treatment of chronic kidney disease-mineral and bone disorder (CKD-MBD) foreword. Kidney Int Suppl 2017;7(1):1–59.
31. KDOQI Work Group. KDOQI clinical practice guideline for nutrition in children with CKD: 2008 update. executive summary. Am J Kidney Dis 2009;53(3 Suppl 2):S11–104.
32. Burtis CA, Ashwood ER. Tietz textbook of clinical chemistry. Amer Assn for Clinical Chemistry. Elsevier; 1994.
33. Raaijmakers R, Houkes LM, Schröder CH, et al. Pre-treatment of dairy and breast milk with sevelamer hydrochloride and sevelamer carbonate to reduce phosphate. Perit Dial Int 2013;33(5):565–72.

34. Alfrey A. Effect of dietary phosphate restriction on renal function and deterioration. Am J Clin Nutr 1988;47(1):153–6.
35. Jureidini KF, Hogg RJ, van Renen MJ, et al. Evaluation of long-term aggressive dietary management of chronic renal failure in children. Pediatr Nephrol 1990; 4(1):1–10.
36. Furth SL, Abraham AG, Jerry-Fluker J, et al. Metabolic abnormalities, cardiovascular disease risk factors, and GFR decline in children with chronic kidney disease. Clin J Am Soc Nephrol 2011;6(9):2132–40.
37. Harambat J, Kunzmann K, Azukaitis K, et al. Metabolic acidosis is common and associates with disease progression in children with chronic kidney disease. Kidney Int 2017;92(6):1507–14.
38. Kraut JA, Madias NE. Adverse effects of the metabolic acidosis of chronic kidney disease. Adv Chronic Kidney Dis 2017;24(5):289–97.
39. Kraut JA, Madias NE. Retarding progression of chronic kidney disease: use of modalities that counter acid retention. Curr Opin Nephrol Hypertens 2018; 27(2):94–101.
40. Mathur RP, Dash SC, Gupta N, et al. Effects of correction of metabolic acidosis on blood urea and bone metabolism in patients with mild to moderate chronic kidney disease: a prospective randomized single blind controlled trial. Ren Fail 2006;28(1):1–5.
41. Abramowitz MK, Melamed ML, Bauer C, et al. Effects of oral sodium bicarbonate in patients with CKD. Clin J Am Soc Nephrol 2013;8(5):714–20.
42. de Brito-Ashurst I, Varagunam M, Raftery MJ, et al. Bicarbonate supplementation slows progression of CKD and improves nutritional status. J Am Soc Nephrol 2009;20(9):2075–84.
43. Levin A, Stevens PE, Bilous RW, et al, Kidney Disease: Improving Global Outcomes (KDIGO) CKD Work Group. KDIGO 2012 clinical practice guideline for the evaluation and management of chronic kidney disease. Kidney Int Suppl 2013;3(1):1–150.
44. Goraya N, Simoni J, Jo C-H, et al. Treatment of metabolic acidosis in patients with stage 3 chronic kidney disease with fruits and vegetables or oral bicarbonate reduces urine angiotensinogen and preserves glomerular filtration rate. Kidney Int 2014;86(5):1031–8.
45. Goraya N, Simoni J, Jo C-H, et al. A comparison of treating metabolic acidosis in CKD stage 4 hypertensive kidney disease with fruits and vegetables or sodium bicarbonate. Clin J Am Soc Nephrol 2013;8(3):371–81.
46. Bushinsky DA, Hostetter T, Klaerner G, et al. Randomized, controlled trial of TRC101 to increase serum bicarbonate in patients with CKD. Clin J Am Soc Nephrol 2017;13(1):26–35.
47. Goraya N, Wesson DE. Management of the metabolic acidosis of chronic kidney disease. Adv Chronic Kidney Dis 2017;24(5):298–304.
48. Kraut JA, Madias NE. Consequences and therapy of the metabolic acidosis of chronic kidney disease. Pediatr Nephrol 2011;26(1):19–28.
49. Abuelo JG. Treatment of severe hyperkalemia: confronting 4 fallacies. Kidney Int Rep 2018;3(1):47–55.
50. Thomsen RW, Nicolaisen SK, Hasvold P, et al. Elevated potassium levels in patients with chronic kidney disease: occurrence, risk factors and clinical outcomes—a Danish population-based cohort study. Nephrol Dial Transplant 2017. https://doi.org/10.1093/ndt/gfx312.
51. Einhorn LM, Zhan M, Walker LD, et al. The frequency of hyperkalemia and its significance in chronic kidney disease. Arch Intern Med 2009;169(12):1156–62.

52. Palmer BF, Clegg DJ. Hyperkalemia across the continuum of kidney function. Clin J Am Soc Nephrol 2018;13(1):155–7.

53. Hayes C Jr, McLeod M, Robinson R. An extravenal mechanism for the maintenance of potassium balance in severe chronic renal failure. Trans Assoc Am Physicians 1967;80:207–16.

54. Nguyen L, Levitt R, Mak RH. Practical nutrition management of children with chronic kidney disease. Clin Med Insights Urol 2016;9:S13180.

55. Hill LJ, Herald AJ. Kidney-friendly label reading for chronic kidney disease shoppers. J Ren Nutr 2018;28(1):e1–4.

56. Harel Z, Harel S, Shah PS, et al. Gastrointestinal adverse events with sodium polystyrene sulfonate (Kayexalate) use: a systematic review. Am J Med 2013; 126(3):264.e9-e24.

57. Fried L, Kovesdy CP, Palmer BF. New options for the management of chronic hyperkalemia. Kidney Int Suppl 2017;7(3):164–70.

58. Haffner D, Rees L. Growth and puberty in chronic kidney disease. In: Geary DF, Schaefer F, editors. Pediatric kidney disease. Berlin: Springer Berlin Heidelberg; 2016. p. 1425–54.

59. Group ET. Strict blood-pressure control and progression of renal failure in children. N Engl J Med 2009;361(17):1639–50.

60. Vegter S, Perna A, Postma MJ, et al. Sodium intake, ACE inhibition, and progression to ESRD. J Am Soc Nephrol 2012;23(1):165–73.

61. McMahon EJ, Bauer JD, Hawley CM, et al. A randomized trial of dietary sodium restriction in CKD. J Am Soc Nephrol 2013;24(12):2096–103.

62. Nomura K, Asayama K, Jacobs L, et al. Renal function in relation to sodium intake: a quantitative review of the literature. Kidney Int 2017;92(1):67–78.

63. Graudal NA, Hubeck-Graudal T, Jürgens G. Effects of low-sodium diet vs. high-sodium diet on blood pressure, renin, aldosterone, catecholamines, cholesterol, and triglyceride (Cochrane Review). Am J Hypertens 2012;25(1):1–15.

64. Graudal N, Jürgens G, Baslund B, et al. Compared with usual sodium intake, low-and excessive-sodium diets are associated with increased mortality: a meta-analysis. Am J Hypertens 2014;27(9):1129–37.

65. Cogswell ME, Mugavero K, Bowman BA, et al. Dietary sodium and cardiovascular disease risk—measurement matters. N Engl J Med 2016;375(6):580.

66. Hui WF, Betoko A, Savant JD, et al. Assessment of dietary intake of children with chronic kidney disease. Pediatr Nephrol 2017;32(3):485–94.

67. Schaefer F, Doyon A, Azukaitis K, et al. Cardiovascular phenotypes in children with CKD: the 4C study. Clin J Am Soc Nephrol 2017;12(1):19–28.

68. Saland JM, Pierce CB, Mitsnefes MM, et al. Dyslipidemia in children with chronic kidney disease. Kidney Int 2010;78(11):1154–63.

69. Group KK. KDIGO clinical practice guideline for lipid management in chronic kidney disease. Kidney Int Suppl 2013;3:259–305.

70. Gerson A, Hwang W, Fiorenza J, et al. Anemia and health-related quality of life in adolescents with chronic kidney disease. Am J kidney Dis 2004;44(6):1017–23.

71. Perlman RL, Finkelstein FO, Liu L, et al. Quality of life in chronic kidney disease (CKD): a cross-sectional analysis in the Renal Research Institute-CKD study. Am J kidney Dis 2005;45(4):658–66.

72. Fadrowski JJ, Pierce CB, Cole SR, et al. Hemoglobin decline in children with chronic kidney disease: baseline results from the Chronic Kidney Disease in Children prospective cohort study. Clin J Am Soc Nephrol 2008;3(2):457–62.

73. Locatelli F, Mazzaferro S, Yee J. Iron therapy challenges for the treatment of non-dialysis CKD patients. Clin J Am Soc Nephrol 2016;11(7):1269–80.

74. Hattori M. Hemoglobin target in children with chronic kidney disease: valuable new information. Kidney Int 2017;91(1):16–8.
75. Atkinson MA, Kim JY, Roy CN, et al. Hepcidin and risk of anemia in CKD: a cross-sectional and longitudinal analysis in the CKiD cohort. Pediatr Nephrol 2015;30(4):635–43.
76. Ganz T, Nemeth E. Iron balance and the role of hepcidin in chronic kidney disease. Semin Nephrol 2016;36(2):87–93.
77. Chand S, Ward DG, Ng Z-YV, et al. Serum hepcidin-25 and response to intravenous iron in patients with non-dialysis chronic kidney disease. J Nephrol 2015; 28(1):81–8.
78. Akchurin O, Sureshbabu A, Doty SB, et al. Lack of hepcidin ameliorates anemia and improves growth in an adenine-induced mouse model of chronic kidney disease. Am J Physiol Renal Physiol 2016;311(5):F877–89.
79. Akchurin OM, Schneider MF, Mulqueen L, et al. Medication adherence and growth in children with CKD. Clin J Am Soc Nephrol 2014;9(9):1519–25.
80. Agarwal R, Vasavada N, Sachs NG, et al. Oxidative stress and renal injury with intravenous iron in patients with chronic kidney disease. Kidney Int 2004;65(6): 2279–89.
81. Lukaszyk E, Lukaszyk M, Koc-Zorawska E, et al. Iron status and inflammation in early stages of chronic kidney disease. Kidney Blood Press Res 2015;40(4): 366–73.
82. Querfeld U, Dietrich R, Taira R, et al. Magnetic resonance imaging of iron overload in children treated with peritoneal dialysis. Nephron 1988;50(3):220–4.
83. Soliman AT, Al Dabbagh MM, Habboub AH, et al. Linear growth in children with iron deficiency anemia before and after treatment. J Trop Pediatr 2009;55(5): 324–7.
84. Bandhu R, Shankar N, Tandon OP. Effect of iron on growth in iron deficient anemic school going children. Indian J Physiol Pharmacol 2003;47(1):59–66.
85. Soliman AT, De Sanctis V, Yassin M, et al. Growth and growth hormone - insulin like growth factor -I (GH-IGF-I) axis in chronic anemias. Acta Biomed 2017; 88(1):101–11.
86. Skordis N, Kyriakou A. The multifactorial origin of growth failure in thalassaemia. Pediatr Endocrinol Rev 2011;8(Suppl 2):271–7.
87. Sachdev H, Gera T, Nestel P. Effect of iron supplementation on physical growth in children: systematic review of randomised controlled trials. Public Health Nutr 2006;9(7):904–20.
88. Dewey KG, Domellof M, Cohen RJ, et al. Iron supplementation affects growth and morbidity of breast-fed infants: results of a randomized trial in Sweden and Honduras. J Nutr 2002;132(11):3249–55.
89. Perng W, Mora-Plazas M, Marin C, et al. Iron status and linear growth: a prospective study in school-age children. Eur J Clin Nutr 2013;67(6):646–51.
90. Lozoff B, Castillo M, Clark KM, et al. Iron-fortified vs low-iron infant formula: developmental outcome at 10 years. Arch Pediatr Adolesc Med 2012;166(3): 208–15.
91. KDIGO. KDIGO clinical practice guideline for anemia in chronic kidney disease. Kidney Int Suppl 2012;2:279–335.
92. Akchurin M, Kaskel F. Update on inflammation in chronic kidney disease. Blood Purif 2015;39(1–3):84–92.
93. Mastrangelo A, Paglialonga F, Edefonti A. Assessment of nutritional status in children with chronic kidney disease and on dialysis. Pediatr Nephrol 2014; 29(8):1349–58.

94. Akchurin M, Kogon AJ, Kumar J, et al. Approach to growth hormone therapy in children with chronic kidney disease varies across North America: the Midwest Pediatric Nephrology Consortium report. BMC Nephrol 2017;18(1):181.

95. Mak RH, Cheung WW, Zhan JY, et al. Cachexia and protein-energy wasting in children with chronic kidney disease. Pediatr Nephrol 2012;27(2):173–81.

96. Fouque D, Kalantar-Zadeh K, Kopple J, et al. A proposed nomenclature and diagnostic criteria for protein-energy wasting in acute and chronic kidney disease. Kidney Int 2008;73(4):391–8.

97. Abraham AG, Mak RH, Mitsnefes M, et al. Protein energy wasting in children with chronic kidney disease. Pediatr Nephrol 2014;29(7):1231–8.

98. Klahr S, Levey AS, Beck GJ, et al. The effects of dietary protein restriction and blood-pressure control on the progression of chronic renal disease. N Engl J Med 1994;330(13):877–84.

99. Steiber AL, Kopple JD. Vitamin status and needs for people with stages 3-5 chronic kidney disease. J Ren Nutr 2011;21(5):355–68.

100. Seikaly MG, Salhab N, Gipson D, et al. Stature in children with chronic kidney disease: analysis of NAPRTCS database. Pediatr Nephrol 2006;21(6):793–9.

101. André J-L, Bourquard R, Guillemin F, et al. Final height in children with chronic renal failure who have not received growth hormone. Pediatr Nephrol 2003; 18(7):685–91.

102. Al-Uzri A, Matheson M, Gipson DS, et al. The impact of short stature on health-related quality of life in children with chronic kidney disease. J Pediatr 2013; 163(3):736–41.e1.

103. Furth SL, Stablein D, Fine RN, et al. Adverse clinical outcomes associated with short stature at dialysis initiation: a report of the North American Pediatric Renal Transplant Cooperative Study. Pediatrics 2002;109(5):909–13.

104. Weaver DJ, Somers MJ, Martz K, et al. Clinical outcomes and survival in pediatric patients initiating chronic dialysis: a report of the NAPRTCS registry. Pediatr Nephrol 2017;32(12):2319–30.

105. Wong CS, Gipson DS, Gillen DL, et al. Anthropometric measures and risk of death in children with end-stage renal disease. Am J kidney Dis 2000;36(4): 811–9.

106. Greenbaum LA, Muñoz A, Schneider MF, et al. The association between abnormal birth history and growth in children with CKD. Clin J Am Soc Nephrol 2011;6(1):14–21.

107. Tönshoff B. Pathogenesis, evaluation and diagnosis of growth impairment in children with chronic kidney disease. In: Niaudet P, editor. UpToDate. Waltham (MA): UpToDate Inc; 2018.

108. Tönshoff B, Powell DR, Zhao D, et al. Decreased hepatic insulin-like growth factor (IGF)-I and increased IGF binding protein-1 and-2 gene expression in experimental uremia. Endocrinology 1997;138(3):938–46.

109. Tönshoff B, Blum WF, Wingen A-M, et al. Serum insulin-like growth factors (IGFs) and IGF binding proteins 1, 2, and 3 in children with chronic renal failure: relationship to height and glomerular filtration rate. The European Study Group for nutritional treatment of chronic renal failure in childhood. J Clin Endocrinol Metab 1995;80(9):2684–91.

110. Frystyk J, Ivarsen P, Skjærbæk C, et al. Serum-free insulin-like growth factor I correlates with clearance in patients with chronic renal failure. Kidney Int 1999;56(6):2076–84.

111. Abithol CL, Zilleruelo G, Montane B, et al. Growth of uremic infants on forced feeding regimens. Pediatr Nephrol 1993;7(2):173–7.

112. Rees L, Jones H. Nutritional management and growth in children with chronic kidney disease. Pediatr Nephrol 2013;28(4):527–36.

113. Rees L, Azocar M, Borzych D, et al. Growth in very young children undergoing chronic peritoneal dialysis. J Am Soc Nephrol 2011;22(12):2303–12.

114. Morris K, Sharp J, Watson S, et al. Non-cardiac benefits of human recombinant erythropoietin in end stage renal failure and anaemia. Arch Dis Child 1993;69(5): 580–6.

115. Jabs K. The effects of recombinant human erythropoietin on growth and nutritional status. Pediatr Nephrol 1996;10(3):324–7.

116. Mahan JD, Warady BA, Committee C. Assessment and treatment of short stature in pediatric patients with chronic kidney disease: a consensus statement. Pediatr Nephrol 2006;21(7):917–30.

117. Greenbaum LA, Hidalgo G, Chand D, et al. Obstacles to the prescribing of growth hormone in children with chronic kidney disease. Pediatr Nephrol 2008;23(9):1531–5.

118. Gil S, Aziz M, Adragna M, et al. Near-adult height in male kidney transplant recipients started on growth hormone treatment in late puberty. Pediatr Nephrol 2018;33(1):175–80.

119. Troutt JS, Rudling M, Persson L, et al. Circulating human hepcidin-25 concentrations display a diurnal rhythm, increase with prolonged fasting, and are reduced by growth hormone administration. Clin Chem 2012;58(8):1225–32.

Long-Term Outcomes of Kidney Transplantation in Children

Pamela D. Winterberg, MD*, Rouba Garro, MD

KEYWORDS

- Pediatric • Kidney transplantation • Outcomes

KEY POINTS

- Patient survival is excellent following kidney transplantation in children (90%–95% at 10 year).
- Long-term kidney transplant outcomes are dependent on excellent adherence to follow-up and immunosuppressive regimens.
- Adolescent and young adult recipients have the highest risk for graft loss at 5 years.
- Life-long immunosuppression increases the risk for infections and malignancies in children with kidney transplant.
- Weight gain and immunosuppressive medications increase the risk for cardiometabolic complications (hypertension, dyslipidemia, and diabetes).

KIDNEY TRANSPLANTATION IN CHILDREN

The most common causes of end-stage renal disease (ESRD) in children are congenital, cystic, and hereditary diseases, which combined account for 38% of incident cases.[1] The most common disorders in this category are congenital obstructive uropathies (9.5%) and renal hypoplasia/dysplasia (10%). Primary glomerular disease is the second-most common cause, accounting for 25% of new cases, predominantly due to focal segmental glomerulosclerosis (FSGS). Secondary glomerulonephritis and vasculitis account for 12% of new cases, of which lupus nephritis is the most common. The underlying cause of ESRD also varies by age of presentation (**Fig. 1**A). As expected, congenital/hereditary/cystic disorders are the most common underlying cause of ESRD among the youngest age groups, whereas primary and secondary glomerular diseases are the leading cause among adolescents.[1]

Disclosure Statement: The authors have no financial interests or conflicts of interest to disclose.
Division of Pediatric Nephrology, Emory University School of Medicine, Children's Pediatric Institute, 2015 Uppergate Drive NE, 5th Floor, Atlanta, GA 30322, USA
* Corresponding author.
E-mail address: pdwinte@emory.edu

Pediatr Clin N Am 66 (2019) 269–280
https://doi.org/10.1016/j.pcl.2018.09.008
0031-3955/19/© 2018 Elsevier Inc. All rights reserved.

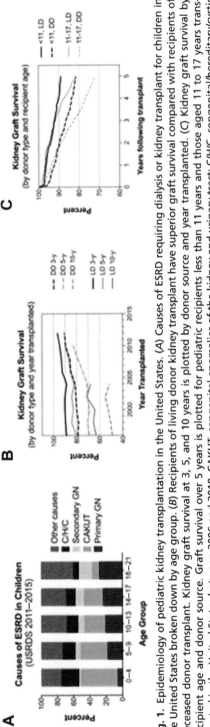

Fig. 1. Epidemiology of pediatric kidney transplantation in the United States. (*A*) Causes of ESRD requiring dialysis or kidney transplant for children in the United States broken down by age group. (*B*) Recipients of living donor kidney transplant have superior graft survival compared with recipients of deceased donor transplant. Kidney graft survival at 3, 5, and 10 years is plotted by donor source and year transplanted. (*C*) Kidney graft survival by recipient age and donor source. Graft survival over 5 years is plotted for pediatric recipients less than 11 years and those aged 11 to 17 years transplanted in the United States between 2006 and 2010. CAKUT, congenital anomalies of the kidney and urinary tract; C/H/C, congenital/hereditary/cystic disorders; DD, deceased donor; GN, glomerulonephritis; LD, living donor. (*Data from* [*A*] The United States Renal Data System (USRDS). Annual data report: epidemiology of kidney disease in the United States. Bethesda (MD): National Institutes of Health, National Institute of Diabetes and Digestive Kidney Diseases. 2017; and [*B*, *C*] Hart A, Smith JM, Skeans MA, et al. OPTN/SRTR 2015 annual data report: kidney. Am J Transplant 2017;17(suppl 1):21–116.)

Kidney transplantation is the preferred treatment for ESRD in children and confers improved survival, skeletal growth, heath-related quality of life, and neuropsychological development compared with dialysis.[1]

Timing of Transplant

Transplantation is initially considered when renal replacement therapy is imminent. Because of increased risk of graft loss and mortality in very young children, most pediatric centers perform kidney transplantation once children achieve a weight greater than 10 to 15 kg, which is typically around the age of 2 years. The underlying cause for kidney failure, the rapidity of decline in kidney function, and the age and size of the patient determine whether an individual can receive a preemptive kidney transplant without preceding dialysis, which may provide a graft survival advantage.[2] On average, 30% of pediatric kidney transplant recipients in the United States receive preemptive transplant, and an additional 24% receive dialysis treatment for less than 1 year before transplant.[3]

Donor Source

Patients can receive kidney transplants from living or deceased donors. Historically, living-related donor transplants were more common in children than deceased-donor transplants. The high historical rate of living donation was likely driven by parents' understanding of the benefit of living donation for their child, such as superior long-term graft survival (**Fig. 1**B) and ability to schedule the procedure.[4,5] However, the rate of living donor transplants in children has been declining since 2002, with only 34% of pediatric recipients in 2015 receiving living donor kidney transplants compared with 50% in 2004.

The transplant community has consistently supported timely access to deceased-donor kidney grafts for pediatric candidates with an allocation system that has historically emphasized younger donors and shorter waiting times over HLA matching. As a result, the absolute number and proportion of deceased-donor kidney transplants in pediatric recipients have been steadily increasing over the past 20 years accompanied by a decrease in the absolute number of living-donor transplants.[6] It is unclear at this time if the trend in fewer living donor transplants is a direct consequence of policy change or due to increasing prevalence of comorbidities in parents that preclude them from donating (eg, obesity and diabetes).[7]

Patient Survival

The success of kidney transplantation in children with ESRD now results in 10-year patient survival of 90% to 95%. Therefore, the long-term management of these patients is focused on maintaining quality of life and minimizing long-term side effects of immunosuppression. Optimal management of pediatric kidney transplant recipients includes preventing rejection and infection, identifying and reducing the cardiovascular and metabolic effects of long-term immunosuppressive therapy, supporting normal growth and development, and managing a smooth transition into adulthood (**Fig. 2**).

DETERMINANTS OF GRAFT SURVIVAL

In general, the estimated half-life for transplanted kidneys in children is 12 to 15 years; therefore, children with ESRD often require more than one kidney transplant in their lifetime. The adolescent age group (11–17 years), which accounts for greater than 50% of the pediatric kidney transplant waiting list, has worse 5-year graft survival compared with pediatric recipients under the age of 11 years (**Fig. 1**C).[3] Overall, living donor transplants have improved long-term outcomes compared with deceased

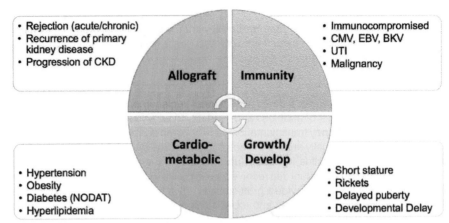

- Rejection (acute/chronic)
- Recurrence of primary kidney disease
- Progression of CKD

Allograft

Immunity

- Immunocompromised
- CMV, EBV, BKV
- UTI
- Malignancy

Cardio-metabolic

Growth/ Develop

- Hypertension
- Obesity
- Diabetes (NODAT)
- Hyperlipidemia

- Short stature
- Rickets
- Delayed puberty
- Developmental Delay

Fig. 2. Long-term outcomes of pediatric kidney transplant. Issues facing pediatric kidney transplant recipients include those pertaining directly to the health of the allograft (eg, rejection, recurrence), immune deficiency due to medications (eg, viral infections, malignancy), growth and development in the context of organ failure (eg, bone disease, transition to adulthood with chronic medical condition), and cardiometabolic comorbidities from immunosuppression (eg, obesity, hypertension). Optimal care of the pediatric kidney transplant recipient addresses these issues in a multidisciplinary fashion.

donor transplants with 10-year graft loss of 38% versus 52%, respectively (see **Fig. 1**B).[3] Long-term graft survival is affected by several factors, including the quality of the donated kidney (eg, living vs deceased donor, number of HLA mismatches, delayed graft function, donor age and size), the presence of preexisting HLA antibodies (presensitization), recipient race/ethnicity, recipient age (eg, adolescence), as well as subsequent graft injury from recurrence of primary disease (eg, FSGS), allograft infections, and acute or chronic rejection episodes.[8]

Rejection

Children with kidney transplants require life-long immunosuppressive therapy to prevent rejection of the allograft. The most common medication regimen in the United States includes the combination of corticosteroid (eg, prednisone), a calcineurin inhibitor (or CNI, most commonly tacrolimus), and an antimetabolite such as mycophenolate mofetil (MMF). Cyclosporine and azathioprine are less commonly used for maintenance immunosuppression. Some centers offer steroid-sparing or CNI-sparing regimens as well.

With modern immunosuppressive therapy, rates of acute rejection episodes within the first 12 months for pediatric kidney transplant in the United States are reported at 11%.[3] Chronic allograft rejection, however, is a leading cause of graft loss in children. Late and multiple episodes of acute rejection are associated with worse long-term allograft survival. Therefore, early identification and treatment of acute rejection are paramount to improve long-term outcomes.

The diagnosis of acute rejection is not always straightforward in pediatric kidney transplant recipients. Small children who have adult-sized allografts have a large renal reserve relative to their muscle mass. Therefore, significant renal injury may occur with little to no change in the serum creatinine. Children with acute rejection can present with low-grade fever and mild hypertension, but can also be asymptomatic. Therefore, most transplant centers follow serum creatinine closely with serial laboratory testing to establish baseline kidney function in order to detect early changes in graft function. Some centers also perform surveillance biopsies to detect and treat subclinical rejection.

Suspected nonadherence contributes to approximately 44% of graft losses and 23% of late acute rejection episodes reported in the literature for adolescent kidney transplant recipients.[9] Pretransplant patterns of medication and dialysis treatment adherence may predict posttransplant behavior. Social, behavioral, and psychiatric interventions should be initiated before transplant and maintained after transplant for those patients with identified or anticipated issues with nonadherence.

INFECTION AND IMMUNITY

Although modern immunosuppression regimens have reduced the rate of acute rejection, infectious complications have become more frequent.[10–12] In particular, pediatric transplant recipients are at risk for developing virus-related complications due to immunologic naiveté at the time of transplantation and primary infection under immunosuppressive therapy.

Common Viral Illnesses

Children with kidney transplants often have more severe and prolonged illness from even common viral pathogens (eg, respiratory syncytial virus, influenza, adenovirus) secondary to their immunocompromised status. Therefore, pediatric transplant recipients are recommended to receive annual influenza vaccination and to remain up-to-date on all other non–live viral vaccine schedules, including those for the prevention of human papilloma virus (HPV), meningococcal, and pneumococcal diseases. Caregivers and close household contacts should also be fully immunized, and there are no restrictions for these otherwise healthy contacts to receive live-attenuated vaccines.

Diarrheal illness in children with kidney transplants requires special attention, because graft injury can occur even with mild dehydration, and diarrhea often significantly alters the metabolism and absorption of immunosuppressant medications. Therefore, children with kidney transplants presenting with vomiting and/or diarrhea require prompt medical evaluation, including laboratory testing to assess kidney function and drug levels, and often the administration of intravenous fluids. Finally, should diarrhea persist, testing for opportunistic pathogens, such as Giardia, microsporidia, and cryptosporidium, should be considered.

Latent Viruses

Transplant recipients are routinely monitored for the reactivation or primary infection of the latent viruses, cytomegalovirus (CMV), Epstein-Barr virus (EBV), and BK polyoma virus (BKV) using detection of viral nucleic acid in plasma (viremia). Roughly half of the children are serologically naïve to CMV or EBV at the time of transplant. The combination of a CMV- or EBV-positive donor with a serologically naïve pediatric recipient represents the highest risk for infection and disease after transplant. Early detection of viremia and intervention with antiviral medications and/or reduced immunosuppression are the cornerstones of management for these viruses after transplant.

CMV disease can present with fever, elevated transaminases, diarrhea, and pneumonia. Morbidity and mortality from early disseminated CMV disease have dramatically improved with the use of surveillance testing and effective prophylaxis (eg, valgancyclovir) in the highest-risk recipients.

Primary EBV infection in children with kidney transplant can present similarly to healthy children (eg, pharyngitis, fever, cervical lymphadenopathy, splenomegaly, mononucleosis syndrome). However, children receiving immunosuppression are at increased risk for developing posttransplant lymphoproliferative disease (PTLD) and lymphoma as consequences of EBV infection (see more under Malignancy in later discussion). There is no effective chemoprophylaxis for EBV infection.

BK virus is a polyomavirus that establishes a latent infection of the uroepithelium and is typically asymptomatic in the healthy host. In the transplant recipient, uncontrolled BK virus replication leads to infection of the kidney allograft (BK nephropathy [BKN]) and can result in permanent damage and graft loss. BK virus infection (eg, viremia) can occur early (within the first month) or late (several years) following kidney transplant in children. Definitive diagnosis of BKN is obtained only by renal biopsy, and the incidence in pediatric kidney transplant recipients is estimated to be 4% to 5%.[13,14] Prospective monitoring for BK viremia with preemptive lowering of immunosuppression has been suggested as an effective approach.[15]

Urinary Tract Infection

Urinary tract infection (UTI) is the most common infectious complication following kidney transplant in children, occurring in 15% to 33% of patients.[10,16] Recurrent UTI has been associated with more rapid deterioration in graft function in children.[16,17] Risk factors for febrile UTI include anatomic abnormalities, dysfunctional bladder, presence of foreign material (eg, urinary catheter or stents), and baseline immunosuppression. Parenteral antibiotics are indicated for febrile UTI in pediatric transplant patients. Some children with recurrent UTI are treated with antibiotic prophylaxis, although the benefit of this approach needs to be weighed against the increased risk for bacterial resistance with prolonged antibiotic use.

Malignancy

Long-term use of immunosuppressive medications coupled with decades of remaining life expectancy places the pediatric transplant recipient at increased risk for the development of malignancy during their lifetime. The most common malignancy in childhood transplant recipients is viral-induced lymphoproliferative disease (or PTLD) with a cumulative incidence of 1.8% by 5 years. PTLD in children is often associated with EBV infection, and children who are immunologically naïve to EBV at the time of transplant are at highest risk of developing PTLD.[3] EBV-related lymphoid hyperplasia may present as adenotonsillar hypertrophy, but can also affect the gastrointestinal tract (chronic diarrhea) and kidney allograft. Central nervous system involvement is also described and can be fatal. Early recognition of PTLD via surveillance for significant EBV viremia and prompt detection of lymphadenopathy with appropriate intervention are essential. Chronic, low-grade EBV viremia in transplant recipients without development of PTLD is not uncommon; therefore, serial monitoring and trending of viral load using consistent laboratory methods (eg, whole blood vs plasma, consistent laboratory site) are required to detect changes in viral control when evaluating risk for PTLD.

There are limited data about long-term risk for nonlymphoproliferative malignancy in patients receiving kidney transplant during childhood. In a study of adult survivors of pediatric ESRD in The Netherlands, nearly 41% developed cancer after 30 years following transplant.[18] Nonmelanoma skin cancer was the most common form of malignancy and had very low mortality associated with it. Renal cell carcinoma of the native kidneys was the most common solid tumor reported during childhood following kidney transplant.[19] Given the increased lifetime risk for all cancers, pediatric transplant recipients should be counseled on avoiding additional risk factors for malignancy, including excessive sun exposure (eg, sunscreen use), alcohol consumption, and tobacco use.

Another viral-associated malignancy to consider in pediatric transplant patients is urogenital cancer associated with HPV. As such, all pediatric transplant recipients are encouraged to complete the full HPV vaccine series before sexual maturity.

CARDIOMETABOLIC COMORBIDITIES

Children with ESRD have increased cardiovascular mortality relative to their peers, accounting for nearly 40% of deaths among pediatric ESRD patients.[20,21] Although kidney transplantation leads to a dramatic improvement in renal function and elimination of many traditional risk factors, cardiovascular disease still accounts for more than one-third of deaths among patients who receive transplants before 21 years of age.

Hypertension

Hypertension is common in children after transplant and is likely due to a combination of rapid weight gain, medication side effects (eg, CNI and steroids), and renal injury. An estimated 50% to 65% of pediatric kidney transplant recipients have hypertension at 1 year after transplant.[22–24] In addition to the concerns for long-term cardiovascular risk associated with uncontrolled hypertension, retrospective analyses of pediatric kidney transplant recipients suggest that systolic hypertension independently predicts poor long-term allograft survival.[24,25]

Obesity

Obesity is an emerging challenge in renal transplant recipients, in parallel with the general pediatric population, leading to increased risk of surgical complications, hyperlipidemia, diabetes, and hypertension after transplant.[26] Many children experience rapid weight gain following transplant, likely due to a combination of lifted dietary restrictions imposed during ESRD and appetite stimulation from corticosteroids used to prevent or treat rejection. Up to 50% of pediatric transplant recipients have been classified as obese or overweight in recent studies.[27,28] Furthermore, obesity complicates hypertension management with approximately 80% of obese pediatric transplant recipients having poor control of hypertension at 1 year.[22] Weight gain should be monitored closely following transplant to identify children early at risk for obesity, because increases in body mass index in the first 6 months following transplant are likely to be persistent.[29]

Hypercholesterolemia and hypertriglyceridemia are also common in children with kidney transplant likely due to a combination of drug side effects[30] (eg, cyclosporine, mTOR inhibitors, glucocorticoids) and obesity.[31,32] Therefore, semiannual screening for hypercholesterolemia and hypertriglyceridemia is suggested.[33] Lifestyle modification, including dietary changes and increased physical activity, is typically preferred for young children with hyperlipidemia. Although the use of 3-hydroxy-3-methylglutaryl-coenzyme A reductase inhibitors (statins) is generally considered safe and effective in children over the age of 8 years, few data are available on long-term safety.[34] Omega-3 fatty acids have been reported to be effective at reducing low-density lipoprotein levels in young kidney transplant recipients in small case series.[35]

Diabetes

Hyperglycemia and new-onset diabetes after transplant (NODAT) are serious and increasingly more common metabolic complications following kidney transplantation, with a reported incidence of 3% to 20% in pediatric recipients.[36–38] NODAT is associated with increased morbidity from cardiovascular complications, increased infection risk, and inferior allograft and patient survival following kidney transplantation.[37] The increased incidence of NODAT in the pediatric kidney transplant population has paralleled both the obesity epidemic in the general population and the increased use of CNIs for posttransplant immunosuppression.[39] Management should focus on prevention with close screening for early signs of glucose intolerance, tailoring of immunosuppressant regimen as appropriate, and promotion of lifestyle modifications. Pharmacologic intervention (eg, insulin) is necessary to reduce complications of hyperglycemia and improve overall allograft and patient survival when lifestyle and medication modifications fail to achieve adequate glycemic control.

GROWTH AND DEVELOPMENT
Short Stature and Bone Health

Impaired linear growth in children with chronic kidney disease (CKD) is multifactorial and is mainly due to disturbances in the axis involving growth hormone (GH), insulin-like growth factor (IGF), and IGF-binding protein. Despite satisfactory renal function following transplant, spontaneous catch-up growth is often insufficient. Abnormalities in mineral metabolism, including disturbances in serum calcium, phosphorus, parathyroid hormone, and vitamin D stores, are common in children following kidney transplant and increase the risk for growth delay and osteopenia or rickets.[40–42]

Determinants of growth following transplant include age at the time of transplant, exposure to glucocorticoids, allograft function, and administration of recombinant human growth hormone (rhGH). Children under the age of 6 years have increased growth rates following transplant compared with older children.[43] The degree of growth stunting before transplant is also predictive of final adult height.[44] Therapy with rhGH is effective in improving the growth velocity and final adult height of children following kidney transplant.[45,46] Finally, steroid-sparing immunosuppressive protocols have demonstrated improved linear growth for prepubertal children undergoing kidney transplant.[47]

Bladder Function

Even children with nonurologic causes of ESRD often have lower urinary tract symptoms following transplant, including urinary urgency, bladder pain, incomplete bladder emptying, nighttime or daytime incontinence, and UTIs.[48] Timed voiding and prevention or treatment of functional constipation are important in the management of incontinence and dysfunctional voiding. For those with congenital bladder outlet obstruction, intermittent catheterization is often still required to avoid graft damage and dysfunction.[49] Anticholinergic therapy and intermittent catheterization should be continued following transplantation as medical management of preexisting neurogenic bladder.

Puberty

Onset of puberty is an important milestone during adolescence. Most children achieve normal puberty following transplant, but many may have a delayed onset and shortened duration of pubertal growth spurt, which is predicted by delayed bone age compared with their chronologic age.[50,51]

Psychosocial Development

Transplant recipients are exposed to additional psychosocial stress related to their chronic illness. Developmental delay, issues with body image from drug side effects, difficulty interacting with peers, prolonged school absences, fastidious schedules required for immunosuppressant medication regimens, symptoms of posttraumatic stress, and family disruption due to financial burden or role strain may exacerbate psychosocial difficulties in the pediatric transplant recipient. Collaboration with psychologists, psychiatrists, and social workers is important for the early identification and intensified treatment of high-risk individuals.

Children with emotional or psychiatric disorders often require additional mental health resources, including psychiatric care before and after transplant. Acquisition of coping skills, problem-solving skills, and behavior modification can improve a child's experience with the inherent complexity of dialysis or transplantation medical care. Pharmacotherapy for depression, bipolar disorder, and attention-deficit/hyperactivity disorder are important adjunctive therapies. Reduced clearance with impaired renal function, clearance by dialysis, and interference with the metabolism of immunosuppressive medications should be considered when selecting psychotropic medications in children with ESRD or transplant.

Children with ESRD during infancy can have significant developmental delay due to uremia. In the absence of structural brain abnormalities, psychomotor delay often improves following transplant, with many infants regaining normal developmental milestones.[52] Lower IQ and learning disabilities are most common in children born prematurely and those who had multiple hypertensive crises and/or seizures before transplant.[53] Ongoing evaluation of neurocognitive abilities and appropriate support from school systems are needed to achieve optimal school performance following transplant.

Adolescence and Emerging Adulthood

Adolescence is an important transition period between childhood and adulthood characterized by a quest for independence and autonomy. This rapidly changing and volatile developmental period places adolescent transplant recipients at increased risk for medication nonadherence, acute rejection episodes, and graft loss. Furthermore, it may be difficult for teenagers to accept the cosmetic side effects of immunosuppressant medications, such as weight gain, Cushingoid facial features, acne, and gingival hypertrophy. The accompanying psychological stress and impact on self-image for teenagers can provide a dangerous disincentive to adhere to immunosuppressant medications. Medical management of this population can be challenging and benefits from specialized, multidisciplinary approaches to improve outcomes.

Sexuality-related issues, including prevention of sexually transmitted diseases and family planning, also need to be addressed with teenage transplant patients. Adolescent female transplant recipients have successfully become pregnant while receiving cyclosporine or tacrolimus. The effect of contraception on the metabolism of immunosuppressant medications needs to be considered when counseling adolescent girls about pregnancy prevention. In addition, the teratogenic potential of immunosuppressant medications (notably MMF) and antihypertensive medications (eg, ACE inhibitors) should be explained to the female adolescent and her family.

Transition to Adult Health Care Delivery

The term, emerging adulthood, is used to define the interval of 18 to 25 years of age when young adults appear physically mature, yet brain maturation has not yet completed. This age group is at increased risk for graft failure likely due to a combination of age-related risk behavior and the processes involved in transitioning from pediatric-based to adult-based health care delivery systems.[54] The identification of strategies to facilitate safe transition to adult health care delivery systems and improve outcomes for adolescent transplant recipients has become a priority for the pediatric transplant community.[54–56]

REFERENCES

1. USRDS. United States Renal Data System. 2017 USRDS annual data report: epidemiology of kidney disease in the United States. Bethesda (MD): National Institutes of Health, National Institure of Diabetes and Digestive Kidney Diseases; 2017.

2. Lofaro D, Jager KJ, Abu-Hanna A, et al. Identification of subgroups by risk of graft failure after paediatric renal transplantation: application of survival tree models on the ESPN/ERA-EDTA Registry. Nephrol Dial Transplant 2016;31(2):317–24.

3. Hart A, Smith JM, Skeans MA, et al. OPTN/SRTR 2015 annual data report: kidney. Am J Transplant 2017;17(Suppl 1):21–116.

4. Van Arendonk KJ, Chow EK, James NT, et al. Choosing the order of deceased donor and living donor kidney transplantation in pediatric recipients: a Markov decision process model. Transplantation 2015;99(2):360–6.

5. Van Arendonk KJ, James NT, Orandi BJ, et al. Order of donor type in pediatric kidney transplant recipients requiring retransplantation. Transplantation 2013; 96(5):487–93.

6. Agarwal S, Oak N, Siddique J, et al. Changes in pediatric renal transplantation after implementation of the revised deceased donor kidney allocation policy. Am J Transplant 2009;9(5):1237–42.

7. Keith DS, Vranic G, Barcia J, et al. Longitudinal analysis of living donor kidney transplant rates in pediatric candidates in the United States. Pediatr Transplant 2017;21(2):e12859.

8. Hwang AH, Cho YW, Cicciarelli J, et al. Risk factors for short- and long-term survival of primary cadaveric renal allografts in pediatric recipients: a UNOS analysis. Transplantation 2005;80(4):466–70.

9. Dobbels F, Ruppar T, De Geest S, et al. Adherence to the immunosuppressive regimen in pediatric kidney transplant recipients: a systematic review. Pediatr Transplant 2010;14(5):603–13.

10. Hogan J, Pietrement C, Sellier-Leclerc AL, et al. Infection-related hospitalizations after kidney transplantation in children: incidence, risk factors, and cost. Pediatr Nephrol 2017;32(12):2331–41.

11. Kizilbash SJ, Rheault MN, Bangdiwala A, et al. Infection rates in tacrolimus versus cyclosporine-treated pediatric kidney transplant recipients on a rapid discontinuation of prednisone protocol: 1-year analysis. Pediatr Transplant 2017;21(4): e12919.

12. Ettenger R, Chin H, Kesler K, et al. Relationship among viremia/viral infection, alloimmunity, and nutritional parameters in the first year after pediatric kidney transplantation. Am J Transplant 2017;17(6):1549–62.

13. Smith JM, Dharnidharka VR, Talley L, et al. BK virus nephropathy in pediatric renal transplant recipients: an analysis of the North American Pediatric Renal Trials and Collaborative Studies (NAPRTCS) registry. Clin J Am Soc Nephrol 2007; 2(5):1037–42.

14. Momynaliev KT, Gorbatenko EV, Shevtsov AB, et al. Prevalence and subtypes of BK virus in pediatric renal transplant recipients in Russia. Pediatr Transplant 2012;16(2):151–9.

15. Smith JM, Dharnidharka VR. Viral surveillance and subclinical viral infection in pediatric kidney transplantation. Pediatr Nephrol 2015;30(5):741–8.

16. Weigel F, Lemke A, Tonshoff B, et al. Febrile urinary tract infection after pediatric kidney transplantation: a multicenter, prospective observational study. Pediatr Nephrol 2016;31(6):1021–8.

17. Herthelius M, Oborn H. Urinary tract infections and bladder dysfunction after renal transplantation in children. J Urol 2007;177(5):1883–6.

18. Ploos van Amstel S, Vogelzang JL, Starink MV, et al. Long-term risk of cancer in survivors of pediatric ESRD. Clin J Am Soc Nephrol 2015;10(12):2198–204.

19. Smith JM, Martz K, McDonald RA, et al. Solid tumors following kidney transplantation in children. Pediatr Transplant 2013;17(8):726–30.

20. Parekh RS, Carroll CE, Wolfe RA, et al. Cardiovascular mortality in children and young adults with end-stage kidney disease. J Pediatr 2002;141(2):191–7.

21. McDonald SP, Craig JC, Australian and New Zealand Paediatric Nephrology Association. Long-term survival of children with end-stage renal disease. N Engl J Med 2004;350(26):2654–62.

22. Hooper DK, Williams JC, Carle AC, et al. The quality of cardiovascular disease care for adolescents with kidney disease: a Midwest Pediatric Nephrology Consortium study. Pediatr Nephrol 2013;28(6):939–49.

23. Dobrowolski LC, van Huis M, van der Lee JH, et al. Epidemiology and management of hypertension in paediatric and young adult kidney transplant recipients in The Netherlands. Nephrol Dial Transplant 2016;31(11):1947–56.

24. Suszynski TM, Rizzari MD, Gillingham KJ, et al. Antihypertensive pharmacotherapy and long-term outcomes in pediatric kidney transplantation. Clin Transplant 2013;27(3):472–80.

25. Mitsnefes MM, Khoury PR, McEnery PT. Early posttransplantation hypertension and poor long-term renal allograft survival in pediatric patients. J Pediatr 2003;143(1):98–103.

26. Terrace JD, Oniscu GC. Paediatric obesity and renal transplantation: current challenges and solutions. Pediatr Nephrol 2016;31(4):555–62.

27. Friedman AN, Miskulin DC, Rosenberg IH, et al. Demographics and trends in overweight and obesity in patients at time of kidney transplantation. Am J Kidney Dis 2003;41(2):480–7.

28. Boschetti SB, Nogueira PC, Pereira AM, et al. Prevalence, risk factors, and consequences of overweight in children and adolescents who underwent renal transplantation–short- and medium-term analysis. Pediatr Transplant 2013;17(1):41–7.

29. Foster BJ, Martz K, Gowrishankar M, et al. Weight and height changes and factors associated with greater weight and height gains after pediatric renal transplantation: a NAPRTCS study. Transplantation 2010;89(9):1103–12.

30. Habbig S, Volland R, Krupka K, et al. Dyslipidemia after pediatric renal transplantation-The impact of immunosuppressive regimens. Pediatr Transplant 2017;21(3):e12914.

31. Wilson AC, Greenbaum LA, Barletta GM, et al. High prevalence of the metabolic syndrome and associated left ventricular hypertrophy in pediatric renal transplant recipients. Pediatr Transplant 2010;14(1):52–60.

32. Chen J, Liverman R, Garro R, et al. A single center retrospective review of pediatric kidney transplant outcomes according to banff grade and cellular rejection treatment. Poster presented at American Transplant Congress; 5/2/17, 2017; Chicago, IL.

33. Hooper DK, Kirby CL, Margolis PA, et al. Reliable individualized monitoring improves cholesterol control in kidney transplant recipients. Pediatrics 2013;131(4):e1271–9.

34. Braamskamp MJ, Wijburg FA, Wiegman A. Drug therapy of hypercholesterolaemia in children and adolescents. Drugs 2012;72(6):759–72.

35. Filler G, Weiglein G, Gharib MT, et al. Omega3 fatty acids may reduce hyperlipidemia in pediatric renal transplant recipients. Pediatr Transplant 2012;16(8):835–9.

36. Mehrnia A, Le TX, Tamer TR, et al. Effects of acute rejection vs new-onset diabetes after transplant on transplant outcomes in pediatric kidney recipients: analysis of the Organ Procurement and Transplant Network/United Network for Organ Sharing (OPTN/UNOS) database. Pediatr Transplant 2016;20(7):952–7.

37. Koshy SM, Guttmann A, Hebert D, et al. Incidence and risk factors for cardiovascular events and death in pediatric renal transplant patients: a single center long-term outcome study. Pediatr Transplant 2009;13(8):1027–33.

38. Prokai A, Fekete A, Kis E, et al. Post-transplant diabetes mellitus in children following renal transplantation. Pediatr Transplant 2008;12(6):643–9.

39. Garro R, Warshaw B, Felner E. New-onset diabetes after kidney transplant in children. Pediatr Nephrol 2015;30(3):405–16.

40. Shroff R, Knott C, Gullett A, et al. Vitamin D deficiency is associated with short stature and may influence blood pressure control in paediatric renal transplant recipients. Pediatr Nephrol 2011;26(12):2227–33.

41. Bonthuis M, Busutti M, van Stralen KJ, et al. Mineral metabolism in European children living with a renal transplant: a European society for paediatric nephrology/european renal association-European dialysis and transplant association registry study. Clin J Am Soc Nephrol 2015;10(5):767–75.

42. Ebbert K, Chow J, Krempien J, et al. Vitamin D insufficiency and deficiency in pediatric renal transplant recipients. Pediatr Transplant 2015;19(5):492–8.

43. Franke D, Thomas L, Steffens R, et al. Patterns of growth after kidney transplantation among children with ESRD. Clin J Am Soc Nephrol 2015;10(1):127–34.

44. Englund MS, Tyden G, Wikstad I, et al. Growth impairment at renal transplantation-a determinant of growth and final height. Pediatr Transplant 2003;7(3):192–9.

45. Gil S, Vaiani E, Guercio G, et al. Effectiveness of rhGH treatment on final height of renal-transplant recipients in childhood. Pediatr Nephrol 2012;27(6):1005–9.

46. Berard E, Andre JL, Guest G, et al. Long-term results of rhGH treatment in children with renal failure: experience of the French Society of Pediatric Nephrology. Pediatr Nephrol 2008;23(11):2031–8.

47. Tsampalieros A, Knoll GA, Molnar AO, et al. Corticosteroid use and growth after pediatric solid organ transplantation: a systematic review and meta-analysis. Transplantation 2017;101(4):694–703.

48. Van der Weide MJ, Cornelissen EA, Van Achterberg T, et al. Lower urinary tract symptoms after renal transplantation in children. J Urol 2006;175(1):297–302 [discussion: 302].

49. Luke PP, Herz DB, Bellinger MF, et al. Long-term results of pediatric renal transplantation into a dysfunctional lower urinary tract. Transplantation 2003;76(11):1578–82.

50. Tainio J, Qvist E, Vehmas R, et al. Pubertal development is normal in adolescents after renal transplantation in childhood. Transplantation 2011;92(4):404–9.

51. Ghanem ME, Emam ME, Albaghdady LA, et al. Effect of childhood kidney transplantation on puberty. Fertil Steril 2010;94(6):2248–52.

52. Mendley SR, Zelko FA. Improvement in specific aspects of neurocognitive performance in children after renal transplantation. Kidney Int 1999;56(1):318–23.

53. Qvist E, Pihko H, Fagerudd P, et al. Neurodevelopmental outcome in high-risk patients after renal transplantation in early childhood. Pediatr Transplant 2002;6(1):53–62.

54. Foster BJ. Heightened graft failure risk during emerging adulthood and transition to adult care. Pediatr Nephrol 2015;30(4):567–76.

55. Harden PN, Walsh G, Bandler N, et al. Bridging the gap: an integrated paediatric to adult clinical service for young adults with kidney failure. BMJ 2012;344:e3718.

56. Kreuzer M, Prufe J, Oldhafer M, et al. Transitional care and adherence of adolescents and young adults after kidney transplantation in Germany and Austria: a binational observatory census within the TRANSNephro trial. Medicine (Baltimore) 2015;94(48):e2196.

Printed and bound by CPI Group (UK) Ltd, Croydon, CR0 4YY

07/10/2024

01040505-0006